OBESITY

OBESITY

New Directions in Assessment and Management

Senior Editors
Theodore B. VanItallie, MD
Artemis P. Simopoulos, MD

Associate Editors
Stephen Pernice Gullo, PhD
Walter Futterweit, MD

Foreword by
Albert J. Stunkard, MD

The Charles Press, Publishers
Philadelphia

The Charles Press, Publishers
Post Office Box 15715
Philadelphia, PA 19103
(215) 545-8933

Published in cooperation with the American Institute of Life-Threatening Illness and Loss, New York, New York

Library of Congress Cataloging-in-Publication Data

Obesity: new directions in assessment and management / edited by
    Theodore VanItallie and Artemis Simopoulos.
        p.   cm.
    Includes bibliographical references and index.
    ISBN 0-914783-74-2
    1. Obesity. I.   VanItallie, Theodore B. 1919-   . II Simopoulos,
Artemis P., 1933-   .
    [DNLM: 1. Obesity — therapy. 2. Obesity — complications. 3. Body
Weight.   WD 210 01243 1994]

RC628.0286   1994
616.3 ' 98—dc20
DNLM / DLC
for Library of Congress   94-29964
                                                                        CIP

Printed in the United States of America

ISBN 0-914783-74-2

Senior Editors

Theodore B. VanItallie, MD
Professor Emeritus of Medicine
St. Luke's-Roosevelt Hospital Center
Columbia University College of
Physicians and Surgeons
New York, New York

Artemis P. Simopoulos, MD
President, Center for Genetics,
Nutrition and Health
Washington, DC
Series Editor, World Review of
Nutrition and Dietetics
Basel, Switzerland

Associate Editors

Stephen Pernice Gullo, PhD
President, Institute for Health and
Weight Sciences, Center for Healthful Living;
Director of Health Planning and Services
The American Institute of Life-Threatening
Illness and Loss
New York, New York

Walter Futterweit, MD, FACP
Clinical Professor of Medicine
Mt. Sinai School of Medicine
New York, New York

Contributors

Janet D. Allan, PhD, RNC, FAAN
Associate Professor of Nursing
University of Texas at Austin
Austin, Texas

David B. Allison, PhD
Obesity Research Center
St. Luke's-Roosevelt Hospital Center
Columbia University College of Physicians
and Surgeons
New York, New York

George L. Blackburn, MD, PhD
Associate Professor of Surgery
Harvard Medical School
Director, Nutrition Support Service
New England Deaconess Hospital
Boston, Massachusetts

Rocco L. Brunelle, MS
Statistician, Eli Lilly and Company
Indianapolis, Indiana

Carlo C. DiClemente, PhD
Professor of Psychology
University of Houston
Houston, Texas

Walter Futterweit, MD, FACP
Clinical Professor of Medicine
Mt. Sinai School of Medicine
New York, New York

Sharon L. Gallagher, RD, CDE
Department of Dietetics
New England Deaconess Hospital
Boston, Massachusetts

Robert J. Garrison, MS
Chief of Field Studies and Biometry
Division of Epidemiology and Clinical Applications
National Heart, Lung and Blood Institute
Bethesda, Maryland

David J. Goldstein, MD, PhD
Research Physician, Eli Lilly and Company
Department of Pharmacology and Toxicology
Indiana University School of Medicine
Department of Pediatrics
Methodist Hospital of Indiana
Indianapolis, Indiana

Stephen Pernice Gullo, PhD
President, Institute for Health and Weight Sciences
Center for Healthful Living
Director of Health Planning and Services
The American Institute of Life-Threatening Illness and Loss
New York, New York

Michael Hamilton, MD
Director, Duke University Diet and Fitness Center
Durham, North Carolina

Susan B. Head, PhD
Associate Director of Research
Duke University Diet and Fitness Center
Durham, North Carolina

Stanley Heshka, PhD
Research Associate, Obesity Research Center
St. Luke's-Roosevelt Hospital Center
Columbia University College of Physicians and Surgeons
New York, New York

Susan L. Holman, MS
Statistician, Eli Lilly and Company
Indianapolis, Indiana

Ronette L. Kolotkin, PhD
Director, Behavioral Program
Duke University Diet and Fitness Center
Durham, North Carolina

JoAnn E. Manson, MD, DrPH
Channing Laboratory, Department of Medicine
Brigham and Women's Hospital
Harvard Medical School
Boston, Massachusetts

John C. Norcross, PhD
Professor and Chair
Department of Psychology
University of Scranton
Scranton, Pennsylvania

Ellen S. Parham, PhD, RD
Professor of Human and Family Resources
Northern Illinois University
Dekalb, Illinois

Amy E. Peterson, MS, RD
Department of Dietetics
New England Deaconess Hospital
Boston, Massachusetts

Stephen D. Phinney, MD, PhD
Division of Clinical Nutrition
School of Medicine
University of California at Davis
Davis, California

Martha G. Pontes, RN, MAA-HCA, MBA
Formerly, Nutrition Support Service
New England Deaconess Hospital
Boston, Massachusetts

James O. Prochaska, PhD
Professor of Psychology
University of Rhode Island
Kingston, Rhode Island

Alvin H. Rampey, Jr., PhD
Manager, Statistical and Mathematical
Sciences Division
Eli Lilly and Company
Indianapolis, Indiana

Jane M. Rees, MS, RD
Director, Nutrition Services and Education
Division of Adolescent Medicine
Lecturer, Department of Pediatrics
University of Washington School of Medicine
Seattle, Washington

Paul J. Roback, MS
Statistician, Eli Lilly and Company
Indianapolis, Indiana

Mary L. Rowan, MS, RD
Department of Dietetics
New England Deaconess Hospital
Boston, Massachusetts

David E. Schteingart, MD
Professor of Internal Medicine
Division of Endocrinology and Metabolism
University of Michigan Medical Center
Ann Arbor, Michigan

Artemis P. Simopoulos, MD
President, Center for Genetics, Nutrition and Health
Washington, DC
Series Editor, World Review of Nutrition and Dietetics
Basel, Switzerland

Caren G. Solomon, MD
Division of Preventive Medicine
Department of Medicine
Brigham and Women's Hospital
Harvard Medical School
Boston, Massachusetts

Albert J. Stunkard, MD
Professor Emeritus of Psychiatry
Director, Obesity Research Group
University of Pennsylvania School of Medicine
Philadelphia, Pennsylvania

Michael E. Swiander, MA
Department of Clinical Psychology
Fordham University
Bronx, New York

Gary D. Tollefson, MD, PhD
Executive Director, Lilly Research Laboratories
Eli Lilly and Company
Indianapolis, Indiana

Theodore B. VanItallie, MD
Professor Emeritus of Medicine
St. Luke's-Roosevelt Hospital Center
Columbia University College of Physicians and Surgeons
New York, New York

Walter C. Willett, MD, DrPH
Professor of Epidemiology and Nutrition
Harvard School of Public Health
Boston, Massachusetts

Michael G. Wilson, MS
Statistician, Eli Lilly and Company
Indianapolis, Indiana

Gary K. Zammit, PhD
Director, Sleep Disorders Institute
St. Luke's-Roosevelt Hospital Center
Assistant Professor of Clinical Psychology
Columbia University College of Physicians and Surgeons
New York, New York

Barnett Zumoff, MD
Chief, Division of Endocrinology and Metabolism
Beth Israel Medical Center
Professor of Medicine
Mt. Sinai School of Medicine
New York, New York

Contents

Foreword

The United States has traditionally been thought of as a land of great abundance. This notion of abundance has permeated the national consciousness and "the more abundant life" is widely considered to be a commendable objective.

In this country, abundance is also associated with the notion of generosity — a perception that has found expression in the size of our automobiles, television screens, refrigerators and our supermarkets. One has only to compare the size of our soft-drink cans with those dispensed in Britain and Japan.

A particularly distressing offshoot of this attitude of generosity is the oversized portions of foods served in American homes and restaurants as well as the number and size of snacks consumed between meals. Generosity on this scale has contributed to the production of large numbers of generously sized people and a national prevalence of severe overweight unequalled in the industrialized world.

Many factors contribute to human obesity, particularly genetic inheritance. But it requires a culture of abundance to elicit serious obesity even in genetically susceptible individuals. Accordingly, the prevention or treatment of obesity requires measures to help predisposed individuals protect themselves against obesity-promoting forces in the environment. These forces include the abundance and ready availability of highly palatable, calorie-dense foods and of labor-saving devices of all kinds. Another approach receiving renewed attention is to counteract metabolic vulnerability to obesity by the use of pharmacologic agents.

This book provides a wealth of information about the adverse effects of overweight on health and longevity and focuses on innovative theories dealing with the pathogenesis of this disorder. In addition, it offers a thorouhly detailed discussion of the newest approaches used in treatment and overall management of obesity.

Ass. w abundance.

Clearly, abundance has its costs as well as its benefits. For society, the costs include waste, environmental pollution, and notably, widespread obesity with its attendant risks and its negative impact on the quality of life and its duration. To cope with the growing problem of obesity we need a more discerning and judicious management of our food environment, both at the societal and individual levels. The task before us is a daunting one. Yet, as this book testifies, many advances have been made in our understanding of the problem of obesity. There is reason to hope that such progress will continue at an accelerating pace during the coming decade.

Albert J. Stunkard, MD

Introduction

The varied contributions included in this study of obesity and the problems involved in its treatment and management exemplify well the paradox that exists in the field today — we know much more about obesity than we once did, yet surprisingly, little progress has been made in either the prevention or the treatment of this widespread disorder. Indeed, we are not even sure how to define obesity. One reason for this uncertainty is the lack of agreement among epidemiologists about the level of body mass index (BMI) that is optimal for health and longevity at any given age. This key issue is forthrightly addressed in three separate chapters. After a thorough analysis of the evidence, Caren Solomon and her associates have concluded that in the United States, average weights are considerably higher than optimal for minimum mortality. In the following chapter, Artemis Simopoulos reviews highlights in the history of body weight standards. The most recent event in this history is the weight table issued as part of the 1990 U.S. Dietary Guidelines. This table allows a substantial increase in body weight for both men and women after age 35. As Simopoulos notes, the 1990 USDA-DHHS table appears to ignore the findings of recent, well-conducted longitudinal studies such as the Framingham Heart Study and the Nurses' Health Study. Moreover, this table seems to accept a substantial weight increase at precisely the time when young adults who are at high risk of becoming obese should not be gaining any weight. Based on experience with the Framingham offspring cohort, Robert Garrison has determined that for prevention of cardiovascular disease, maintenance of a BMI of less than 22 kg/m^2 (well below average) is highly desirable.

Contrary to these findings, the Dietary Guidelines for Americans, issued in 1990 by a committee of the U.S. Department of Agriculture (USDA) and the Department of Health and Human Services (DHHS), affirms that for Americans aged 35 years and older, body mass indexes can safely exceed the mean BMI value for middle-aged and older men and women derived from the second National Health and Nutrition Examination Survey (NHANES II) conducted between 1976 and 1980.

Evidence that "central adiposity" may be more sensitive and specific than the BMI as an indicator of health and mortality risk compounds the problem of arriving at a reasonably precise definition of obesity.

In addition to adverse effects on health, obesity can also have a severely damaging effect on the quality of life. In their chapter, Ronette Kolotkin and her co-workers show that a high BMI is associated with difficulties in mobility and in carrying out activities of daily living. For example, severely overweight men "experience more problems than less heavy persons in most aspects of their lives — health, sexual life, social/interpersonal life, work, self-esteem — and they experience particular distress in their ability to get around and perform everyday tasks."

As to the causes of obesity, we suffer from an embarrassment of riches. We now recognize that obesity has a strong genetic component. However, so many genetically determined mechanisms have been proposed that it will take many years of research to sort them out. In his chapter, Barnett Zumoff points out that nearly all of the hormonal abnormalities of obesity are reversible with weight loss. One apparent exception is hyperendorphinemia, a condition found to persist after therapeutic weight loss in four of the five studies that have examined this question. Hence, endorphin abnormality is yet another factor (perhaps genetic in origin) that could play a role in the causation of obesity.

In his indepth discussion of sleep disorders associated with obesity, Gary Zammit looks at sleep apnea, central alveolar hypoventilation and nocturnal eating syndrome as well as at the state of current treatment options.

Stephen Phinney calls attention to the interesting observation that obese humans exhibit abnormal patterns of polyunsaturated fatty acids (PUFA) in serum phospholipids (PL). This abnormality persists following major weight loss. He suggests that the pattern of PUFA in serum and liver PL in obese humans and certain animal models of obesity may reflect an accelerated flux of substrate through the pathway producing arachidonic acid (20:4ω6). As he points out, "A paucity of PL 20:4ω6 can increase hepatic lipogenesis, impair insulin secretion, cause peripheral insulin resistance and contribute to sodium retention." Phinney makes a persuasive case for further testing of the hypothesis that certain obesity-related risk factors ("Syndrome X") may arise from a disturbance in 20:4ω6 cycling.

Despite the earlier belief that obesity is "glandular" in origin, Walter Futterweit, in his comprehensive review of the endocrine aspects of obesity, points out that the endocrinopathies that manifest as obesity are rare. However, he also emphasizes that it is the treating physician's responsibility to exclude them.

A considerable amount of modern-day research in obesity is concerned with the heritability of fatness and with various phenotypic factors that could promote accumulation of excess fat. As David Allison points out in his discussion of methodologic issues in obesity, biometric genetics is fundamentally the study of the causes of phenotypic variation. Allison shows how lack of attention to various pitfalls in biometric genetic studies can lead to incorrect or anomalous results. As examples, he cites the unreliability of querying twins about their preference for single foods rather than employing a strategy of aggregation. When subjects are asked to respond to a questionnaire consisting of a number of related items instead of just one, their responses can be combined into a single index. When this aggregative approach is used, "true" variance accumulates more rapidly than error variance.

Allison also discusses the problem of "over-control," which entails controlling for a variable that is actually an integral link in the causal chain in which one is interested. A notable example can be found in certain epidemiologic studies that "control for" intermediate risk factors associated with obesity such as hypertension, glucose intolerance, and hyperlipidemia. When such over-control is exerted, it is not surprising that the positive association between obesity and subsequent all-cause mortality can be greatly attenuated.

Other pitfalls described by Allison are ones that result from failure to consider carefully the implications of a selected model, and in particular, its underlying assumptions. It is not enough to assume the validity of a given model just because it fits the data well. As Allison emphasizes, it is important to rule out competing models that might fit the data equally well.

The treatment of obesity is given a good deal of attention in this book. Theodore VanItallie emphasizes that weight reduction treatment "continues to be undertaken by physicians and nonphysicians with little or no understanding of, or attention to, the effect of energy restriction on body composition and, more particularly, on the body's fat-free mass (FFM) and intracellular protein status." He points out that if rates of weight loss are reasonably restrained by the treating physician during prolonged weight reduction therapy, few adverse side effects are likely to occur and FFM will be better preserved.

The need is surely urgent to develop and apply principles of dietary treatment that are grounded in up-to-date knowledge about the physiology of weight loss. However, weight-reduction regimens (however sound) are of little use if they are not adhered to. It is essential, therefore, to find better ways of helping patients control energy intake and expenditure so as to achieve and maintain a healthier weight.

In this regard, Jane Rees reminds us that "self-efficacy" is "one of the few patterns consistently associated with success in changing food-related behaviors." It follows that weight-control programs should be designed to enhance self-efficacy. According to Rees, there are a number of ways of approaching this goal. They include the use of sophisticated counseling techniques to convey nutrition messages effectively, the teaching of eating and exercise skills, and the replacement of unhealthy eating behaviors that provide immediate gratification with corresponding healthy behaviors that are also gratifying. Moreover, she emphasizes the need to establish weight goals that are reasonable and to work toward these goals incrementally. Stephen Gullo proposes a totally new approach to weight control — food control theory and training — that emphasizes the importance of control and cognitive restructuring Food control theory, as described by Gullo "contends that effective maintenance of reduced weight is dependent upon the management of the physiologic, sociocultural and cognitive variables which prompt a return to problem foods and behavior...and lead to an eventual loss of control over food."

In their chapter, John Norcross and his co-authors recommend the use of a "transtheoretic analysis in weight control." They stress that in this model, individuals move through stages utilizing specific processes of change. In their terminology, the stages progress from "precontemplation" to "contemplation" to "action," and finally to "maintenance." Patients who are trying to lose weight often need professional help in order to make a successful transition from one stage to the next. The Norcross group found that in progressing from one stage to another, certain commonly employed processes of change can be identified. For example, to move from contemplation to action, threat minimization is emphasized. In the authors' experience, contingency control best bridges the action and maintenance stages.

George Blackburn and his colleagues report on the comparison of patient retention rate of a weight management program employing an interdisciplinary team approach (physician, dietitian, nurse and behavior therapist) with the retention rate experienced in a traditional hospital outpatient system where physicians refer patients to dietitians for nutrition counseling. Compared to the clinic offering only counseling, the clinic utilizing the interdisciplinary team achieved a significantly higher patient retention rate. Clearly, the interdisciplinary approach resulted in greater patient satisfaction.

According to some surveys, 20 to 30 percent of obese persons who seek treatment are "compulsive eaters" (CEs). More females than males are CEs. In her contribution, Ellen Parham considers the applicability of the "addiction-as-disease" (AAD) model to CEs. According to Parham, "the AAD model assumes that addiction is the product of a defect, usually thought to be genetic, that alters the individual's response to the substance [certain foods] under question." She reviews evidence that specific foods may be psychoactive and cites some examples suggesting that the taste preference and food consumption of binge-eaters (herein equated with compulsive eaters) could be in part the product of abnormalities in control of serotonin and several other neurotransmitters. Although these and other commonalities exist between compulsive eating and dependence on psychoactive substances, Parham states that "there are major flaws in the analogy in regard to consideration of food as intoxicating [and] the evidence for tolerance and for withdrawal is extremely weak." She concludes that "there is a real potential that application of that [AAD] model may worsen the condition [and that] as food cannot truly be considered psychoactive, attempts to define compulsive overeating as addiction may be inhibiting understanding of the problem."

Janet Allan presents a fascinating study of the patterns and processes of weight management among working- and middle-class black women. She found that most black women did not regard being overweight as unhealthy; what troubled them the most was the adverse effects on appearance — not being able to wear "nice clothes or just not looking good." Many black women, although obese by prevailing weight standards, did not define themselves as overweight. Allan noted that in her cohort there were class differences in the use of particular methods for weight loss. For example, more middle-class women than working-class women turned to exercise, new eating patterns and a new lifestyle. Thus, it seemed that the women who were most successful at weight control were those who were well-educated and who recognized that they were overweight. The most obese women had the greatest difficulty in losing a substantial amount of weight and in maintaining their reduced weight. Allan concludes by emphasizing the importance of examining weight management within the context of lifestyle, and of paying particular attention to the opportunities and barriers that confront women as they attempt to lose weight.

In this book, the pharmacotherapy of obesity is considered from three differing perspectives. David Schteingart discusses the short-term effectiveness of a nonprescription anorexic agent, phenylpropanolamine (PPA), at a dose of 75 mg per day as an adjunct in the dietary management of obesity. He reports on a study showing that when PPA was taken along with a calorie-reduced diet, weight loss was greater than with diet plus placebo. Over an 8-week period, the mean cumulative weight loss was 2.59 kg when PPA was used (51 subjects) and 1.07 kg when placebo was used (50 subjects).

Stanley Heshka reviews the long-term effectiveness of the serotonin agonist dexfenfluramine (dFF) in weight control, citing among other sources the experience over 1 year of a large multicenter study of dF in nine European countries. In that study, mean weight loss of "completers" (those who remained in the study) amounted to 9.8 kg in the dFF group and 7.1 kg in the placebo group. Heshka concludes that dFF is a promising medication for use in a program of long-term weight loss and maintenance. In his words, "The immediate side effects are mild and the weight loss...seems to be achieved without strenuous effort on the part of the subject."

Finally, in a third view of pharmacotherapy, David Goldstein and his co-workers report on their examination of the "fluoxetine obesity long-term clinical trial database" to identify baseline variables associated with a successful long-term treatment effect. They evaluated the weight loss patterns from 1026 patients studied in four double-blind, placebo-controlled trials lasting at least 36 weeks. A greater proportion of fluoxetine-treated patients (8.6 percent) than placebo-treated patients (5.4 percent) achieved a successful weight loss pattern. To cite their findings, "The baseline predictors associated with a long-term treatment effect on weight loss are age, smoking status, and plasma uric acid concentrations. Patients who were older, did not smoke, and had higher uric acid concentrations lost the most weight over comparable placebo-treated patients."

In the concluding chapter, Artemis Simopoulos discusses the evolutionary aspects of diet and the contributions made by relatively recent dietary changes to the increasing prevalence of obesity and chronic diseases in Western societies. Compared to early man, modern man consumes less protein, fewer fruits and vegetables, and much more sugar and saturated fat. As she points out, fructose from calorie sweeteners alone now accounts for about 8 percent of total calories. Fructose is known to promote fatty acid synthesis and fat storage under certain dietary circumstances.

The paleolithic diet contained roughly equal amounts of omega-6 and omega-3 polyunsaturated fatty acids. Currently the ratio of omega-6 to omega-3 PUFA from vegetable and animal sources is reported to be between 20 and 25 to 1. Moreover, owing to the widespread use of hydrogenation of liquid vegetable oils in margarine manufacture, trans fatty acids (reported to raise LDL cholesterol, lower HDL cholesterol, increase platelet aggregation, and raise plasma triglyceride concentration) now constitute 5 to 7 percent of the energy contributed by fat to the daily diet.

Evidence is accumulating that reduced sensitivity to insulin is the primary metabolic defect from which many of the undesirable metabolic disturbances associated with obesity follow. Indeed, there is a growing belief that in many instances a decrease in insulin sensitivity precedes obesity — although excess fat (particularly in the visceral region) itself produces and/or exacerbates insulin resistance. Simopoulos carefully reviews recent evidence indicating that certain dietary PUFA are readily incorporated into cell membranes, increasing membrane fluidity, the number of insulin receptors, and responsiveness to insulin. Saturated fatty acids (SFA) and trans fatty acids (TFA) have the opposite effect. In humans, the ratio of omega-6/SFA in serum phospholipids correlates with insulin sensitivity.

Simopoulos suggests that the current U.S. diet, high in saturated and trans fatty acids, could contribute to the development of impaired insulin sensitivity, particularly in individuals genetically predisposed to obesity. (There appear to be many such individuals in the U.S population.) Thus, by changing the physical properties of the surrounding lipid milieu in cell membranes (and perhaps in other ways as well), long-chain PUFA could modulate the function of insulin receptors as well as certain mechanisms of glucose transport.

It will be recalled that Stephen Phinney and his co-authors have suggested that a reduced concentration of 20:4ω6 in the serum phospholipid may be a marker for predisposition to obesity. In their view, 20:4ω6 plays a significant role in energy balance regulation. When insufficient 20:4ω6 is available in liver cells, lipogenesis becomes enhanced and the liver shunts carbohydrate-derived calories from glycogen or oxidation into fat storage. Thus, one can visualize that in an individual with a reduced membrane 20:4ω6, a high carbohydrate intake would promote fat accumulation and increase body weight.

In recent years, considerable attention has been given to the complementary roles, in the causation of obesity, of physical inactivity and a dietary environment characterized by an abundance of readily available, palatable, calorie-dense foods. On the other hand, as Simopoulos reminds us, an important modulating factor has been neglected — diet composition — and particularly the fatty acid composition of the diet's fat moiety. Variations in dietary fatty acid composition can alter tissue composition and thereby influence important metabolic processes, including energy partitioning and insulin sensitivity. More research is clearly needed on the potential for good or harm of certain key constituents of the diet, such as fructose, trans fatty acids and omega-3 and omega-6 polyunsaturated fatty acids.

Theodore B. VanItallie, MD
Artemis P. Simopoulos, MD

OBESITY

1

Body Weight and Mortality

Caren G. Solomon, MD, Walter C. Willett, MD, DrPH
JoAnn E. Manson, MD, DrPH

The relationship between obesity and mortality has been the subject of considerable controversy. Morbid obesity is clearly associated with decreased longevity,[1] but the consequences of mild overweight have varied in different studies. Moreover, estimates of optimal weight in terms of longevity have been controversial. The importance of these issues is underscored by the observation that an estimated 34 million Americans are obese, as defined by a weight approximately 20 percent or more above desirable levels.[2]

The lack of a direct relationship between weight and mortality in many studies could reflect some unknown protective effect of obesity,[3] or could result from methodologic problems. We have previously reviewed the potential effects of important biases on attenuating the relationship between adiposity and mortality.[4] Disease, even subclinical disease, may cause weight loss and thus underestimation of the association between relative weight and mortality; analyses based on short duration of follow-up or those which do not eliminate early mortality are particularly susceptible to this problem. Cigarette smoking, a major risk factor for both cardiovascular and cancer mortality, is also associated with relative leanness. In addition, control for metabolic consequences of obesity, including hypertension and glucose intolerance, which are themselves cardiovascular risk factors, results in underestimation of the true association between overweight and mortality.

Other potential confounders should also be noted. Physical inactivity is both a correlate of obesity and an independent risk factor for coronary disease and all-cause mortality.[5] Socioeconomic status tends to vary inversely with both weight and mortality in the United States,[6] though it may vary directly with weight in other populations.[7] In addition, chronic depression is also associated with leanness secondary to weight loss, as well

1

as excess mortality. All of the above factors are relevant to the interpretation of any study addressing the association between weight and mortality.

Insurance company studies have the advantage of including a generally healthy population, minimizing confounding by pre-existing disease. Two such studies, the 1959 Build and Blood Pressure Study[8] and the 1979 Build Study,[9] each with over 4 million participants, reported increasing mortality with increasing relative weight, and optimal longevity at weights lower than average. The 1979 study suggested a J-shaped relationship between obesity and mortality, but failed, as did the earlier study, to control for smoking. Importantly, whereas mortality among overweight subjects increased with duration of follow-up, the mortality associated with low relative weights was most marked early on, and diminished with prolonged follow-up, suggesting the possibility of bias from subclinical disease even in this relatively healthy cohort.

The generalizability of results from this insured population was supported by results of an American Cancer Society study[10] which involved 750,000 men and women apparently healthy at baseline. Again a J-shaped relationship was noted between obesity and mortality. Subjects 30 to 40 percent above average weight had 50 percent greater mortality than those of average weight, and those more than 40 percent above average weight had almost 90 percent greater mortality. The lowest mortality occurred at 10 to 20 percent below average weight. Separate analyses for smokers and nonsmokers confirmed that leanness was associated with a much greater risk in smokers, who tended to die from smoking-associated malignancies. Among nonsmokers, leanness was associated with lower mortality than overweight; only the leanest women—those less than 80 percent of average weight—had mortality rates slightly greater than women of average weight.

While some studies have suggested that a U-shaped curve describes the relationship between relative weight and mortality[11-14] bias from cigarette smoking and chronic or preclinical disease appears to explain the apparent excess mortality at the lowest relative weights. Quadratic associations between body mass index (BMI) and mortality appear stronger in smokers than nonsmokers,[13,14] although increased risks among the lean have also been reported in nonsmokers.[15] Among participants in the Harvard Alumni Health Study, stratification by smoking status revealed direct associations between BMI and mortality in never-smokers and past smokers, in contrast to a U-shaped association in current smokers. The importance of length of follow-up in this cohort was demonstrated by the observation of a U-shaped association between BMI and mortality in the first 13 years of follow-up, a J-shaped association in the next 7 years, and a direct association after 20 years of follow-up.[16]

A recent study involving 8828 Seventh-day Adventist men[17] is particularly illustrative, insofar as smoking is rare in this population, and leanness is generally a result of choice, rather than underlying illness. Data from this population suggest that mortality increases linearly with BMI. No increase in mortality was seen even among 439 subjects with BMI < 20 kg/m^2. As compared with men in the leanest quintile (BMI ≤ 22.3 kg/m^2), relative risk of all-cause mortality among the most obese men was approximately 1.4 (95 percent confidence interval [CI]: 1.3 to 1.6), after adjustment for several potential confounders, including physical activity level and dietary pattern. The fact that the men in the most obese quintile in this study had a BMI greater than 27.5 kg/m^2—an index only slightly above average in the general population—suggests a significant risk with even mild obesity.

Observations in this population also argue against social class as an explanation of the higher mortality seen in the obese, as education level varied minimally with BMI. Control for social factors in a large Swedish study likewise did not significantly attenuate the approximately twofold relative risk of mortality in obese subjects.[18] Among Finnish males, control for social class actually resulted in a slight increase in the risk associated with obesity and slight attenuation of the risk associated with leanness.[7]

Of several studies that have failed to find associations between obesity and mortality, it is notable that none had sample sizes comparable to the largest studies discussed above. Power in all was insufficient to exclude significant mortality differences among weight quintiles.[4]

OBESITY AND CAUSE-SPECIFIC MORTALITY

Coronary Heart Disease

Obesity is associated with several coronary risk factors, including hypertension,[19] dyslipidemia,[20] and diabetes.[21] Thus it is not surprising that much of the excess mortality observed in the obese is a result of coronary disease. Increasing relative weight has been associated with increasing coronary morbidity[22,23] as well as mortality in several studies, with on average nearly twice the risk of coronary mortality among the most obese as among the nonobese.[8,10,17] While the relationship between obesity and mortality is attenuated by controlling for the associated cardiac risk factors noted above, there is good evidence for an independent effect of obesity on cardiac mortality.[24] The adverse impact of overweight may be explained, at least in part, by its association with insulin resistance and hyperinsulinemia,[25] recently shown to be an independent risk factor for coronary disease.

The relationship between obesity and coronary mortality becomes more pronounced with longer duration of follow-up. Both the insurance company studies and the American Cancer Society Study reported greater relative risks of coronary mortality in the obese in the later years of the studies. Consistent with these data, later analyses from the Framingham

Heart Study[24] suggested a stronger relationship between weight and myocardial infarction than did earlier analyses based on shorter follow-up.[26]

Stroke

Mortality due to stroke is also more common in the obese. In the Build Study,[9] men who were 25 percent or more overweight had approximately 1.3 times the risk of mortality from stroke of those of average weight. Among Seventh-day Adventists,[17] there was a significant trend toward increasing risk of fatal cerebrovascular disease with increasing BMI, such that men with BMI > 27.5 had a relative risk of 1.7 (95 percent CI: 1.2 to 2.3) compared with those with BMI $\leq$ 22.3 kg/m^2.

Cancer

Obesity has also been associated with increased risk of mortality from certain types of cancer. Overweight males have been reported to have higher rates of colorectal and prostate cancer, and overweight women to have higher rates of endometrial, gallbladder, cervical, and ovarian cancer.[10] Some data have suggested an increase in mortality from breast cancer with obesity; while data from the Nurses Health Study[27] and other cohorts have suggested an inverse association between obesity and premenopausal breast cancer incidence, and little association between obesity and postmenopausal breast cancer incidence. The tendency to later diagnosis in obese women may result in a more direct relationship between relative weight and breast cancer mortality.

In many studies, cancer mortality is also high in the underweight, and explains much of the excess mortality seen in this group. Cancers of the lung,[10,12,28] bladder,[10] and stomach,[12] in particular, have been more common in the lean. This observation likely reflects, at least in part, the confounding effects of cigarette smoking, or the effects of pre-existing disease on body weight. Exclusion from analysis of smokers, or those dying in the first few years of follow-up, has generally attenuated the risk of mortality in the underweight.

Other Diseases

Obesity has also been associated with increased risk of mortality from other causes. Among participants in the Build Study,[9] mortality from diabetes mellitus was increased 1.25 times among those 5 to 15 percent overweight, 2 times among those 15 to 25 percent overweight, and more than 5 times among those 25 percent or more overweight. Similar results were reported in the American Cancer Society Study.[10] Risk of mortality from gastrointestinal disease was higher in the overweight than in those of average weight, though it was also higher in the very lean.[9]

OBESITY IN FEMALES

Some studies have suggested the possibility of a gender difference in the relationship between obesity and mortality. Among participants in the Lipid Research Clinic Program, for example, an association between BMI and mortality was noted only in males.[14] However, null results of analyses restricted to women appear most likely a result of insufficient power to detect associations, resulting from inadequate numbers of endpoints in women.

Data from studies including large numbers of women have indicated J-shaped relationships between obesity and mortality in women as well as men.[9,10,29] Among participants in the Nurses Health Study, a large prospective cohort study involving 115,886 women apparently healthy at baseline, there was a strong association between BMI and cardiovascular disease.[29] As compared with women whose BMI was less than 21 kg/m^2, the age- and smoking-adjusted relative risk of nonfatal myocardial infarction or fatal coronary disease for women with BMI 25 to < 29 was 1.8 (95 percent CI: 1.2 to 2.5), and that for women with BMI $\geq$ 29 was 3.3 (2.3 to 4.5). While a J-shaped curve described the relationship between BMI and all-cause mortality over 14 years of follow-up, exclusion of smokers and of women who died or did not maintain a stable weight in the first 4 years of follow-up revealed lowest mortality risk among the leanest women (BMI < 21 kg/m^2).

EARLY BMI AND SUBSEQUENT MORTALITY

Studies demonstrating a stronger relationship between obesity and mortality with longer follow-up have suggested a protracted impact of obesity on mortality risk. Consistent with these observations are data indicating a significant effect of adolescent obesity on later coronary disease and mortality. Among 508 subjects participating in the Harvard Growth Study (1922 to 1935), men whose BMI measured above the 75th percentile between ages 13 and 18 had a relative risk of all-cause mortality of 1.8 (95 percent CI: 1.2 to 2.7) and of coronary heart disease mortality of 2.3 (95 percent CI: 1.4 to 4.1) as compared with men whose adolescent BMI was between the 25th and 50th percentile. Adjustment for adult BMI did not have a major impact on these relative risk estimates. While associations between adolescent BMI and all-cause and cause-specific mortality were not observed in women, statistical power was limited due to a much smaller number of endpoints in this group.[30]

Similarly, in a nested case-control study involving 7658 members of the Dutch male birth cohort,[28] cardiovascular mortality over 32 years of follow-up increased with increasing BMI at age 18 over 19 to 19.99 kg/m². Mortality from cancer, in contrast, was more common among those very lean at age 18; this remained true even after a decade of follow-up, which would likely eliminate effects of pre-existing disease. However, the potential importance of smoking as a confounder is clear from demographic data suggesting a very high prevalence of smoking in this population, and the observation that exclusion of deaths due to lung cancer markedly attenuated the risks associated with underweight.

An effect of obesity even earlier in life has likewise been suggested. Among 13,146 people whose weights were recorded between ages 5 and 18, the risk of mortality over the next 40 to 52 years increased linearly with prepubertal relative weight.[31]

Also, there is evidence that weight gain may have a significant influence on mortality independent of early BMI. Data from the Nurses Health Study has shown a significantly increased risk of fatal and nonfatal coronary heart disease with weight gain of 10 kg or more after the age of 18, controlling for baseline BMI.[29]

OBESITY IN THE ELDERLY

While it is well accepted that early-life obesity increases later risk of mortality, the mortality risk associated with obesity in the elderly is complicated. Bias from confounding by pre-existing disease is particularly relevant in this age group, among whom leanness is often a consequence of weight loss from underlying illness. Also, it is important to recognize that BMI in this age group may be a poor measure of adiposity; low BMI often reflects loss of lean body mass, which may result from underlying illness and/or inactivity, another risk factor for mortality. The reported increase in "optimal" weight (that associated with lowest mortality) at older ages[32] appears to be explained by these confounding factors.

To eliminate effects of underlying illness, which may be chronic and prolonged (e.g., cardiac and pulmonary disease), it may be necessary to exclude from analysis the first 10 or even 20 years of follow-up—not very practical with an elderly cohort. Alternatively, analyses may be limited to those whose weight has been stable for the past 10 or more years.

Among studies reporting a negligible risk of mortality with obesity in the elderly was the National Health and Nutrition Survey (NHANES), which involved 4710 subjects aged ≥ 55 years. Significant obesity (BMI > 30 kg/m²) was associated with a relative risk of mortality of only 1.2 (95 percent CI: 1.0 to 1.4) among males aged 55 to 64 years, and 1.1 (95 percent CI: 1.0 to 1.2) among males aged 65 to 74 years, as compared with those with BMI between 22 and 30 kg/m².[33] Obesity in women ≥ 55 years conferred no increase in relative risk of mortality. In contrast, leanness (BMI < 22 kg/m²) was associated with an increased risk of mortality in both sexes. However, this study excluded only mortality in the first year of follow-up, inadequate to control for the effects of underlying illness. In addition, this study inappropriately controlled for blood pressure, classified ex-smokers as nonsmokers, and had limited follow-up (maximum of 12 years) and also infrequent endpoints in females.

Other data suggest that obesity remains an important risk factor for mortality in the elderly. Long-term follow-up of 1723 nonsmokers in the Framingham study[34] demonstrated an association between mortality and BMI at age 65 not unlike the association between earlier BMI and mortality. Males with BMI at or above the 70th percentile (28.5 kg/m^2) had a relative risk of mortality of 1.7 (95 percent CI: 1.1 to 2.5), as compared with males with BMI between 23.0 and 25.2 kg/m^2. Similarly, women with BMI at or above the 70th percentile (28.7 kg/m^2) had a relative risk of mortality of 2.0 (95 percent CI: 1.4 to 2.8), as compared with those with BMI between 24.1 and 26.1 kg/m^2.

While this study confirmed an adverse impact of obesity even at older ages, it also raised the question of an increased mortality risk with leanness in this age group. Even with exclusion of all subjects who reported smoking in the 10 years before age 65, males with BMI < 23 and females with BMI < 24.1 had relative risks of mortality of 1.7 (95 percent CI: 1.0 to 2.9) and 1.4 (95 percent CI: 1.0 to 2.0), respectively, as compared with the referent groups above. However, these increased relative risks were attenuated and not statistically significant after exclusion of the first 4 years of follow-up from the analysis; as noted, exclusion of a longer time period would be necessary to control more completely for confounding by pre-existing illness.

It is notable that the leanest subjects among the generally healthy population of Seventh-day Adventists continued to have lower mortality than more obese subjects throughout the lifespan.[17] Relative risks of obesity did diminish with age in this cohort, but the higher mortality rates in the elderly suggest that attributable risks associated with obesity in this age group likely increased.

RACIAL DIFFERENCES IN THE OBESITY-MORTALITY RELATIONSHIP

Recent studies have begun to address the relationship between obesity and mortality among ethnic groups other than Caucasians. Earlier literature suggested that body mass index might be unrelated to mortality in black males.[6] However, these null findings appear likely to have been a function of inadequate power to detect true associations. More recent studies have reported a significant association of obesity with all-cause[35] and coronary mortality[36] in black males, with relative risk estimates associated with obesity comparable to estimates in whites.

The association between obesity and mortality in black females remains unclear. No association has been observed in several studies.[35,37,38] As above, insufficient statistical power may underlie null findings. Obesity in this population has been linked to diabetes and hypertension,[39] known risk factors for coronary mortality.

The association between obesity and mortality among other ethnic groups remains less well-defined. Studies among Mexican Americans[40] and Pima Indians,[41] two populations with a high prevalence of obesity, have not revealed clear correlations between body weight and mortality, though there is evidence of an increased mortality risk among Pima men with BMI greater than 40 kg/m^2.[41]

OTHER MEASURES OF OBESITY

The studies discussed thus far used BMI or relative weight as indicators of obesity. However, neither of these measures directly reflects adiposity, nor distribution of adiposity, which may be especially important in mediating cardiovascular risk. Among the elderly, in particular, low BMI may reflect loss of lean body mass, rather than an absence of excessive adipose tissue. This limitation has been suggested as one explanation for the inconsistent associations observed across studies between these measures and mortality risk.

Several studies have evaluated measures of central adiposity, a known correlate of insulin resistance,[25] as predictors of mortality. Abdominal circumference has been associated with mortality in some but not other populations.[36,37]

Increased waist-to-hip ratio (WHR), a common measure of central obesity, has been associated with hypertension, diabetes, dyslipidemia, and coronary heart disease.[42] Consistent with these data, others have shown a significant association between WHR and cardiovascular mortality. In a retrospective study of 105,062 U.S. Army veterans followed for 23 years, baseline WHR was a significant predictor of premature mortality from ischemic heart disease and cerebrovascular disease.[43]

Recently, data on 41,837 participants in the Iowa Women's Health Study, aged 55 to 69 years, indicated that waist-hip ratio was significantly and directly associated with all-cause mortality at 5-year follow-up.[44] Among never-smokers, women with WHR in the highest quintile had a relative risk of mortality 2.2 times that of women with WHR in the lowest quintile (95 percent CI: 1.7 to 2.8). The relative risk of mortality increased 1.6-fold (95 percent CI: 1.47 to 1.74) with each 0.15 unit increase in WHR. In this population, BMI had little effect on all cause-mortality after controlling for waist-hip ratio.

CONCLUSIONS

When adjustment is made for effects of smoking and preclinical disease, the preponderance of evidence suggests that even mild overweight is probably associated with some increase in mortality risk, and that average weights are higher than optimal. The excess risks of being underweight appear to be largely if not entirely artifactual, due to inadequate control of confounding by chronic or subclinical illness and/or cigarette smoking. Measures of central adiposity may provide additional information on mortality risk, particularly among older individuals, though further studies are needed.

While this review focuses only on mortality, the morbidity associated with obesity is also important in assessing the true impact of body weight. Risks of hypertension,[19] dyslipidemia,[20] diabetes,[21] gallstones,[45] musculo-skeletal diseases,[46] and nonfatal coronary disease[29] and cancer[2] increase with increasing weight. Thus the evidence is compelling that avoidance of even moderate obesity will maximize health and longevity.

NOTES

1. Drenick EJ, Bale GS, Seltzer F, Johnson DG (1980). Excessive mortality and causes of death in morbidly obese men. JAMA 243:443-445.
2. VanItallie T (1979). Obesity: adverse effects on health and longevity. Am J Clin Nutrition 32:2732-2733.
3. Bradley PJ (1982). Is obesity an advantageous adaptation? Int J Obesity 6:43-52.
4. Manson JE, Stampfer MJ, Hennekens CH, Willett WC (1987). Body weight and longevity: a reassessment. JAMA 257:353-358.
5. Beasley JW (1987). Body weight and longevity. JAMA 257:1895.
6. Tyroler HA, Knowles MG, Wing SB, Logue EE, Davis CE, Heiss G, Heyden S, Hames CG (1984). Ischemic heart disease risk factors and 20-year mortality in middle-age Evans County black males. Am Heart J 108:738-746.
7. Rissanen A, Heliovaara M, Knekt P, Aromaa A, Reunanen A, Maatela J (1989). Weight and mortality in Finnish men. J Clin Epidemiol 42:781-789.
8. Build and blood pressure study (1959). Chicago: Society of Actuaries.
9. Build study (1979). Chicago: Society of Actuaries and Association of Life Insurance Medical Directors of America.
10. Lew EA, Garfinkel L (1979). Variations in mortality by weight among 750,000 men and women. J Chron Dis 32:563-576.
11. Keys A (1980). Seven countries: a multivariate analysis of death and coronary heart disease. Cambridge: Harvard University Press.
12. Waaler HT (1983). Height, weight, and mortality: the Norwegian experience. Acta Med Scand 679 S:1-51.
13. Dyer AR, Stamler J, Berkson DM (1975). Relationship of relative weight and body mass index to 14-year mortality in the Chicago Peoples Gas Company Study. J Chron Dis 28:109-123.

10 *Obesity*

14. Wilcosky T, Hyde J, Anderson JJB, Bangdiwala S, Duncan B (1990). Obesity and mortality in the Lipid Research Clinics Program Follow-Up Study. J Clin Epidemiol 43:743-752.
15. Rissanen A, Knekt P, Heliovaara M, Aromaa A, Reunanen A, Maatela J (1991). Weight and mortality in Finnish women. J Clin Epidemiol 44:787-795.
16. Lee I-M, Manson JE, Hennekens CH, Paffenbarger RS, Jr (1933). Body weight and mortality: a 27-year follow-up of middle-aged men. JAMA 270:2823-2828.
17. Lindsted K, Tonstad S, Kuzma JW (1991). Body mass index and patterns of mortality among Seventh-day Adventist men. Int J Obesity 15:397-406.
18. Alleback P, Bergh C (1992). Height, body mass index and mortality: Do social factors explain the association? Public Health 106:375-382.
19. Wittemann JC, Willett WC, Stampfer MJ, Colditz GA, Sacks FM, Speizer FE, Rosner B, Hennekens CH (1989). A prospective study of nutritional factors and hypertension among U.S. women. Circulation 80:1320-1327.
20. Farinaro E, Cortese C, Rubba P, DiMarino L, Mancini M (1979). Overweight and plasma lipoprotein abnormalities in a random sample of the Neapolitan population. In Mancini M, Lewis B, Contaldo F, Eds, Medical complications of obesity. London: Academic Press.
21. Colditz GA, Willett WC, Stampfer MJ, Manson JE, Hennekens CH, Arky RA, Speizer FE (1990). Weight as a risk factor for clinical diabetes in women. Am J Epidemiol 132:501-513.
22. Rabkin SW, Mathewson FAL, Hsu PH (1977). Relation of body weight to development of ischemic heart disease in a cohort of young North American men after a 26-year observation period: the Manitoba Study. Am J Cardiol 39:452-458.
23. Keys A, Aravanis C, Blackburn H, Van Buchem FS, Buzina R, Djordjevic BS, Fidanza F, Karvonen MJ, Menotti A, Puddu V, Taylor HL (1972). Coronary heart disease: overweight and obesity as risk factors. Ann Intern Med 77:15-27.
24. Hubert HB, Feinleib M, McNamara PM, Castelli WP (1983). Obesity as an independent risk factor for coronary disease: a 26-year follow-up of participants in the Framingham Heart Study. Circulation 67:968-977.
25. Lonnroth P (1988). Potential role for adipose tissue in the development of insulin resistance in obesity. Acta Med Scand Suppl 723:91-94.
26. Truett J, Cornfield J, Kannel WB (1967). A multivariate analysis of the risk of coronary heart disease in Framingham. J Chron Dis 20:511-526.
27. London SJ, Colditz GA, Stampfer MJ, Willett WC, Rosner B, Speizer FE (1989). Prospective study of relative weight, height, and risk of breast cancer. JAMA 262:2853-2858.
28. Hoffmans MDA, Kromhout D, De Lezenne Coulander C (1989). Body mass index at the age of 18 and its effects on 32-year mortality from coronary heart disease and cancer. J Clin Epidemiol 42:513-520.
29. Manson JE, Colditz GA, Stampfer MJ, Willett WC, Rosner B, Monson RR, Speizer FE, Hennekens CH (1990). A prospective study of obesity and risk of coronary heart disease in women. N Engl J Med 322:882-889.
30. Must A, Jacques PF, Dallal GE, Bajema CJ, Dietz WH (1992). Long-term morbidity and mortality of overweight adolescents: a follow-up of the Harvard Growth Study of 1922 to 1935. N Engl J Med 327:1350-1355.
31. Nieto FJ, Szklo M, Comstock GW (1992). Childhood weight and growth rate as predictors of adult mortality. Am J Epidemiol 136:201-213.
32. U.S. Department of Agriculture (1990). Nutrition and your health: dietary guidelines for Americans. Washington, DC: U.S. Government Printing Office.
33. Tayback M, Kuminyika S, Chee E (1990). Body weight as a risk factor in the elderly. Arch Intern Med 150:1065-1072.

34. Harris T, Cook EF, Garrison R, Higgins M, Kannel W, Goldman L (1988). Body mass index and mortality among nonsmoking older persons: The Framingham Heart Study. JAMA 259:1520-1524.
35. Wienpahl J, Ragland DR, Sidney S (1990). Body mass index and 15-year mortality in a cohort of black men and women. J Clin Epidemiol 43:949-960.
36. Stevens J, Keil JE, Rust PF, Verdugo RR, Davis CE, Tyroler HA, Gazes PC (1992). Body mass index and body girth as predictors of mortality in black and white men. Am J Epidemiol 135:1137-1146.
37. Stevens J, Keil JE, Rust PF, Davis CE, Gazes PC (1992). Body mass index and body girths as predictors of mortality in black and white women. Arch Intern Med 152:1257-1262.
38. Johnson JL, Heineman EF, Heiss G, Hames CG, Tyroler HA (1986). Cardiovascular disease risk factors and mortality among black women and white women aged 40-64 years in Evans County, Georgia. Am J Epidemiol 123:209-220.
39. Gillum RF, Grant CT (1982). Coronary heart disease in black populations, II: Risk factors. Mosby/Year Book 104:852-864.
40. Stern MP, Patterson JK, Mitchell BD, Haffner SM, Hazuda HP (1990). Overweight and mortality in Mexican Americans. Int J Obesity 14:623-629.
41. Pettitt DJ, Lisse JR, Knowler WC, Bennett PH (1982). Mortality as a function of obesity and diabetes mellitus. Am J Epidemiol 115:359-366.
42. Donahue RP, Abbott RD, Bloom E, Reed DM, Yano K (1987). Central obesity and coronary heart disease in men. Lancet 1:821-824.
43. Terry RB, Page WF, Haskell WL (1992). Waist hip ratio, body mass index, and premature cardiovascular disease mortality in U.S. army veterans during a 23-year follow-up study. Int J Obesity 16:417-422.
44. Folsom AR, Kaye SA, Sellers TA, Hong C-P, Cerhan JR, Potter JD, Prineas RJ (1993). Body fat distribution and 5-year risk of death in older women. JAMA 269:483-487.
45. Stampfer MJ, Maclure KM, Colditz GA, Manson JE, Willett WC (1992). Risk of symptomatic gallstones in women with severe obesity. Am J Clin Nutr 55:652-658.
46. Leach RE, Baumgard S, Boom J (1973). Obesity: its relationship to osteoarthritis of the knee. Clin Orthop 93:271-273.

2

Body Weight Reference Standards

Artemis P. Simopoulos, MD

The prevalence of overweight and obesity depends on the definition used. This chapter reviews the scientific evidence for the body weight reference standards that have been used in the United States and the current data from national surveys and long-term prospective studies. Also presented is evidence that body weight reference standards should be based on measures of morbidity and mortality rates in the U.S. population and not on measures based on statistical definitions.

The first evaluation of body weight as a factor in health and the first tables based on height and weight were published in the Transactions of the London Medico-Chirurgical Society in 1847. In April 1850, Dr. Thomas King Chambers referred to these tables in his Gulstonian Lectures delivered before the President and Fellows of the Royal College of Physicians, published in *The Lancet*.[1] The tables gave the average weight at various heights and an attempt was made to define the weight of a healthy man. Since then many attempts have been made to define the range in weight for height at various ages for men and women that is associated with the lowest morbidity, mortality, or increased longevity.[2-4]

THE USE OF BODY WEIGHT TABLES IN THE UNITED STATES

In the U.S., the use of weight tables associated with life expectancy dates back at least to the Medico-Actuarial-Mortality Investigation published in 1913.[5] In 1940 Tannenbaum[6] published his paper on the relationship of body weight to cancer incidence. It was based on a review of the data from the Medico-Actuarial-Mortality Investigation, the Medical Impairment Study, the records of the Metropolitan Life Insurance Company, and the New York Life Insurance Company. Tannenbaum concluded:

> Although the results of experimental work with animals and the analysis of insurance statistics strongly suggest that body weight is a factor affecting

cancer incidence, there are many considerations that must be critically studied and evaluated before the fundamental nature of the relationship is fully understood.

What is the practical significance of this apparent relationship of weight to cancer inception and incidence? If further critical, comprehensive studies should confirm the results reported here, it would appear that an important prophylactic measure has been brought to the attention of the medical profession. By establishing and maintaining weight levels at a minimum, compatible with general good health (possibly 10 to 20 pounds [4.5 to 9 kg] below present normal levels), cancer may be prevented in a considerable number of persons in whom it would otherwise develop; at least, the cancer process might be delayed in time of appearance. Such a regimen is already known to affect beneficially other pathologic conditions, such as diabetes, heart disease, cerebral hemorrhage and other degenerative diseases.[6]

Thus the relationship of overweight to cancer incidence in human beings and the effects of energy restriction and fat intake in experimental animals were recognized as early as the first half of this century. A number of studies suggest that overweight or obesity are associated with cancer of the breast and endometrium in postmenopausal women and cancer of the prostate and colon in men.[7-9]

In 1942 and 1943, Metropolitan Life developed an "ideal weight table"[2,3] to encourage people to keep their weight at or below the average for the insured population examined. In 1959, the company developed the Desirable Body Weight Table based on the Build and Blood Pressure Study of 1959.[10] It is this table (Table 1) that was used by the Framingham Heart Study (FHS) investigators as a reference to derive the Metropolitan Relative Weight[11] (Tables 2 and 3). The FHS remains the longest prospective heart study that is representative of the U.S. population. It was based on the population of Framingham, Massachusetts, which has morbidity and mortality statistics comparable to the U.S. population as a whole.

In the early 1980s, two very important papers were published: H.B. Hubert's "Obesity as an independent risk factor for cardiovascular disease: A 26-year follow-up of participants in the Framingham Heart Study,"[12] and R.J. Garrison's "Cigarette smoking as a confounder of the relationship between weight and long-term mortality: The Framingham Heart Study."[13] Garrison provided proof that validated the concept of the desirable body weight. The range of the desirable body weight was similar to the 1959 Metropolitan Body Weight Table and provided the data to resist the inclusion of the 1983 Metropolitan Body Weight Table in the U.S. Dietary Guidelines for Americans, published in 1980[14] for the first time and again in 1985.[15] In the 1990 Dietary Guidelines,[16] however, a new table appeared called "Healthy Weights" which was not based on any scientific data and has been severely criticized.[17]

Table 1. Desirable Body Weight Ranges

Height without Shoes	Men (pounds)	Women (pounds)
	Weight without Clothes	
4'10"		92-121
4'11"		95-124
5'0"		98-127
5'1"	105-134	101-130
5'2"	108-137	104-134
5'3"	111-141	107-138
5'4"	114-145	110-142
5'5"	117-149	114-146
5'6"	121-154	118-150
5'7"	125-159	122-154
5'8"	129-163	126-159
5'9"	133-167	130-164
5'10"	137-172	134-169
5'11"	141-177	
6'0"	145-182	
6'1"	149-187	
6'2"	153-192	
6'3"	157-197	

Note: For women 18 to 25 years, subtract 1 pound for each year under 25. Adapted from the 1959 Metropolitan Life Desirable Weight Table.

BODY WEIGHT, HEALTH AND LONGEVITY

In 1982, in order to define precisely the relation of body weight to health and longevity, a two-day workshop at the National Institutes of Health was cosponsored by the Nutrition Coordinating Committee and the Centers for Disease Control to collate and put into perspective new information about body weight, health, and longevity; to ascertain the reliability of the available data and their relevance to health and longevity; to examine the relation of body weight to body composition and size of frame; and to clarify the terminology and concepts about body weight in a way that might be helpful to practicing physicians, public health workers, and clinical investigators. The workshop concluded:

> In the United States, the weight associated with the greatest longevity tends to be below the average weight of the population under consideration, if such weights are not associated with a history of significant medical impairment.

Table 2. Desirable Weight Ranges for Women Aged 25 and Over

Height (ft/in)	Weight Range (lb)	Weight[1] (MRW = 100)	Weight[2] (MRW = 110)	Weight (MRW = 120)
4'9"	90-118	100	110	120
4'10"	92-121	103	113	124
4'11"	95-124	106	117	127
5'0"	98-127	109	120	131
5'1"	101-130	112	124	134
5'2"	104-134	116	128	139
5'3"	107-138	120	132	144
5'4"	110-142	124	136	149
5'5"	114-146	128	141	154
5'6"	118-150	132	145	158
5'7"	122-154	136	150	163
5'8"	126-159	140	154	168
5'9"	130-164	144	158	173
5'10"	134-169	148	163	177
BMI (all heights)		21.32	23.47	25.58

Note: For women between the ages of 18 to 25 years, subtract 1 pound for each year under 25.

[1] Midpoint of medium frame range used to compute Metropolitan Relative Weight (MRW) is actual weight / midpoint of medium frame range x 100.
[2] In the U.S. adult population over 40 years of age, 80 percent of men and 70 percent of women have weights that exceed an MRW of 110, and consequently are at increased risk for cardiovascular disease. The average weight of the adult U.S. population is above MRW 120; an individual with a weight over MRW 120 is considered "obese."

From AP Simopoulos, Obesity and body weight standards. Annu Rev Public Health 7:481, 1986. Data are adapted from the 1959 Metropolitan Life Desirable Weight Table. Weight is measured in pounds, without clothing and height is measured without shoes.

Overweight persons tend to die sooner than average-weight persons, especially those who are overweight at younger ages. The effect of being overweight on mortality is delayed and may not be seen in short-term studies. Cigarette smoking is a potential confounder of the relationship between obesity and mortality. Studies on body weight, morbidity, and mortality must be interpreted with careful attention to the definitions of obesity or relative weight used, preexisting morbid conditions, the length of follow-up, and confounders in the analysis. The terminology of body weight standards should be defined more precisely and cited appropriately. An appropriate database relating body weight by sex, age, and possibly frame size to mor-

Table 3. Desirable Weight Ranges for Men Aged 25 and Over

Height (ft/in)	Weight Range (lb)	Weight[1] (MRW = 100)	Weight[2] (MRW = 110)	Weight (MRW = 120)
5'1"	105-134	117	129	140
5'2"	108-137	120	132	144
5'3"	111-141	123	135	148
5'4"	114-145	126	139	151
5'5"	117-149	129	142	155
5'6"	121-154	133	146	160
5'7"	125-159	138	152	166
5'8"	129-163	142	156	170
5'9"	133-167	146	161	175
5'10"	137-172	150	165	180
5'11"	141-177	155	170	186
6'0"	145-182	159	175	191
6'1"	149-187	164	180	197
6'2"	153-192	169	186	203
6'3"	157-197	174	191	209
BMI (all heights)		21.66	23.83	26.00

[1] Midpoint of medium frame range used to compute Metropolitan Relative Weight (MRW) is actual weight / midpoint of medium frame range x 100.
[2] In the U.S. adult population over 40 years of age, 80 percent of men and 70 percent of women have weights that exceed an MRW of 110, and consequently are at increased risk for cardiovascular disease. The average weight of the adult U.S. population is above MRW 120; an individual with a weight over MRW 120 is considered "obese."

From AP Simopoulos, Obesity and body weight standards. Annu Rev Public Health 7:481, 1986. Data are adapted from the 1959 Metropolitan Life Desirable Weight Table. Weight is measured in pounds, without clothing and height is measured without shoes.

bidity and mortality should be developed to permit the preparation of reference tables for defining the desirable range of body weight on morbidity and mortality statistics.

Based on the studies reviewed at the workshop in 1982, the desirable body mass index (BMI) for men is 22 (mean) with a range of 20 to 25, and for women 21.5 (mean) with a range of 19 to 26. It is the BMI that is associated with the lowest mortality.

THE NATIONAL CENTER FOR HEALTH STATISTICS
DEFINITION OF DESIRABLE BODY WEIGHT

The National Center for Health Statistics also uses the term "Desirable Body Weight," but BMI is determined statistically on the basis of the weights and heights of the U.S. population from the National Health and Nutrition Examination Survey (NHANES). It is thus a statistical determination, not a measure that has been shown to be associated with decreased morbidity or mortality. Overweight is defined as a BMI greater than or equal to the 85th percentile of men or women 20 to 29 years of age. Severe overweight is defined as a BMI greater than or equal to the 95th percentile from NHANES. Based on data from NHANES II,[18] men are considered overweight if their BMI is greater than or equal to 27.8, and "severely overweight" is defined as a BMI greater than or equal to 31.1. For women the BMI cut-off points are 27.3 and 32.2, respectively. Using the average weight at 20 to 29 years of age as the "desirable BMI" is inappropriate since data from epidemiologic and other longitudinal studies indicate a continuous increase in weight during the age period from 20 to 29, which leads to an overestimation of desirable weight and an underestimation of obesity in the population.

THE 1990 DIETARY GUIDELINES AND WHY THE
"HEALTHY WEIGHT" TABLE SHOULD BE WITHDRAWN

Despite the conclusions of the 1982 NIH workshop and the data from the FHS, the 1985 NIH Consensus Conference set the desirable BMI at 27.8 for men and 27.3 for women as the upper limit of the normal range based on the NHANES II statistical definition. Yet the FHS data showed that a unit change in the BMI increases mortality from cardiovascular disease.[12] Since then, other prospective studies of short duration[19] and further analyses of the FHS have shown that the relative risks of nonfatal myocardial infarction and fatal coronary heart disease combined, as adjusted for age and cigarette smoking, are lowest at a BMI of 21 or less, increased to 1.8 at a BMI of 23 to < 25, and rose to 3.3 at a BMI of 25 to < 29. Yet despite all this evidence the 1990 U.S. Dietary Guidelines recommended an increase in the range of the body weight table. This table, referred to as "Healthy Weights," has an upper BMI range of 27, a level at which both morbidity and mortality from cardiovascular disease are higher than indicated on the table included in the previous two editions of the U.S. Dietary Guidelines.

At the higher weight ranges recommended in the 1990 Dietary Guidelines, the population is already overweight and at a BMI of 27, it is already obese. Considering the difficulties involved in treating obesity, the emphasis should be on the prevention of obesity and initiating treatment at lesser degrees of obesity. Another problem with the 1990 Dietary Guidelines table is the fact that it permits an increase in body weight above age 35, just at the age (25 to 44) when women who are overweight have been shown to have the highest incidence of major weight gain of any subgroup.[20] Williamson and co-workers[20] using the NHANES data for the definition of obesity, showed that the incidence of major weight gain over a 10-year period was twice as high in women as in men, and was highest in persons aged 25 to 34 years. Based on these findings, special emphasis is needed for young women who are overweight. Obesity prevention should begin early since persons in their 20s and 30s are at highest risk of becoming overweight. In the Williamson study, the incidence of obesity would have been much higher if a BMI range of 20 to 25 had been used instead of the NHANES cut-off points of ≥ 7.8 for men and 7.3 for women.[20]

THE PREVALENCE OF OBESITY IN WOMEN
AND SOME ETHNIC GROUPS

Both the incidence and the prevalence of obesity depend on the definition of obesity, whether it is a statistical determination or a measure based on morbidity and mortality. The prevalence is disproportionately high in certain population groups, especially women, the poor, and members of some ethnic minorities.[21] Black women are more at risk than any other population group. Obesity, particularly trunk obesity, is more prevalent in black women than white women after adolescence, regardless of socioeconomic status, but black women of lower socioeconomic status are at highest risk for obesity. There is an approximate 2:1 prevalence of overweight in black women compared to white women.[22,23] The NHANES data suggest higher calorie intake in black females than white females during adolescence (12 to 20 or 12 to 24 years of age in both surveys).[22,23] Adolescence is the period when the adult pattern of excess weight gain begins to emerge among black females.

RANGE OF BODY WEIGHT REFERENCE STANDARDS
FOR THE TREATMENT OF OBESITY

The weight loss necessary to improve the metabolic state varies with the particular disease entity and the individual involved. We must understand and take into account the genetic predisposition to obesity and the fact that obesity or weight gain during the young adult years has dire consequences. Genetic predisposition should lead to early identification of individuals at risk and to specific recommendations for the prevention of the genetic expression. The development of reference standards as a guide to prevention is essential. It should be the line not to cross. If the line is crossed and the person becomes obese, his or her target weight should be decided by the physician based on family history, the existence of other disease, the individual's personality and ability to respond to the various treatment modalities, including diet, exercise, and pharmacologic programs. In obesity, as in any disorder, treatment needs to be tailored to the individual.

BODY WEIGHT REFERENCE STANDARDS FOR THE PREVENTION OF OBESITY

The range in weight for the prevention of obesity shown in Tables 1 and 2 is based on the 1959 Metropolitan Life Insurance table and the review of studies in the 1982 workshop. Taking into consideration the data from the prospective Framingham Heart Study and the study by Manson and co-workers,[19] a range of between 20 to 25 for men and between 19 to 25 for women is the desirable BMI range (Table 4).

CONCLUSION

The prevalence of obesity continues to increase in the U.S. population. There is a need to develop reference standards based on data indicating the weight range that is associated with the lowest mortality rates by age and sex. In the meantime, the desirable body weight table (Table 1) based on the long-term prospective Framingham Heart Study data and other short-term prospective studies should be used. This table was used in the 1980 and 1985 Dietary Guideline for Americans. The 1990 Dietary Guidelines for Americans —Healthy Weight Table is not based on scientific data and should be abandoned. For the prevention of obesity, the recommended

Table 4. Mean Body Mass Index (BMI) for Men and Women Aged 30 to 39, 40 to 49, and 50 to 62

	Men kg/m^2 (1 SD)	Women kg/m^2 (1 SD)
Desirable BMI mean	22.0	21.5
Desirable BMI range	20-25	19-26
Olympic sprinters	23.0	23.0
Olympic marathon runners	20.0	20.0

From the 1959 Metropolitan Life Desirable Weight Table (mean of midpoint of medium frame; range of all heights and frames for all ages).

range in body mass index is 20 to 25 for men, and 19 to 25 for women. For the treatment of obesity, therapy and weight goals should be targeted to the individual.

NOTES

1.   Chambers TK (1993). On corpulence. Obesity Res 1(1):57-84.
2.   Ideal weight for women (1942). New York: Metropolitan Life Insurance Co.
3.   Ideal weight for men (1943). New York: Metropolitan Life Insurance Co.
4.   Abraham S, Johnson CL, Najjar MF (1979). Weight and height of adults 18-74 years of age, United States, 1971-74. DHEW Publication (PHS) 79-1659 (Vital and Health Statistics, series 11, no. 211). Hyattsville, MD: National Center for Health Statistics.
5.   Medico-Actuarial Mortality Investigation (1913). New York: Association of Life Insurance Medical Directors and Actuarial Society of America.
6.   Tannenbaum A (1940). Relationship of body weight to cancer incidence. Arch Pathol 30:509.
7.   Simopoulos AP (1985). Fat intake, obesity and cancer of the breast and endometrium. Med Oncol Tumor Pharmacother 2:125-135.
8.   Simopoulos AP (1987). Nutritional cancer risks derived from energy and fat. Med Oncol Tumor Pharmacother 4:227-239.
9.   Simopoulos AP (1990). Energy imbalance and cancer of the breast, colon and prostate. Med Oncol Tumor Pharmacother 7:109-120.
10. Build and Blood Pressure Study, vol 1 (1959). Chicago: Society of Actuaries.
11. Simopoulos AP (1986). Obesity and body weight standards. Annu Rev Public Health 7:481-492.
12. Hubert HB, Feinleib M, McNamara PM, Castelli WP (1983). Obesity as an independent risk factor for cardiovascular disease: a 26-year follow-up of participants in the Framingham Heart Study. Circulation 67:968-977.
13. Garrison RJ, Feinleib M, Castelli WP, McNamara PM (1983). Cigarette smoking as a confounder of the relationship between relative weight and long-term mortality: the Framingham Heart Study. JAMA 249:2199-2203.
14. U.S. Department of Agriculture (1980). Nutrition and your health: dietary guidelines for Americans. (Home and Garden Bulletin no. 232, 1/e.) Washington, DC: U.S. Department of Health and Human Services.
15. U.S. Department of Agriculture (1985). Nutrition and your health: dietary guidelines for Americans. (Home and Garden Bulletin no. 232, 2/e.) Washington, DC: U.S. Department of Health and Human Services.
16. U.S. Department of Agriculture (1990). Nutrition and your health: dietary guidelines for Americans. (Home and Garden Bulletin no. 232, 3/e.) Washington, DC: U.S. Department of Health and Human Services.
17. Willett WC, Stampfer M, Manson J, VanItallie T (1991). New weight guidelines for Americans: justified or injudicious? Am J Clin Nutrition 53:1102-1103.
18. Najjar MR, Rowland M (1987). Anthropometric reference data and prevalence of overweight, United States, 1976-80. DHHS Publication (PHS) 87-1688 (Vital and Health Statistics, series 11, no. 238). Hyattsville, MD: National Center for Health Statistics.
19. Manson JE, Colditz GA, Stampfer MJ, et al. (1990). A prospective study of obesity and risk of coronary heart disease in women. N Engl J Med 322:882-889.

20. Williamson DF, Kahn HS, Remington PL, et al. (1990). The 10-year incidence of overweight and major weight gain in U.S. adults. Arch Intern Med 150:6665-6672.
21. Methods for voluntary weight loss and control (1992). National Institutes of Health Technology Assessment Conference Statement. Bethesda, MD: Office of Medical Applications of Research, National Institutes of Health.
22. Gartside PS, Khoury P, Glueck CJ (1984). Determinants of high-density lipoprotein cholesterol in blacks and whites: the second National Health and Nutrition Examination Survey. Am Heart J 108:641-653.
23. Dietary intake findings, United States, 1971-1974 (1977). DHEW Publication (HRA) 77-1647 (Vital and Health Statistics, series 11, no. 202). Hyattsville, MD: National Center for Health Statistics.
24. Simopoulos AP, Herbert V, Jacobson B (1993). Genetic nutrition: designing a diet based on your family medical history. New York: Macmillan.

3

The Role of Adiposity in the Prevention of Cardiovascular Disease

Robert J. Garrison, MS

It has been conclusively demonstrated that cardiovascular disease that continues to ravage middle-aged and older Americans is "largely" preventable (Farquhar et al. 1990). However, the primary prevention of cardiovascular disease would require large changes in the quality and quantity of diets, including substantial reductions in fat and sugar consumption, as well as major changes in exercise habits and the elimination of cigarette smoking. While national average saturated fat consumption appears to be declining gradually over the last decade (Human Nutrition Information Service 1985) and cigarette smoking has declined more rapidly, there is little evidence that sedentary lifestyles are becoming less prevalent. Furthermore, while health education efforts have clearly succeeded in increasing the level of knowledge about lifestyles which promote optimal cardiovascular health (Farquhar et al. 1990), the pervasive knowledge of the need for such health behaviors has not resulted in the necessary changes in large numbers of Americans (Fortmann et al. 1990).

At the beginning of this century the lives of most Americans differed in many respects from those of the typical American who will live in the next century. The most conspicuous difference was the relatively high energy demands in the occupations of most men. Of note also was the nature of daily patterns of activity for most women who spent their days doing household labor. As sedentary occupations became common and a proclivity toward household labor-saving devices appeared in mid-century, energy requirements became substantially lower for most Americans. However, Americans continued to eat as they were taught to eat at the family dining table. The consequence was a rise in obesity that is probably unmatched in size and absolute numbers of afflicted individuals in the history of man. The consequences of this rise in obesity are only recently

22

being fully understood, but the epidemic of obesity and its intractable nature are appreciated. In addition to overnutrition and sedentary lifestyles, the high fat content of most diets and the high prevalence of cigarette smoking contributed to the epidemic. Thus, there is compelling evidence that the cardiovascular disease epidemic is the result of lifestyles that are either out of balance (energy) or abusive in the consumption of high-fat foods and tobacco. While the seeds of cardiovascular disease can be sown differently for each individual, it is clear that with few exceptions, the pathological patterns and their sequelae can be prevented in all but a few individuals.

During the first half of the twentieth century, as the epidemic was building, complications of atherosclerosis appeared to afflict a disproportionate number of the middle and upper classes in the United States. Writing in *The Lancet* in 1910, William Osler commented that "we are all familiar that angina pectoris is an affliction of the better classes and not often seen except in private practise." Osler, a physician, continued his description of the epidemiology of angina pectoris by stating that an outstanding feature of the disease was the "frequency of the disease in our profession" and that "angina may almost be called 'morbus medicorum.'" This early view of the sociodemographics of coronary disease contrasts sharply with results of the Physicians' Health Study (Steering Committee of the Physicians' Health Research Group 1989), a randomized clinical trial involving 22,071 physicians in the U.S. conducted between 1983 and 1988. This study documented that the coronary disease death rates in physicians are only about 15 percent of that in the general population. Also, it is becoming apparent that physicians constitute only one distinct subgroup that has markedly lower cardiovascular disease mortality. There is substantial evidence that sociodemographic distribution of cardiovascular disease has changed rapidly over the last few decades in the U.S. with declines in cardiovascular disease mortality rates in some groups, but not in others (Feldman et al. 1989). These structural changes in the cardiovascular disease epidemic seem to confirm what is known about the lifestyle-based causes of cardiovascular disease. For example, the cigarette smoking rate in physicians dropped precipitously after the 1964 Surgeon General's Report on Smoking and Health and now appears to be one of the lowest among major occupational groups.

Another prominent change in the nature of the cardiovascular disease epidemic is the mortality associated with the major manifestations of cardiovascular disease. U.S. mortality rates from stroke and coronary heart disease have declined substantially in the later half of this century (Thom 1989). The mortality decline results from the joint impact of the reduction in cigarette smoking, more efficacious and more prevalent treatment for hypertension and improved tertiary treatment for clinically recognized cardiovascular disease. While it is difficult to quantify the impact of each of these changes on mortality, it is worth noting that the differential impact of the primary, secondary and tertiary prevention on the character of the cardiovascular disease epidemic is of major importance.

Primary prevention of lifestyle characteristics and health behaviors that are deleterious is the optimum strategy for preventing the mortality associated with cardiovascular disease. Decreases in cigarette smoking in the U.S. during the last three decades have without doubt made a major contribution to the reduction in stroke and coronary heart disease death rates and, while major proportions of the population continue to smoke, and, as noted above, subgroups of the population continue to resist change, the success of health education in contributing to this change is substantive and widely recognized. The advantages of primary prevention of cardiovascular disease is that the disease process is altered or eliminated early in the pathological process without the need for expensive medical intervention or the use of medication. Also, as implied by the use of the term "primary," no actual case of disease develops and therefore no continuing burden of prevalence cases exists in the population. Thus, a strong case can be made for the need to find efficacious methods of primary prevention of cardiovascular disease. Such methods need to focus on the lifestyle characteristics such as sedentary behavior, overnutrition and cigarette smoking, which are the underpinnings of the cardiovascular disease epidemic.

The important contribution of medication for hypertension to reduction of the mortality from cardiovascular disease is difficult to quantify but is undoubtedly large. Effective drugs for the treatment of hypertension are now available to most individuals with high blood pressure and compliance rates remain high. The National High Blood Pressure Education Program, which encouraged detection and treatment of hypertension, was the first of several national programs which rely on the medical model. While the success of such prevention programs is widely acknowledged and their cost is relatively low, the need for such measures could be greatly reduced if adequate primary prevention was practiced (Kannel 1987).

Tertiary prevention of cardiovascular disease, defined as medical or surgical life-saving intervention applied to individuals who have clinically manifest disease, has become a major focus and contributor to mortality decline as technical advances have proceeded during the last 20 years. It has also contributed to the rapid rise in health care costs in the U.S. during the last two decades. Furthermore, such interventions do not usually constitute a cure for the identified cardiovascular malady since individual patients often remain part of the prevalence pool that contributes to the future disease burden, requiring additional medical or surgical treatment. Thus, certain features of the cardiovascular disease epidemic, particularly the declining mortality rates, have created the illusion that the cardiovascular disease epidemic is diminishing. The few studies that are designed to measure trends in the cardiovascular disease morbidity incidence rates have concluded that there is little evidence that rate of occurrence of new cases of cardiovascular disease, nonfatal and fatal combined, has changed dramatically in the last half of the twentieth century. This is not unexpected since, with the exception of cigarette smoking, there is little change in the overall prevalence of the fundamental lifestyle-driven substrates of risk determination.

Cardiovascular disease is the most pervasive health problem in the United States. The numerous manifestations or clinical expressions of the disease include coronary heart disease, cerebral vascular disease and other diseases of the heart and vascular system. These cardiovascular maladies caused over 900,000 of the 2.15 million deaths that occurred in the U.S. during 1991 (National Center for Health Statistics 1991), a far greater number than were caused by cancer, which accounted for 514,000 deaths that year. As high as the death rates from these diseases are, there are other, more sobering statistics that characterize the twentieth century epidemic of cardiovascular disease in the West. For example, it has been estimated that nearly 8 million Americans had symptomatic coronary heart disease (Adams and Benson 1991) that caused about 2 million hospital admittances during 1990. A large proportion of these hospital admissions involve the application of new and expensive life-saving technologies. One of the more common surgical interventions is the coronary artery bypass graft. A total of 407,000 of these procedures were performed in 1990 at an average cost of $32,000 each (Wittels et al. 1990). Such procedures, while undoubtedly saving thousands of lives each year, have contributed substantially to the enormous cost of the cardiovascular disease epidemic.

Most of the manifestations of cardiovascular disease have a very well understood etiology with atherosclerosis, or fatty deposits in the linings of the vasculature, being the underlying pathology for coronary heart disease and most cerebrovascular disease. While the progression and consequences of the atherosclerosis are highly variable between individuals, the process of fat deposition in the vasculature is known to begin in the teenage years (Newman et al. 1986; Solberg and Strong 1983) and progress to pathological levels in most adults (Ross 1986). The progression of atherosclerosis is primarily influenced by lifestyle choices of the individual. The fat content of the diet, the quantity of nutrition, the amount of exercise and cigarette smoking all play important roles, with possibly differing impacts on different individuals. While it is difficult to show direct independent effects of each of these lifestyle variables in human studies, because direct assessment of atherosclerosis is difficult, strong supportive evidence for this view of atherogenesis comes from the rapidly increasing understanding of lipoprotein metabolism in humans. The body of evidence from observational and experimental studies of lipoprotein metabolism presents the best evidence of the lifestyle-based pathology of atherosclerosis, and thus the ultimate preventability of most cardiovascular disease.

The most compelling documentation of the preventability of cardiovascular disease comes from information generated from epidemiologic studies about the relationship of various lipoprotein cholesterol levels, such as high-density lipoprotein cholesterol (HDL-C) and low-density lipoprotein cholesterol (LDL-C) and lifestyle variables. Adiposity, whether it results from sedentary habits or overnutrition, appears to dominate interindividual variation of both LDL-C and HDL-C levels. These findings are particularly noteworthy in young adults who are just beginning to increase their fat mass. In young adults in the Framingham Offspring Study, a unit increase in body mass index (BMI) (approximately 5 pounds of body fat) was shown to result in a 10 mg/dl increase in LDL-C (Anderson et al. 1987). Similarly, HDL-C decreases were found to be strongly associated with increases in BMI and the total "lipoprotein profile"; the combination of the two lipoproteins is substantially negatively influenced when body fat increases. Studies have also shown that physical activity increases have a very salutary impact on HDL-C levels, independent of any change in adiposity levels (Dannenberg et al. 1989). LDL levels, in contrast, are particularly sensitive to the *quality* of the diet. The higher the percentage of saturated fat in the diet, the higher the LDL cholesterol is likely to be (Grundy et al. 1988). All of these findings point to the conclusion that the lifestyle variables and particularly eating and exercise behavior have strong relationships with lipoprotein metabolism dysfunction, the fundamental cause of atherosclerosis.

The consequences of atherosclerosis seem to be very diverse, given how relatively homogeneous and complete is the exposure of the population to the atherogenic lifestyle. It is obvious that two individuals with equivalent adiposity exposures do not necessarily experience the same overt cardiovascular disease consequences. The reasons for such disparities are not as well understood as the underlying causes of atherosclerosis, but it is important to acknowledge their importance. First, there are several well-documented (Slack and Evans 1966; Snowden et al. 1982; Goldstein et al. 1973), genetically determined causes of the diversity of response. Certain genotypes have easily discernible alterations in lipoprotein metabolism that have drastic impact on propensity for atherogenesis (Goldstein et al. 1973). Information about more subtle differences in lipoprotein structure and function is rapidly expanding and continues to contribute to the evidence that similar overnutrition in different individuals can have very diverse impact on the pace and extent of atherosclerosis. Also, the hypertensive response to overnutrition, characterized by adiposity and elevated salt intake, appears to have a strong genetic determination (Bondjers et al. 1991; Folkow 1990). Genetic differences are the most likely explanation for the fact that some fat individuals never develop hypertension, while many others do (Carter and Kannel 1990).

The second major explanation for the diversity of responses to atherosclerosis is what could be characterized as trigger mechanisms. These are the environmental stressors that cause an acute event, that in the atherosclerotic milieu are often the first indication of pathology. Often this acute event is the formation of a thrombus that causes ischemia and consequent damage to the heart, brain or other organ. Cigarette smoking has often been considered a trigger mechanism for myocardial infarction and stroke because chemicals in cigarette smoke are thought to directly enhance clotting (Mustard and Murphy 1963). Other trigger mechanisms include emotional stress (Sime et al. 1980; Williams et al. 1982) and physical stress (Boyer et al. 1960).

Thus, an examination of the vast literature that attempts to find the causes of the cardiovascular disease epidemic yields a very clear conclusion that a prevention strategy should target overnutrition and sedentary lifestyle as the fundamental driving forces behind this burdensome and tragic epidemic. While mechanisms are well understood and "risk factors" thoroughly described, the target or optimum levels of adiposity and exercise that would minimize the risk of cardiovascular disease, and "largely" prevent it, continue to be debated. Such standards are at least as necessary as those for "hypertension" or "hypercholesterolemia," especially if there is to be movement away from the medical model of prevention.

Adiposity "standards" for adult men and women, while they have traditionally been based on long-term mortality studies, can be developed using a strategy that takes advantage of large cross-sectional data bases that have measured adiposity and an array of other health-related attributes during middle age. The Framingham Offspring Study provides one such opportunity (Garrison and Kannel 1993).

Between 1971 and 1975 a second Framingham cohort was enrolled for study. This cohort consists of the offspring (and their spouses) of the original cohort who were adults at the time of initiation of the study. These study participants are often referred to as the Framingham offspring cohort (Kannel et al. 1979). The offspring study eligibility roster was established from information obtained at the first biennial examination of the original cohort, when participants were asked to list the names and birth dates of their children. This information was updated and addresses and phone numbers were obtained at the later biennial examinations. Finally, in 1970, a computer file was constructed which contained the names and addresses of all surviving children.

The children who had both parents in the original Framingham cohort were the first to be invited to the offspring study examination. Spouses of these offspring were also enrolled whenever possible and the children of other members (without spouses) in the original cohort were also invited to participate. When recruitment was completed the offspring cohort consisted of 5,124 men and women aged 9 to 72 years. Most participants (92.1

percent) were from 20 to 54 years old at the time of their initial examination between 1971 and 1975.

This initial examination was intended to screen participants for existing cardiovascular disease and obtain baseline measurements of body weight, plasma lipoprotein levels, blood pressure and a medical history. Those who participated in this initial examination were invited to a second, much more extensive evaluation beginning in 1979, approximately 8 years following the initial examination. Since 1979 the offspring cohort has been invited to participate in quadrennial evaluations.

The offspring cohort members were asked to come to the Framingham clinic in the morning without having eaten breakfast. No remuneration was given to participants (including travel costs), but a light snack was provided to those who requested it after blood was drawn for testing. A 12-lead electrocardiogram was performed by a technician prior to an extensive physician-administered physical examination. The physician also performed two measurements of the systolic and diastolic blood pressure, and completed the medical history interview which included questions about medication use, cigarette smoking and alcohol consumption. A nurse measured skinfold thickness at 1 inch below the right scapula, as well as stature and weight. The fasting blood specimen was used to measure the cholesterol content of the high- and low-density lipoprotein fractions using Lipid Research Clinic methodology and total cholesterol and plasma glucose was measured using standard laboratory methods (Garrison et al. 1979).

Table 1 lists the mean values and standard deviations of right subscapular skinfold (RSS) thickness and the cardiovascular disease (CV) risk factors as well as the age-adjusted regression coefficient for the regression of each CV risk factor on RSS for 20- to 39-year-old men and women. As indicated by the p-values in this table, all CV risk factors are found to be statistically significantly related to RSS in both men and women in this group of young adults. With the exception of total plasma cholesterol, where the regression coefficient for men is more than two times greater than for women, relationships appear to be very similar in women and men. This similarity holds despite consistently more adverse mean values of the CV risk factors in men. Note that while the strength and shape of the relationships vary, all measures show an association with adiposity that is in an unfavorable direction. The decile of RSS that had the lowest average (highest for HDL cholesterol) was determined and a summary threshold based on the maximum decile for which any CV risk factor had a minimum value was determined. This resulted in a healthy adiposity threshold of RSS < 12 for men and RSS < 15 for women.

When men and women with RSS at or above these levels were excluded there remained only 89 men and 380 women nonsmokers (ages 20 to 59) who could be considered to have healthy adiposity status. The dark bars of Figures 1 and 2 show the BMI distribution of these individuals rounded to

Table 1. Mean and Standard Deviation of CV Risk Factors and RSS and the Age-adjusted Regression of each CV Risk Factor on RSS by Sex in 20- to 39-year-old Adults

	Men				Women			
	Mean	*SD*	*β*	*p*	*Mean*	*SD*	*β*	*p*
SBP (mmHg)	121.70	(12.3)	.434	**	110.40	(11.1)	.292	**
BBP (mmHg)	78.80	(8.80)	.245	**	72.70	(8.10)	.182	**
TC (mmol/l)	4.92	(.903)	.022	**	4.68	(.810)	.010	*
HDL (mmol/l)	1.16	(2.69)	-.007	**	1.42	(.296)	-.008	**
LDL (mmol/l)	3.18	(.845)	.015	*	2.86	(.757)	.014	**
GL (mmol/l)	5.43	(.610)	.011	*	5.07	(.496)	.009	**
RSS (mm)	19.80	(8.8)			18.90	(10.4)		

Men: n=357; women: n=403. Data from the Framingham Offspring Study.
* p < .01
** p < .001

the nearest BMI integer value. The mean BMI for this group of men and women, respectively, is 22.6 and 21.2. The comparison of these distributions with the BMI distribution of the entire sample allows an estimate of the probability of having an unhealthy adiposity level for each individual unit of BMI as shown in Figure 3. The body adiposity percentage (BAP) curve appears to rise more rapidly in men than women as BMI increases but reaches a plateau with probabilities of over .90 in both sexes at BMI = 25.

Thus, the BAP curves show that men and women with BMI above 24.5 have a very high probability (above .90) of having adiposity in excess of that which is consistent with optimum health. Furthermore, individuals with a BMI greater than 22 have a high (above .50) probability of unhealthy adiposity levels. Individuals at these levels are strong candidates for careful evaluation by skinfold measurements or other adiposity assessment methods to determine whether they have unhealthy adiposity levels. Even men with a BMI as low as 21 should be considered for more careful evaluations. Thus, the estimates from this white sample suggest that only in the 24 percent of men and 34 percent of women, those with a BMI between 22 and 24, would further evaluation than the simple calculation of BMI be necessary. It should be noted, however, that these estimates could vary widely in subgroups with different racial and age composition.

Given the recent documentation that most attempts to lose weight are unsuccessful (NIH Technology Assessment Conference Panel 1993), findings such as these might be taken as entirely unrealistic. However, arguments can be made that the large number of moderately obese middle-aged individuals might appropriately be targeted for weight loss as they make

Men - Age 20-59

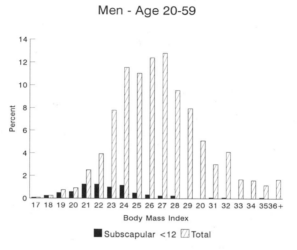

Figure 1. Body mass index of 89 nonsmoking men 20 to 59 years old with healthy adiposity status (filled bars) and all men aged 20 to 59 (hatched bars).

Women - Age 20-59

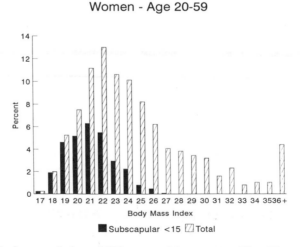

Figure 2. Body mass index of 380 nonsmoking women 20 to 59 years old with healthy adiposity status (filled bars) and all women aged 20 to 59 (hatched bars).

Men and Women, Age 20-59

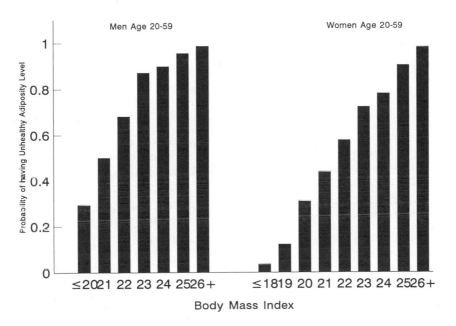

Figure 3.   The probability of having an unhealthy adiposity level for each unit (rounded to the nearest integer) of BMI for nonsmoking men and women 20 to 59 years old.

up a very large "at risk" group where success in even a relatively small proportion of subjects would be expected to relieve a substantial burden of overt disease, suffering and medical resources. There is also a possibility that such individuals have less ingrained obesity-promoting lifestyles and would be more amenable to changes to lower their adiposity levels.

Since cardiovascular diseases are the major cause of morbidity, disability and death and are a dominant and growing focus of medical resources in North America, it seems most appropriate that the measures of health used in this report all are established "risk factors" for clinically recognizable cardiovascular disease. While the use of these risk factors to define "health" may seem arbitrary, the fact is that these attributes are the focus of most current health screening efforts in asymptomatic individuals. The availability of large samples, such as in this study, for detailed biochemical studies and noninvasive testing, should result in better definitions of health, involving many different organ systems, in the future.

Thus, prevention strategies that seek to "largely" prevent cardiovascular disease will need to address overnutrition, the fundamental force that promotes high adiposity levels and is responsible for a large and growing portion of cardiovascular disease morbidity and mortality in the United States.

REFERENCES

Adams PF, Benson V (1991). Current estimates from the National Health Interview Survey—National Center for Health Statistics. Vital and Health Statistics-NCHS, 10-181. Atlanta: U.S. Department of Health and Human Services.

Anderson KM, Wilson PWF, Garrison RJ, Castelli WP (1987). Longitudinal and secular trends in lipoprotein cholesterol measurements in a general population sample: the Framingham offspring study. Atherosclerosis A68:59-66.

Bondjers G, Glukhova M, Hansson GK, Postnov YV, Reidy MA, Schwartz SM (1991). Hypertension and atherosclerosis—cause and effect, or two effects with one unknown cause. Circulation A84(6-2):6-16.

Boyer JT, Fraser JRE, Doyle AE (1960). The hemodynamic effects of cold immersion. Clin Sci 19:539-550.

Carter CL, Kannel WB (1990). Evidence of a rare gene for low systolic blood pressure in the Framingham heart study. Hum Hered 40:235-241.

Dannenberg AL, Keller JB, Wilson PWF, Castelli WP (1989). Leisure time physical activity in the Framingham offspring study: description, seasonal variation and risk factor correlates. Am J Epidemiol 129:76-88.

Farquhar JW, Fortmann SP, Flora JA, Taylor B, Haskell WL, Williams PT, Maccoby N, Wood PD (1990). Effects of community-wide education on cardiovascular disease risk factors. JAMA 264:359-365.

Feldman JJ, Makuc DM, Kleinman JC, Cornoni-Huntley J (1989). National trends in educational differentials in mortality. Am J Epidemiol 129:919-933.

Folkow B (1990). "Structural factor" in primary and secondary hypertension. J Hypertension 16:89-101.

Fortmann SP, Winkleby MA, Flora JA, Haskell WL, Taylor CB (1990). Effect of long-term community health education on blood pressure and hypertension control. Am J Epidemiol 132:629-646.

Garrison RJ, Castelli WP, Feinleib M, Kannel WB, Havlik RJ, Padgett SJ, McNamara PM (1979). The association of total cholesterol, triglycerides and plasma lipoprotein cholesterol levels in first-degree relatives and spouse pairs. Am J Epidemiol 110:313-321.

Garrison RJ, Kannel WB (1993). A new approach for estimating healthy body weights. Int J Obesity 17:417-423.

Goldstein JL, Hazzard WR, Schrott HG (1973). Hyperlipidemia in coronary heart disease. Lipid levels in 500 survivors of myocardial infarction. J Clin Invest 52:1533-1541.

Grundy SM, Barrett-Conner E, Rudel LL (1988). Workshop on the impact of dietary cholesterol on plasma lipoproteins and atherogenesis. Atherosclerosis A8:95-101.

Human Nutrition Information Service (1985). Nationwide Food Consumption Survey: continuing survey of food intakes by individuals, women 19-50 years and their children 1-5 years, 1 day. Hyattsville, MD: U.S. Department of Agriculture.

Kannel WB (1987). Cardiovascular risk factors and "preventive management." Hosp Pract [Off] 22:147-164.

Kannel WB, Feinleib M, McNamara PM, Garrison RJ, Castelli WP (1979). An investigation of coronary heart disease in families: the Framingham offspring study. Am J Epidemiol 110:281-290.

Mustard JF, Murphy EA (1963). Effect of smoking on blood coagulation and platelet survival in man. Br Med J 272:846-849.

National Center for Health Statistics (1991). Monthly Vital Statistics Report—births, marriages, divorces for August 1991. Atlanta: U.S. Department of Health and Human Services.

Newman WP, Freedman DS, Voors AW, Gard PD, Srinivasan SR, Cresanta JL, Williamson GD, Webber LS, Berenson GS (1986). Relation of serum lipoprotein levels and systolic blood pressure to early atherosclerosis. N Engl J Med 314:138-144.

NIH Technology Assessment Conference Panel (1993). Methods for voluntary weight loss and control. Ann Intern Med 119:764-770.

Ross R (1986). The pathogenesis of atherosclerosis—an update. N Engl J Med 314:488-500.

Sime WE, Buell JC, Eliot RS (1980). Cardiovascular responses to emotional stress in post-infarct cardiac patients and matched control subjects. J Human Stress 6:39-46.

Slack J, Evans KA (1966). The increased risk of death from ischaemic heart disease in first-degree relatives of 121 men and 96 women with ischaemic heart disease. J Med Genet 3:239-240.

Snowden CB, McNamara PM, Garrison RJ, Feinleib M, Kannel WB, Epstein FH (1982). Predicting coronary heart disease in siblings—a multivariate assessment: the Framingham heart study. Am J Epidemiol 115:217-222.

Solberg LA, Strong JP (1983). Risk factors and atherosclerotic lesions: a review of autopsy studies. Atherosclerosis A3:187-198.

Steering Committee of the Physicians' Health Research Group (1989). Final report on the aspirin component of the ongoing physicians' health study. N Engl J Med 321:129-135.

Thom TJ (1989). International mortality from heart disease: rates and trends. Int J Epidemiol 18(1-20):1-28.

Williams RB, Lane JD, Kuhn CM, Melosh W, White AR, Schanberg SM (1982). Physiological and neuroendocrine response patterns during different behavioral challenges: differential hyperresponsivity of type A men. Science A218:483-485.

Wittels ET, Hay JW, Gotto AM (1990). Medical costs of coronary artery disease in the United States. Am J Cardiol 65:432-440.

4

Assessing Impact of Weight on Quality of Life

Ronette L. Kolotkin, PhD, Susan B. Head, PhD
Michael Hamilton, MD

Obesity is a chronic, refractory condition, with relapse rates ranging from 50 to 90 percent (Brownell, Marlatt, Lichtenstein and Wilson 1986). The strong, negative impact of obesity on physiological health has been well-established (see Perri, Nezu and Viegener 1992 for a review). However, the impact of obesity on psychological and social functioning has been studied less extensively and is the subject of some debate. While it is generally believed that obesity has adverse effects on many areas of psychosocial functioning (Wadden and Stunkard 1985), the impact of weight on overall quality of life has not been studied directly.

Until recently there has been no direct method of assessing the impact of weight on major areas of psychosocial functioning. This chapter discusses the psychometric properties and clinical utility of a newly developed instrument, the Impact of Weight on Quality of Life (IWQOL) questionnaire. Unlike other quality of life instruments, this questionnaire deals specifically with weight and its effects.

In developing the IWQOL, the authors had several aims in mind: (1) to develop a questionnaire that would reliably and validly measure the extent to which weight affects quality of life; (2) to be able to determine the aspects of quality of life that are most affected by weight; and (3) to measure improvements in quality of life associated with weight loss or other treatment interventions.

This chapter reports on two studies that have been presented separately elsewhere. In the first study we describe item development, assess reliability and compare pre- and post-treatment scores on the IWQOL; in the second study we examine the effects of body mass index (BMI), gender and age on subjects' perceptions of impact of weight on quality of life.

STUDY 1

Method

Subjects

Subjects were 64 male and female outpatients in treatment for obesity at Duke University Diet and Fitness Center (DDFC), a multidisciplinary day treatment program in Durham, North Carolina. The typical length of treatment at the DDFC is 28 days.

Item Development

In the course of their regular treatment, patients (other than those participating in the studies reported here) were asked to describe the effects of being overweight in their everyday lives. Based on their responses, 74 items were written, modified, tested for clarity and categorized into eight scales: Health, Social/Interpersonal Life, Work, Mobility, Self-Esteem, Sexual Life, Activities of Daily Living and Comfort with Food. Scales are scored independently and with the exception of Comfort with Food, the higher the score, the more problems in that particular area.

Procedure

Subjects were administered the questionnaire at three points in time: day 1, day 2 and day 28. Day 1 scores were compared with day 2 scores to determine test-retest reliability using Spearman correlation coefficients. Internal consistency estimates were calculated using Cronbach's alpha based on day 1 scores. To measure treatment outcome, paired t-tests were used comparing day 1 to day 28 scores. Sixty-four subjects completed the questionnaire on day 1, 51 on day 2 and 37 on day 28.

Results

Item test-retest reliabilities averaged .75, ranging from .53 on "little attention to how much I eat" under Comfort with Food, to .92 on "ankles and lower legs swollen" under Health. Scale test-retest reliabilities averaged .89, ranging from .81 on Comfort with Food, to .93 on Social/Interpersonal Life and Self-Esteem. Measures of scale internal consistency averaged .87, ranging from .68 for Comfort with Food, to .93 for Mobility. Post-treatment scores decreased significantly on all eight scales using a Bonferroni corrected significance level of .001. Significantly lower scores suggest improvement in all areas of quality of life except Comfort with Food. Lower scores on this scale indicate *less* comfort with food.

STUDY 2

Method

Subjects

Subjects were 181 outpatients (117 women, 64 men) in treatment for obesity at Duke University Diet and Fitness Center (DDFC).

Procedure

The IWQOL was administered on day 1 of the treatment program. In this study, the relationships between impact of weight and BMI, gender and age were examined. Several analyses were performed: (1) the effect of BMI was examined for the total sample and by gender using Spearman rank correlation coefficients; (2) scores for men and women were compared using paired t-tests; (3) scores for men and women were compared again, after controlling for BMI using a multiple regression analysis; (4) subjects were divided into three levels of BMI by tertiles (< 32.6, 32.7 to 39.8, > 39.9) and scores were compared by gender within tertiles using paired t-tests; (5) scores were compared within gender across tertiles using multivariate analysis of variance and Bonferroni t-tests for two-group comparisons; and (6) the effect of age on impact of weight was examined for the total sample and by gender after controlling for BMI using multiple regression analysis. The Bonferroni correction for multiple t-tests was used on all comparisons to arrive at an acceptable overall alpha of .05.

Results

BMI and Impact of Weight

For men and the total sample, there was a significant relationship (all p's < .05) between BMI and all aspects of quality of life except Comfort with Food. The highest degree of association occurred in the areas of Activities of Daily Living and Mobility. These results indicate that larger persons experience more problems than less heavy persons in most aspects of their lives—health, sexual life, social/interpersonal life, work, self-esteem—and they experience particular distress in their ability to get around and perform everyday tasks.

When women were examined separately, the association between BMI and quality of life held true for only five of the eight scales (all p's < .05). No linear relationship existed for women between BMI and effects of weight on Self-Esteem, Sexual Life and Comfort with Food. Since scores on Self-Esteem and Sexual Life were relatively high, this seems to indicate that the negative impact of weight on these areas remains essentially constant for women, regardless of their size.

Gender and Impact of Weight

Women scored higher than men on all scales but differed significantly from men on only two scales, Self-Esteem and Sexual Life (p's < .05). After controlling for BMI, women scored significantly higher than men on all scales (all p's < .05) except Comfort with Food. Women's scores were especially high on Self-Esteem (p < .0001), indicating that self-esteem is a particularly vulnerable area for women.

In comparisons of men and women within three levels of BMI, women and men differed significantly on Self-Esteem and Sexual Life (p's < .05) within the first tertile (BMI < 32.6). In the second tertile (BMI 32.7 to 39.8), women and men differed significantly only on Self-Esteem (p < .05). In the third tertile (BMI > 39.9) women and men did not differ significantly. In each instance of statistical significance, women scored higher than men, again indicating greater impact of weight for women. It also appears that women experience distress about their sexual life even at relatively low BMIs. Finally, women seem to experience more distress than men in the area of self-esteem, regardless of their amount overweight.

In comparisons within gender across BMI levels for men, mean scores differed significantly across BMI tertiles for all scales (all p's < .05) except Work and Comfort with Food. For the two-group comparisons, there were no significant differences on any scale comparisons between the first and second BMI groups. However, scores differed on four scales (all p's < .05)— Health, Social/Interpersonal Life, Mobility and Activities of Daily Living— in comparisons between the second and third BMIs. In comparisons between the first and third BMIs, scores differed significantly on the same four scales listed above plus Sexual Life (all p's < .05).

There were no significant overall group differences for women on Self-Esteem, Sexual Life and Comfort with Food, indicating that women perceive a negative impact of weight on these areas regardless of differences in amount overweight. In the two-group comparisons there were significant differences on all comparisons on Health, Mobility and Activities of Daily Living (all p's < .05). Additionally, the first and second BMIs differed from the third BMI on Social/Interpersonal Life (p's < .05) and the first differed from the third BMI on Work (p < .05).

Age and Impact of Weight

As age increased, both men and women reported significantly less impact of weight in the areas of Self-Esteem and Social/Interpersonal Life and greater impact on Mobility (all p's < .05). Women and the total sample reported significantly greater impact of weight on Health ($p < .05$) as age increased. There were no significant effects of age on Work, Sexual Life, Activities of Daily Living, or Comfort with Food.

GENERAL DISCUSSION

The results of the studies reported here indicate that the psychometric properties of the IWQOL are well within acceptable limits and support the clinical utility of the instrument for assessing problems of living associated with weight and measuring treatment outcome. Future studies are planned to examine construct validity and establish norms and cut-off scores.

In Study 1, subjects experienced improved quality of life (QOL) in seven areas of functioning after participating in an intensive 1-month treatment program for obesity. Treatment-induced QOL changes are an important, though often ignored, outcome measure of any obesity treatment program. It is our hope that obesity clinicians and researchers will begin to document these types of changes using instruments such as the IWQOL.

In Study 2, we found that women experienced the effects of their weight more profoundly than did men. This finding is consistent with what is generally known about gender differences and body image (Rodin, Silverstein and Striegel-Moore 1984). It would be interesting to determine at what BMI women actually *begin* to experience negative effects of weight on QOL.

The relationship between subjects' actual size (i.e., BMI) and impact of weight on QOL varied according to gender. For men, there was a positive correlation between increasing size and impact of weight on most aspects of QOL. However, a rather complex relationship existed for women regarding BMI and scores on Self-Esteem and Sexual Life. At every level of BMI studied, women scored high on Self-Esteem and Sexual Life, indicating problems in these areas regardless of BMI. It would be interesting to explore the relationship between women's BMI and QOL as it pertains to sexual life and self-esteem in normal weight controls, obese bingers and bulimics.

As age increased, both men and women reported less impact of weight on Self-Esteem and Social/Interpersonal Life and greater impact on Mobility. Regarding the relationship between age and health, women and the total sample reported greater impact of weight with increasing age; however, men did not. The interpretation of this finding is open to speculation.

The Comfort with Food scale is noteworthy in that it is the only scale that produced no significant findings on the dependent measures with the exception of significantly lower post-treatment scores in Study 1. This finding may indicate that through the course of treatment, increased awareness of food and eating habits may actually decrease comfort with food. Psychometrically, the Comfort with Food scale is the weakest, exhibiting adequate but not consistently strong psychometric properties. Perhaps the instability of the scale accounts for the lack of significant findings regarding our dependent variables. We suggest that the Comfort with Food scale be interpreted with caution.

Finally, the IWQOL has implications for the decision of whether or not to treat a specific individual. There is some controversy within the field about whether or not to treat certain overweight individuals given the tendency of many patients repeatedly to relapse and therefore possibly harm themselves physically and/or psychologically (Brownell et al. 1986). Perhaps the IWQOL would be useful in identifying those overweight patients who report significant impairments in quality of life. Treatment, whether aimed at weight loss or not, would have as its goal the improvement in quality of life.

REFERENCES

Brownell KD, Marlatt GA, Lichtenstein E, Wilson GT (1986). Understanding and preventing relapse. Am Psychol 41(7):765-782.

Perri MG, Nezu AM, Viegener BJ (1992). Improving the Long-Term Management of Obesity. New York: John Wiley & Sons.

Rodin J, Silverstein L, Striegel-Moore R (1984). Women and weight: a normative discontent. In TB Sonderegger (Ed.), Psychology and gender: Nebraska symposium on motivation, vol. 32. Lincoln: University of Nebraska Press.

Wadden TA, Stunkard AJ (1985). Social and psychological consequences of obesity. Ann Intern Med 103:1062-1067.

5

Hormonal Abnormalities in Obesity: Cause or Effect?

Barnett Zumoff, MD

Obese persons show numerous hormonal abnormalities. The major findings of these abnormalities have been summarized in comprehensive reviews.[1,2] The purpose here is to describe in detail some of the principal abnormalities, with particular emphasis on the question of whether they are a cause or effect of obesity. Obviously, it would be more exciting if one or more of the hormonal abnormalities of obesity could be shown to be causative than if all of them were simply consequences of obesity, though even hormonal consequences may amplify the overall morbidity of obesity, as we will discuss in the sections on serum estradiol and serum insulin.

The principal tool available to distinguish whether a given hormonal abnormality is cause or effect in obesity is the study of what happens when the obesity is eliminated by weight loss. If a hormonal abnormality then disappears or tends to disappear, it is clearly an effect of obesity, not a cause. On the other hand, if a hormonal abnormality persists after weight loss, the interpretation is not quite so clear. It could mean that the abnormality antedates the obesity and is therefore a possible causative factor, but it could also mean that it is an effect of obesity that has somehow become fixed and resistant to reversal by weight loss; an example of the latter possibility will be discussed in the section on serum estradiol in obese men.

Some of the information to be discussed has been obtained by other investigators, but much has been obtained in our own laboratory.

STUDY POPULATION

In selecting the normal and obese subjects to be studied, we tried to eliminate as many potentially confounding factors as possible. In women, we excluded subjects with historical, physical or laboratory evidence of the

40

polycystic ovary syndrome and subjects who had been pregnant or had taken oral contraceptives within the year prior to study. In both men and women, we excluded significant psychiatric illness, major chronic illness of all kinds and recent acute illness, significant medications within the 6 months prior to the study, and abnormalities of thyroid, kidney, liver, or hematologic function. All the women studied were between the ages of 18 and 47 and were having regular menstrual cycles with a normal interval; all studies were done in the early follicular phase (days 2 to 7).

METHODS IN OUR LABORATORY

All hormone levels were 24-hour mean plasma levels, obtained by sampling blood (through an in-dwelling venous catheter) every 20 minutes, pooling aliquots of the 72 samples, and assaying the pool.[3] This procedure eliminates fluctuations due to the inherent pulsatility of the secretion of nearly all hormones. Obesity was quantified either by percentage deviation from ideal weight (defined as the standard weight-for-height in the U.S. Air Force Table[4]) or by body mass index (weight/height^2 in kg/m^2). We have found that both of these parameters have a correlation of more than .95 with body fat content determined by tritium-water isotope dilution.[5]

HORMONAL DATA

Interesting findings have been obtained in our laboratory with respect to estradiol, estrone, testosterone, gonadotropins, sex hormone-binding globulin (SHBG), and insulin, and elsewhere with respect to growth hormone, prolactin, vasopressin, and β-endorphin, as well as insulin, SHBG, sex hormones, and gonadotropins.

Sex Hormones and Gonadotropins in Obese Men

It has been reported by others[6,7] that obese men have elevated plasma estrogen levels. We, too, found this to be true,[8] and found that the degree of elevation of both estradiol and estrone was proportional to the degree of obesity[9] (Figures 1 and 2). It has also been reported by others that obese men have subnormal plasma testosterone levels.[6,7,10-12] We, too, found this to be true,[13] and found that the degree of subnormality was proportional to the degree of obesity[14] (Figure 3). There has been some controversy about whether obese men also have subnormal plasma levels of *free* testosterone, the biologically active moiety; it has been pointed out by several workers that SHBG levels are low in obesity,[6,11,12] so that one might expect free testosterone levels to be less decreased, or not at all decreased, in obese men. Actually, the controversy has been more verbal than evidentiary: close reading of the literature, including papers by authors who deny the

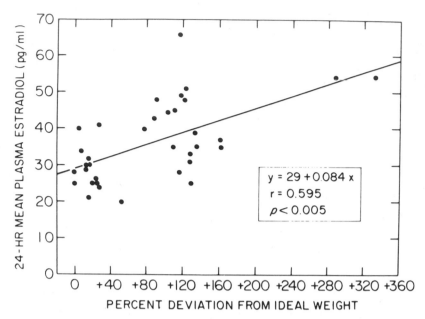

Figure 1.   The 24-hour mean plasma estradiol elevation in obese men was proportional to their degree of obesity. (Reprinted with permission from GW Strain and B Zumoff, Hormonal abnormalities in obesity. Res Staff Phys 31:13PC-24PC,1985.)

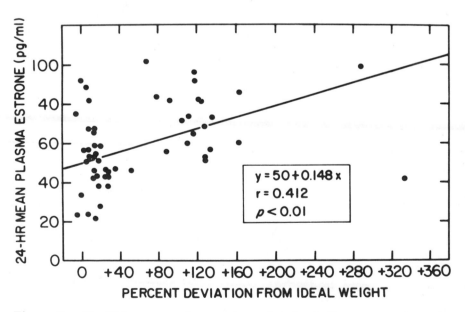

Figure 2.   The 24-hour mean plasma estrone elevation in obese men was proportional to their degree of obesity.

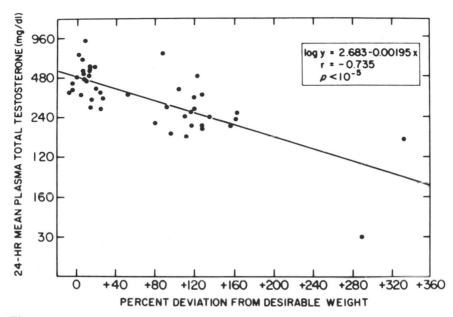

Figure 3. The 24-hour mean levels of plasma total testosterone were decreased in obese men in proportion to the degree of obesity.

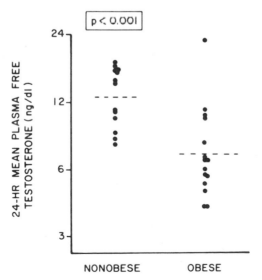

Figure 4. The 24-hour mean levels of plasma free testosterone were significantly lower in obese men than in controls.

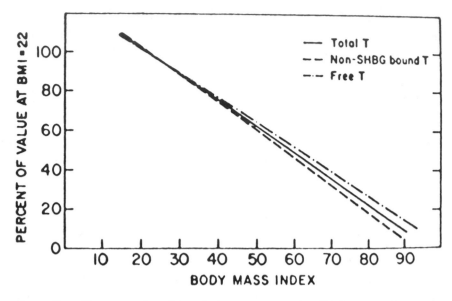

Figure 5. The curves describing the inverse proportionality between decreasing hormone levels and increasing degree of obesity were superimposable for total testosterone, free testosterone, and non-SHBG-bound testosterone. (Reprinted with permission from B Zumoff et al, Plasma-free and non-SHBG-bound testosterone are decreased in obese men in proportion to their degree of obesity. J Clin Endocrinol Metab 71:929-931, 1990.)

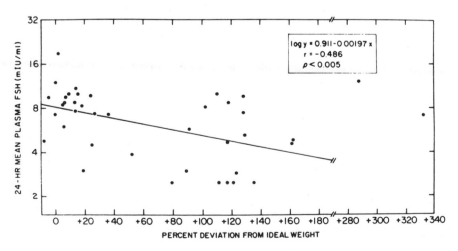

Figure 6. The 24-hour mean plasma FSH decrease in obese men was proportional to their degree of obesity.

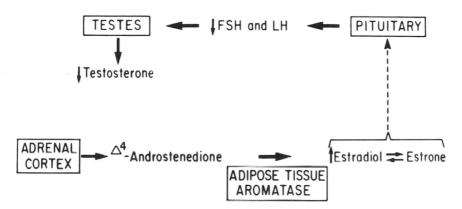

Figure 7. Mechanism of production of hypogonadotropic hypogonadism in obese men.

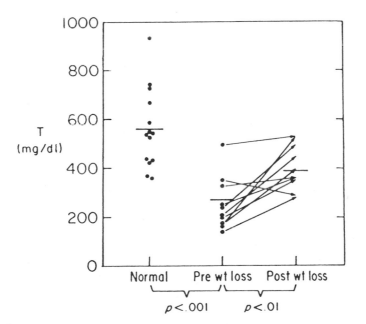

Figure 8. Weight loss increased the subnormal plasma total testosterone levels of obese men toward normal. (Reprinted with permission from GW Strain et al, Effect of massive weight loss on hypothalamic-pituitary-gonadal function in obese men. J Clin Endocrinol Metab 66:1019-1023, 1988.)

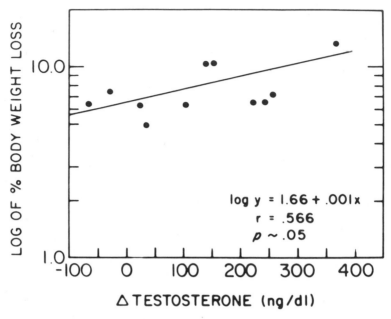

Figure 9.   The degree of recovery of plasma testosterone with weight loss was proportional to the degree of weight loss.

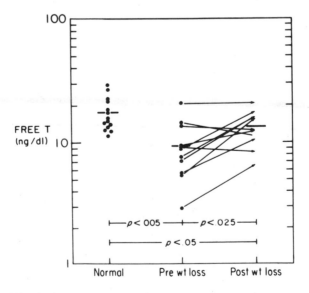

Figure 10.   Weight loss increased the subnormal plasma free testosterone levels of obese men toward normal.

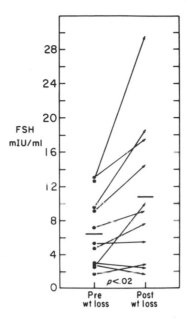

Figure 11. Weight loss increased the subnormal plasma FSH levels of obese men toward normal.

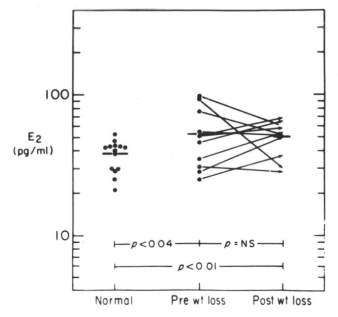

Figure 12. Weight loss had no effect on the elevated plasma estradiol level of obese men. (Reprinted with permission from B Zumoff, Hormonal abnormalities in obesity. Acta Med Scand Suppl 732:153-160, 1987.)

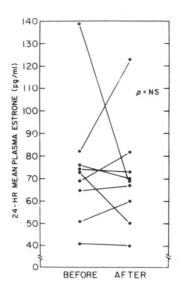

Figure 13. Weight loss had no effect on the elevated plasma estrone levels of obese men. (Reprinted with permission from B Zumoff, Hormonal abnormalities in obesity. Acta Med Scand Suppl 723:153-160, 1987.)

existence of subnormal free testosterone levels in obese men,[6,11,12] shows such subnormal levels in most studies.[6,10-12] Our studies confirmed low total testosterone levels and low SHBG levels, but also clearly demonstrated low free testosterone levels (Figure 4); the percentage decreases of total, free, and non-SHBG-bound (i.e., free plus albumin-bound) testosterone were all identically proportional to the degree of obesity[2,14] (Figure 5). It is of interest that the decreases of free and total testosterone were not accompanied by clinical hypogonadism: libido and potency were normal, as determined by history and measurement of nocturnal penile tumescence, and sperm counts and semen volume were likewise normal.[13]

Whether gonadotropin levels are abnormal in obese men has been controversial: some workers[11,15] have reported subnormal follicle-stimulating hormone (FSH) levels and normal or subnormal luteinizing hormone (LH) levels, but the data have been inconsistent and unconvincing. We found a clear-cut diminution of FSH levels (Figure 6) and normal LH levels,[13] which, of course, are inappropriately low in the face of subnormal testosterone levels (a study by Glass[16] indicates that the LH levels in our subjects should have been about 195 percent of normal to be appropriate for their degree of hypotestosteronemia).

Putting our data together, what we found in obese men was a state of mild hypogonadotropic hypogonadism (HHG), presumably due to partial pituitary suppression by their hyperestrogenemia (Figure 7).

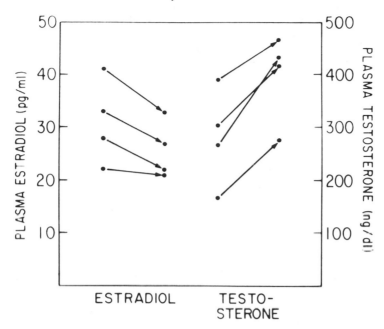

Figure 14. Administration of testolactone to obese men lowered plasma estradiol and raised plasma testosterone levels. (Reprinted with permission from B Zumoff, Hormonal abnormalities in obesity. Acta Med Scand Suppl 723:153-160, 1987.)

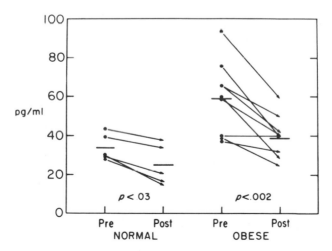

Figure 15. Administration of dexamethasone for 1 week to obese and nonobese men lowered plasma estradiol levels in both groups. (Reprinted with permission from B Zumoff et al, Partial reversal of the hypogonadotropic hypogonadism of obese men by administration of corticosuppressive doses of dexamethasone. Int J Obesity 12:525-531, 1988)

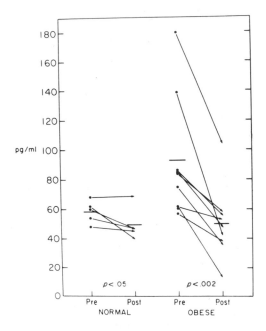

Figure 16. Administration of dexamethasone for 1 week to obese and nonobese men lowered plasma estrone levels in both groups. (Reprinted with permission from B Zumoff et al, Partial reversal of the hypogonadotropic hypogonadism of obese men by administration of corticosuppressive doses of dexamethasone. Int J Obesity 12:525-531, 1988.)

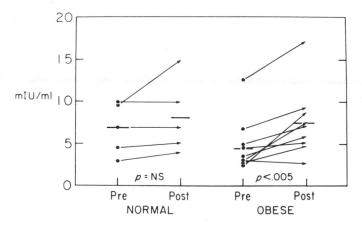

Figure 17. Administration of dexamethasone for 1 week raised the subnormal FSH levels of obese men but had no effect on the levels in nonobese men. (Reprinted with permission from B Zumoff et al, Partial reversal of the hypogonadotropic hypogonadism of obese men by administration of corticosuppressive doses of dexamethasone. Int J Obesity 12:525-531, 1988.)

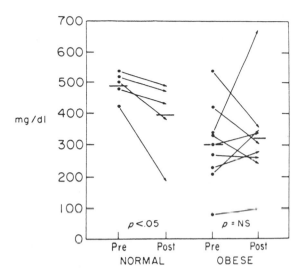

Figure 18. Administration of dexamethasone for 1 week lowered the plasma testosterone levels of nonobese men but had no effect on the levels in obese men; this can be interpreted to mean that there was a balancing off of a tendency to raise the levels in obese men, via an indirect effect, and a tendency to lower the levels in all men, via a direct effect. (Reprinted with permission from B Zumoff et al, Partial reversal of the hypogonadotropic hypogonadism of obese men by administration of corticosuppressive doses of dexamethasone. Int J Obesity 12:525-531 1988.)

It was of interest to see the effect of weight loss on these abnormalities. Stanik and co-workers[17] reported that weight loss normalized the elevated estrogen levels and subnormal testosterone levels of obese men (they did not study gonadotropin levels). We studied 11 men who lost an average of 53 kg, decreasing from a mean of 167 percent above ideal weight to a mean of 93 percent above ideal weight, and then maintained the new, reduced but still obese weight for 6 to 24 months; hormone levels were measured before weight loss and after stabilizing at the new weight.[18] Plasma testosterone rose toward normal (Figure 8), proportionately to the amount of weight lost (Figure 9). Free testosterone remained at a constant proportion of total testosterone and therefore likewise rose toward normal (Figure 10). FSH rose essentially to normal (Figure 11). However, estradiol levels (Figure 12) and estrone levels (Figure 13) did not change. This was unexpected: we had hypothesized that the HHG of obese men was due to hyperestrogenemic suppression of the pituitary, and here weight loss had normalized the HHG without changing the degree of hyperestrogenemia.

A possible reason that we saw no decrease in hyperestrogenemia while Stanik and co-workers observed normalization of estrogen levels is that they reduced their subjects from moderately obese to virtually nonobese, while we reduced ours from extremely obese to still very obese. We hypothesize that the adipose tissues of obese men contain large amounts of dissolved estrogen that can feed back into the blood as adipose tissue is reduced by weight loss and thereby maintain the hyperestrogenemia; when, finally, a nonobese state is reached (as in the study by Stanik), this reservoir function ceases and estrogen levels fall back to normal.

This hypothesis, though plausible, is clearly unproved. In any case, it leaves unexplained why the HHG resolves despite the persistence of the hyperestrogenemia. We have proposed a testable hypothesis[18] to account for that observation, namely that weight loss increases the sensitivity of the pituitary gonadotrophs to stimulation by gonadotropin-releasing hormone (Gn-RH). Support for such a possibility is provided by the observation that the blunted growth hormone response to growth hormone-releasing hormone in obesity[19,20] is normalized after weight loss.[20,21] Studies of the gonadotropin response to Gn-RH stimulation before and after weight loss could determine the validity of our hypothesis, and such studies are planned.

It should be pointed out that two other approaches we have used to eliminate the hyperestrogenemia of obese men, namely depression of tissue aromatase activity by administration of the aromatase inhibitor testolactone (Figure 14) and suppression of the secretion of the estrogen precursor Δ—androstenedione by administration of dexamethasone (Figures 15-18), also result in normalization of HHG.[2,22]

Sex Hormones and Gonadotropins in Obese Women

Our studies excluded women with evidence of polycystic ovary syndrome (PCOS) and thereby deliberately bypassed the fact that obesity can, in some women, induce a PCOS-like condition that is reversible by weight loss.[23-26] Thus it is clear that obesity can cause the type of gonadotropin and sex-hormonal abnormalities that occur in PCOS and that these abnormalities are reversible with weight loss. We are being deliberately vague, since no one really understands what the pathogenetic hormonal sequence is in PCOS, though we suspect that gonadotropin secretory abnormalities may be primary.[27]

Several investigators have reported that obese women show increased aromatization of adrenal androgens (e.g., Δ—androstenedione) to estrogens[28,29] and some have suggested or implied that these women have elevated plasma estradiol levels,[30-32] but none has presented convincing evidence of this. We found essentially normal levels of total estradiol and total estrone (Figure 19) in obese women,[8] but because of their subnormal SHBG levels they had significantly elevated levels of free estradiol[2] (Figure 20), which is the biologically active moiety. Such elevations have been blamed by some authors for the increased risk of breast cancer[33] and

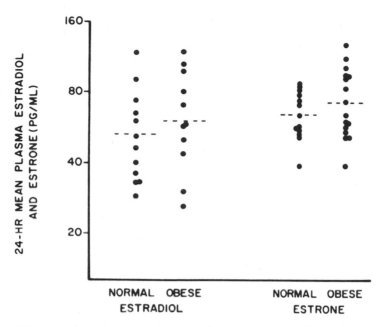

Figure 19. Neither plasma total estradiol nor total estrone showed a significant difference between obese and nonobese women in the follicular stage of the menstrual cycle. (Reprinted with permission from B Zumoff, Hormonal abnormalities in obesity. Acta Med Scand Suppl 723:153-160, 1987.)

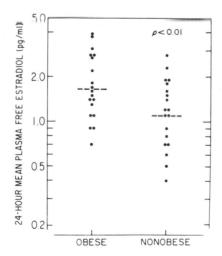

Figure 20. The 24-hour mean plasma free estradiol was significantly higher in obese women than in nonobese women. (Reprinted with permission from B Zumoff, Hormonal abnormalities in obesity. Acta Med Scand Suppl 723:153-160, 1987.)

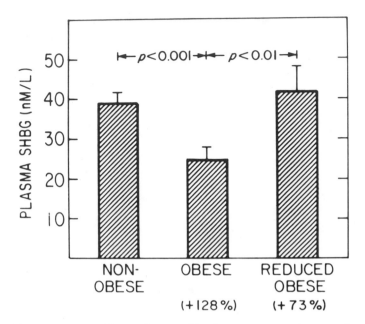

Figure 21.   Plasma SHBG was decreased in obese women and returned to normal with weight loss.

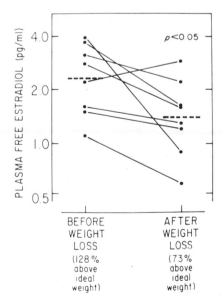

Figure 22.   The elevated plasma free estradiol of obese women was reduced to normal by weight loss. (Reprinted with permission from B Zumoff, Hormonal abnormalities in obesity. Acta Med Scand Suppl 723:153-160, 1987.)

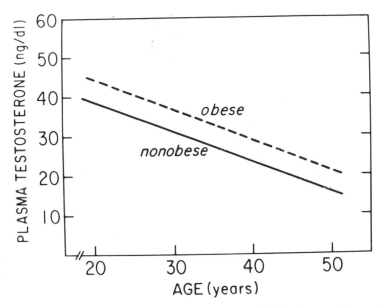

Figure 23. Plasma total testosterone showed parallel declines with age in premenopausal obese and nonobese women; there was no significant difference between the two groups. (Reprinted with permission from B Zumoff, Hormonal abnormalities in obesity. Acta Med Scand Suppl 723:153-160, 1987.)

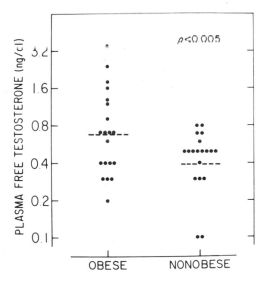

Figure 24. Plasma free testosterone was significantly higher in obese women than in nonobese women. (Reprinted with permission from B Zumoff, Hormonal abnormalities in obesity. Acta Med Scand Suppl 723:153-160, 1987.)

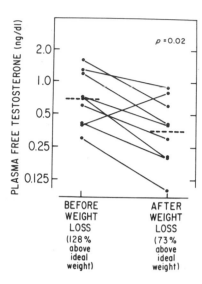

Figure 25.   Weight loss decreased the elevated plasma free testosterone of obese women toward normal. (Reprinted with permission from B Zumoff, Hormonal abnormalities in obesity. Acta Med Scand Suppl 723:153-160, 1987.)

endometrial cancer[34] in obese women. We studied the effect of massive, sustained weight loss (average 35 kg): the levels of SHBG and free estradiol were normalized (Figures 21 and 22).

Turning to the effects of obesity on plasma testosterone in women, we were surprised to observe a phenomenon that seems not to have been reported previously: total testosterone showed an inverse linear correlation with age in nonobese premenopausal women, and a parallel, not significantly different, relationship in obese women (Figure 23); the levels declined by about 50 percent between ages 20 and 50.[2] Because of the low SHBG levels in obese women, however, their free testosterone levels were markedly elevated (Figure 24) (no distinction was made in these studies between women with abdominal ["android"] and femorogluteal ["gynoid"] obesity); massive, sustained weight loss normalized the free testosterone levels in obese women (Figure 25).[2]

Effect of Weight-Losing on the Fasting Serum Insulin Level and Its Relationship to BMI in Men

Obesity is a risk factor for many diseases, among them hypertension,[35,36] coronary disease,[37-40] hyperlipidemias,[41] type II diabetes,[42,43] and breast cancer.[33] In hypertension, hyperlipidemias, and coronary disease, elevated serum insulin levels are found,[44-47] and some believe them to play a caus-

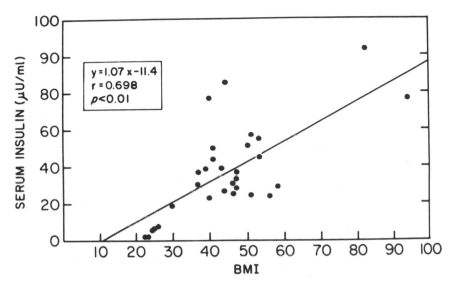

Figure 26. There was a linear increase of the fasting serum insulin level in nondieting, weight-stable obese men, proportional to the degree of obesity.

ative role in these diseases.[48] Obesity has been shown to be associated with hyperinsulinemia,[49-51] and it has been suggested that hormonal abnormality is the mechanism for the predisposing role of obesity in the diseases mentioned.[52] Weight-losing by obese persons is known to improve hypertension,[53,54] hyperlipidemias,[55] and type II diabetes[56,57] and probably decreases the risk of coronary disease.[58,59]

Our approach was to quantify the relationship of the degree of obesity to the degree of basal hyperinsulinemia, which has been studied before,[60] and then to quantify that relationship during the weight-losing process, which has not been reported. We studied 30 healthy men, aged 20 to 50 and ranging in weight from 65 to 300 kg (BMI 23 to 94), under nondieting, weight-stable conditions and again while they were dieting and losing weight (6.9 to 29.5 kg and 2 to 47 BMI units at the time of restudy).

We found a highly significant positive linear relationship between fasting serum insulin levels and BMI over the entire weight range studied[61] (Figure 26), with no discontinuity at the putative borderline of "morbid obesity" (i.e., a BMI of about 45). The slope was 1.07 µU/ml of insulin increase per unit of BMI increase. Weight-losing produced a striking decrease in fasting serum insulin (mean 6.1 µU/ml of insulin decrease per unit of BMI decrease); there was no significant correlation between the amount of weight lost and the decrease in insulin level. The weight-losing men still

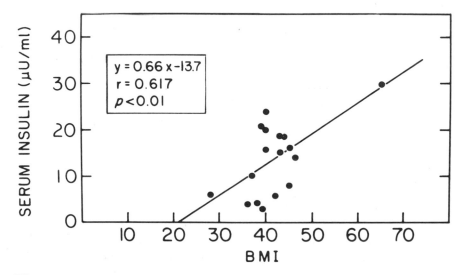

Figure 27. There continued to be a linear proportionality between serum insulin and degree of obesity in dieting, weight-losing men, but values for serum insulin were markedly lower at any given weight.

showed a positive correlation between fasting serum insulin and BMI (Figure 27).

We hypothesize that the increase in fasting insulin with increasing weight in weight-stable obese men is due in part to their higher caloric intake, which is proportional to their degree of obesity,[62] and that the fall in insulin levels during weight-losing is due to the substitution of negative caloric balance for the previous strongly positive balance. The continued relationship between serum insulin and BMI in weight-losing men suggests that there may be some additional factors beyond the increased caloric intake that favors hyperinsulinemia in obesity. One factor that might be considered is β-endorphin, whose plasma levels are uniformly elevated in obese persons[63-80] and do not decrease with weight loss[65,68,70,80] or acute starvation.[81] Endorphin is probably responsible for the accentuated serum insulin response to oral feeding in obese persons[64,68, 82] as inferred from a diminished response when naloxone is infused;[64,82] however, naloxone does not reduce basal serum insulin levels in obese persons,[64,83] and therefore the hyperendorphinemia of obesity is clearly not responsible for the basal hyperinsulinemia. Further studies are needed to elucidate possible nondietary factors.

	Normal	Obese	Naloxone-treated Obese	Obese after Weight Loss or Fasting
Prolactin Levels	Increased by metoclopramide Increased by TRH	Normal basal levels Decreased response to metoclopramide Normal response to TRH	Normalized response to metoclopramide	Normalized response to metoclopramide
Growth Hormone Levels	Increased by GH-releasing hormone arginine L-dopa clonidine hypoglycemia	Normal basal levels Decreased response to all stimuli Better response to pulsed GH-RH than to single injection	Normalized response to all stimuli	Normalized response to all stimuli
Vasopressin Levels	Increased by nicotine metoclopramide hypoglycemia	Normal basal levels Decreased response to all stimuli	Normalized response to all stimuli	Normalized response to all stimuli
β-Endorphin Levels	Increased by corticotropin-releasing hormone (CRH) Decreased by clonidine or dexamethasone	Increased basal levels Decreased response to CRH, clonidine and dexamethasone	No effect on basal levels Effect on stimulation or suppression not studied	Most studies find no decrease of elevated basal levels; some do Most studies find no normalization of dexamethasone suppression, some do

Figure 28. A. Obesity reduces the response of serum prolactin to metoclopramide, but not to thyrotropin-releasing hormone; weight loss or treatment with naloxone normalizes the response to metoclopramide. B. Obesity reduces the response of serum growth hormone to five stimuli; weight loss or treatment with naloxone normalizes the responses to all stimuli. C. Obesity reduces the response of serum vasopressin to three stimuli; weight loss or treatment with naloxone normalizes the response to all stimuli. D. Obesity reduces the upward response of serum β-endorphin to corticotropin-releasing hormone and the downward response to clonidine or dexamethasone; whether weight loss normalizes these responses is controversial in the literature; the effect of naloxone has not been studied.

Effect of Obesity, Naloxone Administration and Weight Loss on Serum Levels and Dynamic Responses of Prolactin, Growth Hormone, Vasopressin and β-Endorphin

Figure 28 summarizes the following relationships: with respect to prolactin, obese persons show a diminution of the normal stimulability with metoclopramide[83] (a dopamine receptor blocker that presumably interferes with pituitary response to hypothalamically secreted dopamine, the principal endogenous inhibitor of prolactin secretion); fasting or weight loss normalizes the response to metoclopramide,[83] as does administration of naloxone,[84] which blocks the effect of β-endorphin. With respect to growth hormone, the normal stimulation by five different agents (L-dopa, arginine, clonidine, insulin-induced hypoglycemia, and growth hormone-releasing hormone) is blunted in obesity;[19,20,21,85,86] weight loss[19,21] or naloxone administration[84] normalizes the responses. With respect to vasopressin, the normal stimulation by nicotine, metoclopramide, or hypoglycemia is blunted in obesity;[87,88] weight loss or naloxone administration normalizes the responses.[88] With respect to β-endorphin, levels are normally stimulated by corticotropin-releasing hormone (CRH) and clonidine and suppressed by dexamethasone; in obesity, basal endorphin levels are elevated and CRH and clonidine stimulation and dexamethasone suppression are all blunted; the effect of weight loss is controversial: most authors report that basal levels are not reduced and blunted responses to CRH and dexamethasone are not normalized;[65,68,70,89] one group has reported normalization of basal levels with weight loss but did not study its effects on the responses to CRH, clonidine, or dexamethasone.[74]

One can conclude from these observations that obesity results in disorders of the hypothalamic regulation of the secretion of prolactin, growth hormone, and vasopressin, and that weight loss or administration of the endorphin antagonist naloxone eliminates the dysregulation. Since weight loss is as effective as naloxone administration in this respect, one might think that weight loss works by reducing the hyperendorphinemia of obesity. However, four out of the five studies that have examined this question have reported that weight loss in obese subjects does not decrease the elevated β-endorphin levels. This is puzzling: the ameliorating effect of naloxone on the peptide hormonal abnormalities in obesity suggests that they are mediated by the hyperendorphinemia, but those same abnormalities are ameliorated by weight loss without decreasing the hyperendorphinemia. A possible explanation is that weight loss may decrease the sensitivity of various CNS hormonal control mechanisms to the effects of β-endorphin.

There are no published data that show such an effect, but there is one published study that shows the inverse, namely *increased* sensitivity to β-endorphin in obesity;[90] this is certainly compatible with the proposal that weight loss *decreases* the sensitivity. Further support for the proposal is provided by a published example of a change in sensitivity to a hypothalamically secreted polypeptide hormone after weight loss, namely the demonstrated increase in sensitivity of pituitary GH secretion to stimulation by growth hormone-releasing hormone.[19,21] In any case, the hypothesis that weight loss decreases CNS sensitivity to β-endorphin is testable and should be investigated.

SUMMARY

Studies in our laboratory and elsewhere have demonstrated numerous abnormalities of steroid and polypeptide hormone secretion in obesity: hyperestrogenemia and hypogonadotropic hypogonadism in obese men; diminished SHBG levels in both sexes; elevated free testosterone and free estradiol in obese women; PCOS-like gonadotropin and sex-hormone abnormalities in obese women; elevated serum insulin in both sexes; blunted stimulability of prolactin, growth hormone, and vasopressin in both sexes; and elevated basal levels and blunted stimulability and suppressibility of β-endorphin in both sexes. All of these abnormalities have been clearly shown to be partly or completely reversible with weight loss, with the exception of the endorphin abnormalities. In that area, four out of the five studies reported show no reversibility with weight loss.

Reversibility of nearly all the hormonal abnormalities of obesity (i.e., all but the hyperendorphinemia) by weight loss suggests that none of them is causative of obesity. Nevertheless, some of the reversible abnormalities may secondarily amplify the morbidity associated with obesity: the hyperinsulinemia may be related to the increased risk of hypertension, hyperlipidemia, coronary disease, and type II diabetes; the elevated levels of free estradiol in obese women may be related to their increased risk of breast and endometrial cancer.

The role of hyperendorphinemia in obesity clearly requires further investigation, since it is the only observed hormonal abnormality that appears to be nonreversible by weight loss, and also since there seems to be increased sensitivity to β-endorphin in obesity. The possibility that endorphin abnormalities may be causal in obesity cannot be ruled out.

NOTES

1. Glass AR, Burman KD, Dahms WT, et al. (1981). Endocrine function in human obesity. Metabolism 30:89-104.
2. Zumoff B (1987). Hormonal abnormalities in obesity. Acta Med Scand Suppl 723:153-160.
3. Zumoff B, Rosenfeld RS, Strain GW, et al. (1980). Sex differences in the 24-hour mean plasma concentrations of dehydroisoandrosterone (DHA) and dehydroisoandrosterone sulfate (DHAS) and the DHA to DHAS ratio in normal adults. J Clin Endocrinol Metab 51:310-333.
4. Strain GW, Zumoff B, Strain JJ, et al. (1980). Cortisol production in obesity. Metabolism 29:980-985.
5. Strain GW, Zumoff B (1994). The relationship of weight-height indices of obesity to body fat content. J Am Coll Nutrition 11:715.
6. Schneider G, Kirschner MA, Berkowitz R, et al. (1979). Increased estrogen production in obese men. J Clin Endocrinol Metab 48:633-638.
7. Kley HK, Solbach HG, McKinnon JC, et al. (1979). Testosterone decrease and estrogen increase in male patients with obesity. Acta Endocrinol 91:553-563.
8. Zumoff B, Strain GW, Kream J, et al. (1981). Obese young men have elevated plasma estrogen levels but obese premenopausal women do not. Metabolism 30:1011-1014.
9. Strain GW, Zumoff B (1985). Hormonal abnormalities in obesity. Resident Staff Physician 31:13PC-24PC.
10. Barbato AI, Landau RL (1984). Testosterone deficiency of morbid obesity. Clin Res 22:647A.
11. Glass AR, Swerdloff RS, Bray GA, et al. (1977). Low serum testosterone and sex hormone-binding globulin in massively obese men. J Clin Endocrinol Metab 45:1211-1219.
12. Amatruda JM, Harman SM, Pourmotabbed G, et al. (1978). Depressed plasma testosterone and fractional binding of testosterone in obese males. J Clin Endocrinol Metab 47:268-271.

13. Strain GW, Zumoff B, Kream J, et al. (1982). Mild hypogonadotropic hypogonadism in obese men. Metabolism 21:871-875.
14. Zumoff B, Strain GW, Miller LK, et al. (1990). Plasma-free and non-SHBG-bound testosterone are decreased in obese men in proportion to their degree of obesity. J Clin Endocrinol Metab 71:929-931.
15. Amatruda JM, Hochstein M, Hsu TH, et al. (1975). Testosterone deficiency of morbid obesity: possible role of the hypothalamus. Clin Res 23:571A.
16. Glass AR (1986). Ketoconazole-induced stimulation of gonadotropin output in men: basis for a potential test of gonadotropin reserve. J Clin Endocrinol Metab 63:1121-1125.
17. Stanik S, Dornfeld LP, Maxwell MH, et al. (1981). The effect of weight loss on reproductive hormones in obese men. J Clin Endocrinol Metab 53:828-832.
18. Strain GW, Zumoff B, Miller LK, et al. (1988). Effect of massive weight loss on hypothalamic-pituitary-gonadal function in obese men. J Clin Endocrinol Metab 66:1019-1023.
19. Williams T, Berelowitz M, Joffe SN, et al. (1984). Impaired growth hormone response to growth hormone-releasing factor in obesity: a pituitary defect reversed with weight reduction. N Engl J Med 311:1403-1407.
20. Kopelman PG, Noonan K, Goulton R, et al. (1985). Impaired growth hormone response to growth hormone releasing factor and insulin-hypoglycemia in obesity. Clin Endocrinol 23:87-94.
21. Tanaka K, Inone S, Numata K, et al. (1990). Very-low-calorie diet-induced weight reduction reverses impaired growth hormone secretion response to growth hormone-releasing hormone, arginine, and L-dopa in obesity. Metabolism 39:892-896.
22. Zumoff B, Strain GW, Miller LK, et al. (1988). Partial reversal of the hypogonadotropic hypogonadism of obese men by administration of corticosuppressive doses of dexamethasone. Int J Obesity 12:525-531.
23. Bates G, Whitworth NS (1982). Effect of body weight reduction on plasma androgens in obese, infertile women. Fertil Steril 38:406-409.
24. Harlass FE, Plymate SR, Farriss BL, et al. (1984). Weight loss is associated with correction of gonadotropin and sex steroid abnormalities in the obese anovulatory female. Fertil Steril 42:649-652.
25. Deitel M, Stone E, Kassam HA, et al. (1988). Gynecologic-obstetric changes after loss of massive excess weight following bariatric surgery. J Am Coll Nutrition 7:147-153.
26. Pasquali R, Antenucci D, Casimirri F, et al. (1989). Clinical and hormonal characteristics of obese amenorrheic hyperandrogenic women before and after weight loss. J Clin Endocrinol Metab 68:173-179.
27. Zumoff B, Freeman R, Coupey S, et al. (1983). A chronobiological abnormality of luteinizing hormone secretion in teenage girls with the polycystic ovary syndrome. N Engl J Med 309:1206-1209.
28. Edman CD, MacDonald PC (1978). Effect of obesity on conversion of plasma androstenedione to estrone in ovulatory and anovulatory young women. Am J Obstet Gynecol 130:456-461.
29. Grodin JM, Siiteri PK, MacDonald PC (1983). Source of estrogen production in postmenopausal women. J Clin Endocrinol Metab 36:207-214.
30. Judd HL, Lucas WE, Yen SSC (1976). Serum 17 β-estradiol and estrone levels in postmenopausal women with and without endometrial cancer. J Clin Endocrinol Metab 43:272-278.
31. Vermeulen A, Verdonck L (1978). Sex hormone concentrations in postmenopausal women. Relation to obesity, fat mass, age, and years postmenopause. Clin Endocrinol 9:59-66.

32. Davidson BJ, Gambone JC, LaGosse LD, et al. (1981). Free estradiol in postmenopausal women with and without endometrial cancer. J Clin Endocrinol Metab 52:404-408.
33. Choi NW, Howe GR, Miller AB (1978). An epidemiological study of breast cancer. Am J Epidemiol 107:510-521.
34. Garfinkel L (1986). Overweight and mortality. Cancer 58:1826-1829.
35. Kannel WB, Brand N, Skinner JJ Jr, et al. (1967). The relation of adiposity to blood pressure and development of hypertension. Ann Intern Med 67:48-59.
36. Stamler R, Stamler J, Riedlinger WF, et al. (1978). Weight and blood pressure: findings in hypertension screening of one million Americans. JAMA 240:1607-1616.
37. Hubert HB, Feinleib M, McNamara PM, et al. (1983). Obesity as an independent risk factor for cardiovascular disease: a 26-year follow-up for participants in the Framingham Heart Study. Circulation 67:968-977.
38. Larsson B, Svardsudd K, Welin L, et al. (1984). Abdominal adipose tissue distribution, obesity, risk of cardiovascular disease and death: a 13-year follow-up of participants in the study of men born in 1913. Br Med J 288:1401-1404.
39. Peiris AN, Sotlemann MS, Hoffman RG, et al. (1989). Adiposity, fat distribution, and cardiovascular risk. Ann Intern Med 110:867-872.
40. Mason JE, Colditz GA, Stampfer MA, et al. (1990). A prospective study of obesity and risk of coronary artery disease. N Engl J Med 322:882-889.
41. Hollister LE, Overall JE, Snow HL (1967). Relationship of obesity to serum triglyceride, cholesterol and uric acid, and to plasma glucose levels. Am J Clin Nutrition 20:777-782.
42. Luft R, Cerasi E, Anderson B (1968). Obesity as an additional factor in the pathogenesis of diabetes. Acta Endocrinol 59:344-352.
43. Rimin AA, Werner LH, Bernstein R, et al. (1972). Disease and obesity in 75,532 women. Obesity Bariatric Med 1:77-84.
44. Welborn TA, Breckenridge A, Dollery CT, et al. (1966). Serum insulin in essential hypertension and in peripheral vascular disease. Lancet 1:1336-1337.
45. Manicardi V, Camelini L, Belloidi G, et al. (1986). Evidence for an association of high blood pressure and hyperinsulinemia in obese men. J Clin Endocrinol Metab 62:1302-1304.
46. Zavaroni I, Bonora E, Pagliara M, et al. (1989). Risk factors for coronary artery disease in healthy persons with hyperinsulinemia and normal glucose tolerance. N Engl J Med 320:702-706.
47. Ducimetiere P, Eschwege E, Papoz L, et al. (1980). Relationship of plasma insulin levels to the incidence of myocardial infarction and coronary heart disease mortality in a middle-aged population. Diabetologia 19:205-210.
48. Reaven GM (1988). Role of insulin resistance in human disease. Diabetes 37:1595-1607.
49. Sims EAH (1982). Mechanisms of hypertension in the overweight. Hypertension Suppl III:43-49.
50. Berglund G, Larson B, Anderson O, et al. (1976). Body composition and glucose metabolism in hypertensive middle-aged males. Acta Med Scand 200:163-169.
51. Bonadonna RC, Groop L, Kraemer N, et al. (1990). Obesity and insulin resistance in humans: a dose-response study. Metabolism 39:452-459.
52. Lucas CP, Estigarribia JA, Darga LL, et al. (1985). Insulin and blood pressure in obesity. Hypertension 7:702-706.
53. Tuck ML, Sowers J, Dornfeld L, et al. (1981). The effect of weight reduction on blood pressure, plasma renin activity, and plasma aldosterone levels in obese patients. N Engl J Med 304:930-933.

54. Reisin E, Abel R, Modan M, et al. (1978). Effect of weight loss without salt restriction on the reduction of blood pressure in overweight hypertensive patients. N Engl J Med 298:1-6.
55. Bray GA (1976). Some metabolic effects of obesity. In The obese patient. Philadelphia: WB Saunders.
56. Bistrian BR, Blackburn GL, Flatt JP, et al. (1976). Nitrogen metabolism and insulin requirements in obese diabetic adults and protein-sparing modified fast. Diabetes 25:494-504.
57. Genuth S (1979). Supplemented fasting in the treatment of obesity and diabetes. Am J Clin Nutrition 32:2579-2586.
58. Ornish D, Brown SE, Scherwitz LW, et al. (1990). Can lifestyle changes reverse coronary artery disease? The Lifestyle Heart Trial. Lancet 336:129-133.
59. Blackenhorn DH, Johnson RL, Mack WJ, et al. (1990). The influence of diet on the appearance of new lesions in human coronary arteries. JAMA 263:1646-1652.
60. Bagdade JD, Bierman EL, Porte D Jr (1967). The significance of basal insulin levels in the evaluation of the insulin response to glucose in diabetic and nondiabetic subjects. J Clin Invest 46:1549-1557.
61. Strain GW, Zumoff B (1992). The effect of weight-losing on the fasting serum insulin level and its relationship to the body mass index in healthy men (unpublished paper).
62. Strain GW, Hershcopf RJ, Zumoff B (1992). Food intake of very obese persons—quantitative and qualitative aspects. J Am Dietetic Assoc 92:199-203.
63. Giugliano D, Salvatore T, Cozzolino D, et al. (1987). Hyperglycemia and obesity as determinants of glucose, insulin, and glucagon responses to beta-endorphin in diabetes mellitus. J Clin Endocrinol Metab 64:1122-1128.
64. Vettor R, Martini C, Cestaro S, et al. (1989). Possible involvement of endogenous opioids in beta-cell hyperresponsiveness in human obesity. Int J Obesity 13:425-432.
65. Giugliano D, Cozzolino D, Tovella R, et al. (1991). Persistence of altered metabolic response to beta-endorphin after normalization of body weight in human obesity. Acta Endocrinol 124:159-165.
66. Giovannini C, Ciucci E, Cassetta MR (1991). Unresponsiveness of the endorphinergic system to its physiological feedback in obesity. Appetite 16:39-43.
67. Scavo D, Barletta C, Vagiri D, et al. (1990). Hyperendorphinemia in obesity is not related to the affective state. Physiol Behav 48:681-683.
68. Giovannini C, Ciucci E, Clementi R, et al. (1990). Beta-endorphin, insulin, ACTH and cortisol plasma levels during oral glucose tolerance test in obesity after weight loss. Horm Metabol Res 22:96-100.
69. Nappi C, Petraglia F, Cudemo V, et al. (1989). Plasma beta-endorphin levels in obese and nonobese patients with polycystic ovarian disease. Eur J Obstet Gynecol Reprod Biol 30:151-156.
70. Slowinska-Srzednicka J, Zgliczynski S, Soszynski P (1988). Effect of clonidine on beta-endorphin, ACTH and cortisol secretion in essential hypertension and obesity. Eur J Clin Pharmacol 35:115-121.
71. Facchinetti F, Bernasconi S, Petraglia F, et al. (1988). Absent β-endorphin response to clonidine in obese children. Horm Metabol Res 20:348-351.
72. Bernasconi S, Petraglia F, Iughetti L, et al. (1988). Impaired β-endorphin response to human corticotropin-releasing hormone in obese children. Acta Endocrinol 119:7-10.
73. Giugliano D, Cozzolino D, Salvatore T, et al. (1988). Altered metabolic responses to epinephrine and beta-endorphin in human obesity. J Clin Endocrinol Metab 67:238-244.

74. Scavo D, Barletta C, Buzzetti R, et al. (1988). Effects of caloric restriction and exercise on β-endorphin, ACTH and cortisol circulating levels in obesity. Physiol Behav 42:65-68.

75. Facchinetti F, Giovannini C, Petragha F, et al. (1988). Plasma β-endorphin resistance to dexamethasone suppression in obese patients. J Endocrinol Invest 11:119-123.

76. Slowinska-Srzednicka J, Zgliczynski S, Soszynski P, et al. (1988). The possible role of beta-endorphin in pathogenesis of obesity and essential hypertension. Clin Exp Hypertension A 10:135-149.

77. Baranowska B, Singh SP, Soszynski P, et al. (1987). The role of opiate, dopaminergic, and adrenergic systems in the hypothalamic-pituitary dysfunction in obesity. Acta Endocrinol 116:221-228.

78. Facchinetti F, Livieri C, Petraglia F, et al. (1987). Dexamethasone fails to suppress hyperendorphinemia of obese children. Acta Endocrinol 116:90-94.

79. Scavo D, Facchinetti F, Barletta C, et al. (1987). Plasma beta-endorphin in response to oral glucose tolerance test in obese patients. Horm Metab Res 19:204-207.

80. Atkinson RL (1987). Opioid regulation of food intake and body weight in humans. Fed Proc 46:178-182.

81. Balon-Perin S, Kolanowski J, Berbinschi A, et al. (1991). The effects of glucose ingestion and fasting on plasma immunoreactive beta-endorphin, adrenocorticotropic hormone and cortisol in obese subjects. J Endocrinol Invest 14:922-925.

82. Vettor R, Martini C, Marino M, et al. (1985). Effects of naloxone-induced opiate receptor blockage on insulin secretion in obesity. Horm Metabol Res 17:374-375.

83. Rojdmark S, Rossner S (1991). Decreased dopaminergic control of prolactin secretion in male obesity: normalization by fasting. Metabolism 40:191-195.

84. Plewe G, Schneider U, Krause U, et al. (1987). Naloxone increases the response of growth hormone and prolactin to stimuli in obese humans. J Endocrinol Invest 10:137-141.

85. Copinschi G, Wegienka LC, Hane S, et al. (1967). Effect of arginine on serum levels of insulin and growth hormone in obese subjects. Metabolism 16:485-491.

86. Laurian L, Oberman Z, Ayalon D, et al. (1975). Underresponsiveness of growth hormone secretion after L-dopa and deep sleep stimulation in obese subjects. Israel J Med Sci 11:482-487.

87. Coiro V, Chiodera P (1987). Effect of obesity and weight loss on the arginine vasopressin response to insulin-induced hypoglycemia. Clin Endocrinol 27:253-258.

88. Chiodera P, Capretti L, Davoli C, et al. (1990). Effect of obesity and weight loss on arginine vasopressin response to metoclopramide and nicotine from cigarette smoking. Metabolism 39:783-786.

89. Zelissen PM, Koppeschaar HP, Erkelens DW, et al. (1991). Beta-endorphin and adrenocortical function in obesity. Clin Endocrinol 35:369-372.

90. Giugliano D, Salvatore T, Cozzolino D, et al. (1987). Sensitivity to β-endorphin as a cause of human obesity. Metabolism 37:974-978.

6

Sleep Disorders Associated with Obesity

Gary K. Zammit, PhD

Sleep is a multidetermined process. Among the primary factors that influence the occurrence, timing, and duration of sleep are age, gender, prior sleep (or sleep debt), the circadian rhythm of sleep and wakefulness, and behavior. However, sleep may also be influenced by food consumption and body weight. In lower animals, it has been shown that an increase in total food consumption following the presentation of a highly palatable diet is associated with an increase in both body weight and total sleep time (TST).[1] It is also known that ventromedial hypothalamic (VMH) lesions that result in weight gain in rats are associated with increases in TST.[2] In humans, little is known about the effect of food consumption or obesity on sleep. Studies have found a strong positive correlation between an adult's body weight and the usual amount of rapid-eye-movement (REM) sleep.[3] There is also an association between the degree of obesity and sleep cycle length, such that the percentage deviation from ideal body weight is significantly correlated with the mean sleep cycle length.[4] There appears to be no difference between normal weight and obese subjects in measures of daytime sleep tendency or postprandial sleepiness,[5] although further studies are needed to address this question.

The most prominent differences between the sleep of normal weight and obese individuals are observed in individuals with sleep pathology. It is well known that certain sleep disorders are commonly associated with obesity. These disorders include the sleep apnea syndrome, central alveolar hypoventilation syndrome (obesity hypoventilation syndrome), and nocturnal eating syndrome. The physical consequences of these disorders, as

The author would like to thank Norma M.T. Brown and Xavier Pi-Sunyer for reviewing the manuscript for this chapter.

well as their dramatic impact on the psychological, social, and occupational functioning of patients, suggests that they are among the most serious problems associated with obesity. This chapter provides an overview of the clinical features and treatments of these disorders.

SLEEP APNEA

Sleep apnea is a sleep-related breathing disorder that is thought to affect between 1 and 10 percent of the general population.[6,7,8] Recent epidemiologic data indicate that 2 percent of women and 4 percent of men between the ages of 30 and 60 years meet the minimum diagnostic criteria for sleep apnea syndrome.[9] This may be a modest estimate of prevalence in the general population, as it appears that the occurrence of the disorder increases with age.[10,11] In studies of people over the age of 65, it has been reported that 24 percent of people living independently, 33 percent of those in acute care inpatient facilities, and 42 percent of those in nursing homes have more than five apneic events per hour of sleep, which is the minimum criterion typically used to diagnose sleep apnea in adults. Male sex and obesity have been found to be strongly associated with the presence of sleep-related breathing disorders such as sleep apnea, with obesity being considered an important risk factor.[9] This is underscored by the finding that approximately two-thirds of patients with sleep apnea are obese.[12] It has been reported that the effect of obesity on the occurrence of sleep apnea is four times greater than that of age, and two times greater than that of gender.[13] One interpretation of these data is that the high prevalence of sleep apnea is an epiphenomenon of obesity, which is one of the primary underlying causes of the disorder. The frequent appearance of sleep apnea in obese patients and its significant impact on health and mortality emphasize the importance of the routine and thorough evaluation of sleep disturbance in obese patients.

Sleep apnea is characterized by multiple respiratory pauses during sleep. These pauses, or apneas, are defined as the complete cessation of airflow at the level of the nose and mouth with a duration of at least 10 seconds.[14] However, the duration of most apneic events exceeds this minimum criterion. The average duration of apneic events in an individual with sleep apnea is between 30 and 40 seconds, and there have been documented events lasting as long as 3 minutes.[15] Partial reductions in airflow are known as hypopneas. Hypopneas are defined as the reduction of airflow at the level of the nose and mouth lasting at least 10 seconds, and associated with oxygen desaturation or evidence of electroencephalographic (EEG) or electromyographic (EMG) arousal. The mean duration of hypopneic events in an individual with sleep apnea tends to be similar to the duration of apneic events.

Apneas and hypopneas result from similar mechanisms that impede airflow during sleep. Consequently, individuals with sleep apnea often have both apneic and hypopneic events during the sleep period. Another pattern of sleep-disordered breathing that has been recently described is known as the upper airway resistance syndrome.[16,17] This disturbance is associated with modest reductions in airflow during sleep that often are not detected by conventional recording methods. An esophageal balloon is required to detect the subtle but greater than expected declines in intraesophageal pressure that are characteristic of upper airway resistance. These changes in respiration can result in EEG arousals during sleep that are similar to those seen in sleep apnea, although events as short as 3 seconds have been reported. Episodes of upper airway resistance may occur in patients with sleep apnea, although the complete upper airway resistance syndrome is known to occur independently of sleep apnea.

There are three types of apneic and hypopneic events.[4] Obstructive events are characterized by the absence or reduction of airflow despite persistent ventilatory effort. These events are due to the complete or partial obstruction of the upper airway. The frequency of events of this type may be high in obesity due to the presence of excess or adipose tissue that compromises upper airway patency, although the specific nature and sites of obstruction are not easily identified. Central events are characterized by the absence or reduction of airflow in association with absent or significantly diminished ventilatory effort. The frequency of these events also may be high in obesity, especially when body mass interferes with lung volume or the efficient mechanical functioning of the diaphragm and respiratory accessory muscles. Mixed events are characterized by the absence or reduction of airflow that are only partly due to reduced ventilatory effort. For example, a single event may begin as a central apnea, but ventilatory effort against a closed airway may appear several seconds prior to the termination of the event.

Individuals with sleep apnea experience multiple respiratory events during sleep. These events often recur throughout the sleep period, and may worsen in severity during rapid-eye-movement (REM) sleep.[15] A minimum of five apneic or hypopneic events per hour of sleep is required in order to diagnose sleep apnea,[18] and at least 40 events should be detected during a normal 8-hour sleep recording. However, most people with sleep apnea have many more events. In patients with obstructive sleep apnea, the average number of apneic events per hour of non-REM sleep is 65 (range 48 to 79), and the average number of apneic events per hour of REM sleep is 42 (range 17 to 90). The recurrence of respiratory events during the sleep period appears to have two main consequences: sleep fragmentation and intermittent transient declines in oxygen saturation. Sleep fragmentation can be so severe that it interferes with sleep architecture, resulting in a reduction in the total minutes and percentage of delta and REM sleep.[19] This is of significance because the greater the degree of sleep fragmentation, the greater the severity of daytime sleepiness associated with sleep apnea.[20,21,22] Oxygen desaturation may contribute to complaints of excessive daytime sleepiness, but is more likely a major contributor to the cognitive deficits seen in some patients with sleep apnea.[23] These deficits include memory and psychomotor impairments.

The diagnosis of sleep apnea syndrome is not made exclusively on the basis of respiratory disturbance during sleep. There are clinical signs and symptoms that define this disorder. Perhaps the two most common signs are snoring and excessive daytime sleepiness. Virtually all patients with obstructive sleep apnea snore, with 94 percent reporting the development of marked snoring before the age of 21,[4] although this is probably less prominent in patients with central sleep apnea. Snoring is frequently loud and interrupted by snorts or other unusual respiratory sounds. It is commonly a source of annoyance or embarrassment, and can be quite disturbing to a bed partner. Many individuals with sleep apnea have been evicted from their bedrooms because of loud snoring, resulting in a situation that interferes with marital and sexual relationships. Some report snoring that is so loud that they have disturbed others in adjoining rooms or apartments. These problems associated with snoring often lead people to seek treatment, and it follows that snoring is one of the most common presenting complaints in patients with sleep apnea.

Excessive daytime sleepiness is considered the primary daytime manifestation of sleep apnea.[24] Subjective complaints of daytime sleepiness are common among individuals with sleep apnea, who often report napping or falling asleep at inappropriate times. When given the opportunity to sleep during the day on the multiple sleep latency test (MSLT), healthy normal subjects have a mean sleep latency of between 10 and 20 minutes, and many subjects will not fall asleep at all. Mean latencies of less than 5 minutes are indicative of a pathological degree of daytime sleepiness.[25] Individuals with sleep apnea have been found to have a mean latency to stage I sleep of 2.6 minutes across four naps, revealing that this group of patients is excessively sleepy during the day.[26] However, it must be kept in mind that there is variability among individuals with respect to the severity of daytime sleepiness and the likelihood that they will report these problems to a physician. Mild symptoms such as fatigue or the tendency to doze in sedentary situations can be the only evidence of daytime sleepiness. These symptoms may not be immediately recognized as a problem,[27] and can be easily dismissed if the patient is not questioned carefully. Severe symptoms of sleepiness can be characterized by reports of difficulty sustaining alertness in virtually any situation, with some patients reporting that they fall asleep at work, while socializing, at meal times, or when operating a motor vehicle. The latter has been documented by studies of actual and simulated driving which show that individuals with sleep apnea perform more poorly than normal controls.[28,29] Severe daytime sleepiness

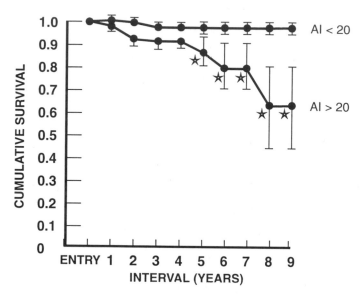

Figure 1.   Probability of cumulative survival for all untreated patients with an apnea index (AI) equal to or less than 20 (top line), or exceeding 20 (bottom line). The difference between the curves at that interval (indicated by stars) is significant (p < .05). Patients with AIs exceeding 20 had a greater mortality. (Reprinted with permission from J He, MH Kryger, FJ Zorick, W Conway and T Roth, Mortality and apnea index in obstructive sleep apnea. Chest 94:9-14, 1988.)

can be debilitating due to its impact on performance, and can result in the risk of accident or injury due to performance failure.

The symptoms of sleep apnea include awakening gasping or choking; awakening for uncertain reasons, often with a sense of anxiety; restless sleep; nonrestorative or unrefreshing sleep; morning headache; morning confusion; mood disturbance, including irritability and dysphoria; and erectile dysfunction in men. Many patients fail to acknowledge these symptoms, minimize the impact that they have on their lives,[23] or attribute them to causes other than sleep disturbance. For example, we have seen one moderately obese patient whose body weight increased during the winter months, at which time he experienced symptoms of low mood, anergia, anhedonia, and a decline in occupational functioning. The recurrent nature of these symptoms led to the diagnosis of seasonal affective disorder which was insufficiently treated with antidepressant medication. However, sleep laboratory studies revealed that the patient had severe obstructive sleep apnea which worsened with weight gain, and which was the primary cause of his psychiatric complaint.

Sleep apnea presents a serious health risk. Hypertension is common. Podszus[30] has reported that the prevalence of systemic hypertension averaged 58 percent among 461 sleep apnea patients evaluated in four studies.[31,32,33,34] The occurrence of hypertension correlates with the risk factors that are commonly associated with sleep apnea, especially age and weight. These findings are complemented by sleep laboratory studies of hypertensive patients with no sleep complaints which show that up to one-half meet minimal criteria for the diagnosis of sleep apnea, and one-third have apnea indices equal to or greater than 20.[35] This has led some authors to suggest that hypertension and sleep apnea may be a significant consequence of obesity.[30] Cardiac arrhythmias also are common. Approximately 48 percent of patients with sleep apnea have cardiac arrhythmias.[36] The most common types of cardiac events observed are premature ventricular contractions and sinus arrest of between 2.5 and 13 seconds in duration.[37] In some patients, transient periods of bradycardia occur during apneic or hypopneic events, followed by tachycardia during periods of respiration. Oxygen desaturation during the night can lead to hypoxemia, and there have been reports of seizures occurring in association with desaturation.[37] The frequent desaturation associated with sleep apnea occasionally results in polycythemia. One evaluation of 1000 patients has found that 7 percent of those with unexplained polycythemia have sleep apnea.[12] One of the most important health risks associated with sleep apnea is increased mortality. Studies have shown that sleep apnea may be associated with an increased mortality risk. In a 9-year longitudinal study of untreated patients with sleep apnea,[38] it was found that those with apnea indices greater than 20 had a high mortality rate, with a cumulative probability of survival of only 0.63, while those with indices below 20 had a cumulative probability of survival of 0.96 (see Figure 1). These data underscore the need for the early evaluation and treatment of sleep apnea.

There are several factors that predispose patients to sleep apnea. The disorder is more common in men, with the male:female ratio estimated at between 3:1 and 20:1.[14,39] Although it may first appear at any age, most cases are identified when patients are between the ages of 40 and 60 years. In women, the disorder is more commonly diagnosed after menopause.[14] As emphasized previously, obesity is a significant risk factor, and is thought to contribute significantly to the development of sleep apnea. There appears to be an association between excess upper body fat and sleep apnea. Recent data have shown a high incidence of sleep apnea in Polynesian and South Pacific island populations, possibly due to an inherited pattern of obesity and excess fat in the upper body.[40] In a sample of predominantly male snorers, the only variable that is associated with sleep apnea is body weight, which accounts for 41 percent of the variance. No other symptom complaint was significantly predictive of sleep apnea.[41] Craniofacial abnormalities (e.g., those associated with Pierre-Robin syndrome) and conditions that compromise airway patency (such as enlarged turbinates, deviated septum, nasal polyps, enlarged tonsils and adenoids) also may be a risk. Disorders such as chronic obstructive pulmonary disease, asthma, interstitial lung disease, and kyphoscoliosis may contribute to or worsen sleep apnea. Finally, alcohol, central nervous system depressant drugs such as the benzodiazepines; and supine body position during sleep can also contribute to sleep apnea.

The treatment of sleep apnea in obese patients commonly begins with the recommendation for weight loss. Several studies have shown that weight reduction through dietary management can result in significant improvement in sleep apnea.[42,43,44,45,46] At least one study has demonstrated that even a slight decline in body weight (5 to 10 percent) can improve symptoms.[47] Gastric surgery is also known to result in symptom improvement.[48] It has been found that sleep apnea, arterial blood gases, pulmonary hypertension, left ventricular dysfunction, lung volume, and polycythemia improve following gastric bypass surgery and subsequent weight loss.[49] Significant reduction in apneic and hypopneic events in these cases is also associated with improvement in sleep architecture, with marked increases in delta and REM sleep.[50,51] However, gastric surgery for the treatment of obesity and sleep apnea has its limitations. One 7-year follow-up study has shown that half of the obese sleep apnea patients who undergo bariatric surgery regain considerable weight, and this is associated with the full return of the symptoms of sleep apnea.[51]

While weight reduction is a universal recommendation for obese patients with sleep apnea, the efficacy of this treatment strategy is generally poor. This is due to the often extended length of time required to achieve a weight at which apneic events are reduced, and the limited ability of patients to maintain weight loss. Consequently, the exclusive use of weight reduction cannot be considered an effective acute or long-term treatment for sleep apnea. It is best used as an adjunct to other treatments, and is most useful in producing long-term health benefits.

The most common treatment for sleep apnea is nasal continuous positive airway pressure (CPAP).[52,53,54] Nasal CPAP is administered by means of a mechanical device that delivers room air to the nasal airway through a nose mask. This device helps to maintain upper airway patency by providing a "pneumatic splint,"[53] although other factors may contribute to its effects. It is highly effective in the treatment of obstructive, central, and mixed sleep apnea. The reduction in the number of apneic and hypopneic events during the sleep period is significant, and many patients may find that respiratory events are virtually abolished. The initial nights of therapy are often associated with a rebound of delta and REM sleep.[55] There is also a long-term improvement in daytime sleepiness[56] and hypertension, as well as cardiovascular, psychological, and cognitive functioning.[57] The CPAP machine must be used nightly in order to maintain its effects, and most studies have found that long-term home use of CPAP is a safe and effective treatment. Major complications with CPAP are rare, with the greatest limiting factor in continued treatment being one of compliance. Compliance and long-term acceptance of CPAP is between 50 and 80 percent,[58,59,60] suggesting that patient education and follow-up are critical if this treatment modality is chosen.

The use of CPAP may not be indicated for all patients. Other devices for the treatment of sleep apnea include the tongue retaining device (TRD), which is an oral appliance that is designed to improve airway patency by advancing the tongue and mandible. The TRD has been found to significantly reduce apneic events in 50 to 60 percent of the patients studied,[61] with improvement rates being greatest in patients with position-dependent apnea. Those patients who were primarily apneic in the supine position, but not in lateral or prone positions, were most likely to respond well to the treatment.[62] Since the development of the TRD, a diverse array of intraoral appliances have been used with varying rates of success, although few studies have shown that these devices reduce the apnea index below 10, and none appear to reduce the index below 5.[63] Other nonsurgical treatments have included the placement of a nasopharyngeal airway to maintain upper airway patency,[64] and positional treatments that enforce lateral sleeping positions in patients with position-dependent sleep apnea (i.e., the placement of a tennis ball sewn into the back of the patient's pajama top).

There are surgical alternatives to the use of nasal CPAP or other mechanical devices. Nasal reconstruction may be indicated in patients with conditions that prevent airflow through the nasal airway, such as nasal congestion, polyps, or deviated septum. Uvulopalatopharyngoplasty (UVPP) is a procedure designed to enlarge the potential airspace in the oropharynx by shortening the uvula and soft palate.[65] It has been found to be successful for approximately 50 percent of unselected patients,[39,66] although success rates have been reported to be higher when preoperative evaluations include endoscopic evaluation of the upper airway with Valsalva's and Muller's maneuvers.[67] The complications associated with UVPP include postoperative bleeding and severe sore throat, as well as long-term problems of nasal reflux and difficulties vocalizing certain sounds.[67] A newer form of upper airway surgery that addresses tissue of the uvula and soft palate is known as laser-assisted uvulopalatoplasty (LAUP). This is a procedure that utilizes laser technology to remove or reduce tissue, producing improvements in airway space that are similar to UVPP. The treatment is typically performed in stages over the course of several brief visits, which reduces discomfort to the patient and minimizes the likelihood of complications. While initial data suggest that LAUP is effective in the treatment of snoring,[68,69] its efficacy in the treatment of sleep apnea has not been determined. More extensive surgical intervention may be indicated when other treatments have failed. These procedures include mandibular osteotomy with genioglossus advancement, hyoid myotomy, or bimaxillary advancement. A high rate of response has been found in patients who undergo the complete sequence of treatment. However, the extensive and complicated nature of the procedures may limit their use and their acceptance by patients.

CENTRAL ALVEOLAR HYPOVENTILATION SYNDROME

Central alveolar hypoventilation syndrome is characterized by ventilatory impairment in patients with normal mechanical properties of the lung.[14] Hypoventilation, arterial oxygen desaturation, and carbon dioxide retention occur during wakefulness and worsen during sleep, at which time hypoxia and hypercapnia can become pronounced. This disorder is also known as Ondine's curse, and when it is associated with obesity it may be called the obesity hypoventilation syndrome or Pickwickian syndrome. Obesity hypoventilation syndrome often occurs in association with sleep apnea, although it may be found in its absence. The disorder is thought to affect a minority of obese individuals but its prevalence in the general population is not known.

The two primary contributors to the development of obesity hypoventilation syndrome are a decrease in central ventilatory drive and a reduction of the mechanical efficiency of the lungs. The latter is often the result of obesity, which results in excessive loads (i.e., weight) on the lungs and respiratory muscles, worsening when the patient is supine.[70,71,72] Upper airway resistance, lung disease, or diaphragmatic dysfunction adds to the mechanical load of impeded respiratory muscles. The mechanical aspects of hypoventilation are further complicated by ventilation-perfusion mismatching which contributes to reduced oxygenation and increases in carbon dioxide levels. The hypoxia and hypercapnia associated with obesity hypoventilation syndrome is thought to be due to reduced carotid body sensitivity to O_2 or to low or absent central chemoresponsiveness to elevations of CO_2.[73] This results in episodes of oxygen desaturation that tend to be longer than those observed in sleep apnea alone. It is common for episodes of hypoventilation to be followed by arousals similar to those that follow apneic and hypopneic events. These arousals may prevent or disrupt episodes of deep sleep, and may result in multiple awakenings during the sleep period. Consequently, the sleep characteristics of patients with obesity hypoventilation syndrome can be similar to those of sleep apnea. The symptoms may include disturbed nighttime sleep and excessive daytime sleepiness. However, it is notable that some patients with severe hypoxia and hypercapnia during sleep fail to arouse or awaken following desaturation (Ondine's curse), and may not report symptoms of disturbed sleep.

According to Hara and Shepard,[74] serious consequences of central alveolar hypoventilation include "left- or right-sided heart failure, cyanosis, plethora, jugular venous distention, cardiac gallops, tricuspid or mitral regurgitant murmurs, rales, hepatomegaly, peripheral edema, mental confusion, polycythemia, and blood gas abnormalities." Electrocardiography may show evidence of "right-heart strain with P-pulmonale, right ventricular hypertrophy, and right axis deviation."

Obesity hypoventilation syndrome is treated with the administration of supplemental oxygen to eliminate hypoxemia, and diuresis to reduce pulmonary and peripheral edema.[74] Supplemental oxygen must be administered with care, as elimination of hypoxemia can result in a further blunting of the respiratory response, which can lead to marked reductions in alveolar ventilation, hypercarbia, and acidosis. Metabolic alkalosis resulting from diuretic use must also be managed. It should be noted that improvement in oxygen saturation is typically not sufficient treatment for obesity hypoventilation syndrome. Reduction of upper airway resistance can be critical. Treatment strategies include the use of nasal CPAP, positive pressure ventilation, and nasopharyngeal or endotracheal intubation. When these measures fail, tracheostomy is often considered as the last recourse. However, even such aggressive forms of managing the patient may be insufficient to reverse the severity of impairments in respiratory physiology. Weight reduction is always recommended as a long-term treatment strategy in treating obese patients with this disorder. In slender Ondine's patients, phrenic nerve pacing may improve ventilation sufficiently to allow sleep, but tracheostomy is often a necessary accompaniment due to upper airway obstruction during pacing.

NOCTURNAL EATING SYNDROME

It has been known for many years that some obese individuals consume significant quantities of food during the sleep period. Stunkard[75] was the first to describe a syndrome characterized by nocturnal hyperphagia, or consumption of at least 25 percent of total daily caloric intake during the period following the evening meal; insomnia occurring three or more times per week; and morning anorexia with negligible or no food intake at breakfast. The prevalence of this pattern of food intake among obese individuals is unknown, but recent evidence suggests that it is common. One study of 110 obese subjects has shown that 50 percent meet criteria for night eating.[76] However, symptoms are infrequently reported by patients unless they are carefully questioned.

Sleep-related eating disorders have been defined in the International Classification of Sleep Disorders.[14] This definition indicates that nocturnal eating (drinking) syndrome "is characterized by recurrent awakenings, with the inability to return to sleep without eating or drinking." Once the expected intake occurs, it is common for the individual to return to sleep without difficulty. While little is known about the nature of nocturnal eating, espe-

cially in the obese, research findings currently suggest that it is a heterogeneous disorder. One group of investigators has studied 19 adult night-eating
patients, 44 percent of which were overweight.[77] They found that nocturnal
eating is commonly associated with impaired judgment and sloppiness
during eating episodes, during which subjects tended to consume high-calorie foods. Impulsive and disinhibited eating behavior was seen during binge
episodes, and patients sometimes reported dreamlike mental imagery during
these episodes.[77] The patient's level of consciousness during eating episodes
and the degree of subsequent recall appear to be variable. However, night
eating in this group was essentially described as an automatic behavior that
typically occurred during an unconscious or semiconscious state. Hunger or
thirst have been rarely reported by these patients, despite the compulsive
and immediate urge to consume food at night.[78]

Another variant of night eating has been described in the morbidly
obese, and appears to be exacerbated by dieting.[79] Obese patients tend to
report hunger and thirst,[80] and seem less likely to demonstrate signs of poor
judgment or sloppiness during binge episodes. While their eating may be
described as impulsive or disinhibited, it appears that these patients are
more likely to be aware of their night eating, and have better recall for eating
episodes. However, they may be reluctant to acknowledge the occurrence
or severity of nighttime binge episodes. Consistent with the report of
Stunkard, these patients tend to restrict food intake in the morning, which
may lead to a cycle of daytime food restriction followed by rebound eating
at night. One study has shown that there is an inverse relationship between
calories consumed during the day and those consumed at night in obese
subjects.[79]

Nocturnal eating syndrome has been observed in bulimic patients, some
of whom have difficulty controlling their weight. Several case reports have
described individuals who consume food during the sleep period,[81,82,83]
many of whom eat in binge episodes. The descriptions of these episodes
are similar to those reported by Shenck, in that they were described as
somnambulistic events during which food was consumed in a disorganized
way, and for which there was little or no memory. However, at least one
report identified an individual who awakened during sleep with craving
for food who could not return to sleep until her urge to eat had been
satisfied. This pattern appears to be most common in obese individuals.

The consequences of nocturnal eating syndrome include daytime fatigue
and sleepiness due to periods of wakefulness at night. However, it is also
possible that this disorder contributes significantly to calorie consumption
and weight gain in obese individuals. It has been suggested that failure to
lose weight despite adherence to dietary restrictions during the day can be
accounted for, in part, by food consumption during the sleep period. These
findings have considerable importance for an understanding of the high
failure and recidivism rates among obese patients in weight reduction

programs. Night eating may worsen sleep-related breathing disorders by interfering with weight loss or contributing to weight gain.

The treatment of night eating syndrome includes the use of sedative-hypnotic medication. Reduction in sleep-related eating has been observed in patients who were administered a benzodiazepine, sometimes in conjunction with an L-dopa/carbidopa combination.[77] Obese patients who consume food during the sleep period may benefit from the application of behavioral techniques, although the efficacy of these methods has not been determined. One technique involves the modification of dietary recommendations to reduce the amount of caloric restriction during the day. This may help to reduce the rebound observed during the sleep period. Another technique involves the use of prepared trays of low-calorie foods that can be consumed during nighttime awakenings. Finally, it is possible that effective treatment of underlying sleep disturbance that may contribute to awakenings, such as sleep apnea, can be useful in sustaining sleep and reducing the number of eating episodes that occur during the sleep period.

NOTES

1. Danguir J (1987). Cafeteria diet promotes sleep in rats. Appetite 8:49-53.
2. Danguir J, Nicolaidis S (1978). Sleep and feeding patterns in the ventromedial hypothalamic lesioned rat. Physiol and Behav 22:735-740.
3. Adam K (1977). Body weight correlates with REM sleep. Brit Med J 1:813-814.
4. Guilleminault C, van den Hoed J, Mitler MM (1978). Clinical overview of the sleep apnea syndromes. In C Guilleminault and WC Dement, Eds, Sleep Apnea Syndromes. New York: Alan R. Liss.
5. Zammit GK, Kolevzon A, Aronoff N, Knight K, Shindledecker R, Ackerman S (1994). Postprandial sleep in obesity. Sleep Res 23:57.
6. Kapunuiai LE, Andrew DJ, Crowell DH, Pearle JW (1985). Estimated prevalence of sleep apnea in adults based on self-report survey apnea scores. Sleep Res 14:175.
7. Lavie P (1983). Incidence of sleep apnea in a presumably healthy working population: a significant relationship with excessive daytime sleepiness. Sleep 6:312-318.
8. Peter JH, Siegrist J, Podszus T, Mayer, J, Selzer K, Wichert P von (1985). Prevalence of sleep apnea in healthy industrial workers. Klin Wochenschr 63:807.
9. Young T, Palta M, Dempsey J, Skatrud J, Weber S, Badr S (1993). The occurrence of sleep-disordered breathing among middle-aged adults. New Eng J Med 328:1230-1235.
10. Ancoli-Israel S, Kripke DF, Klauber MR, Mason WJ, Fell R, Kaplan O (1991). Sleep-disordered breathing in community-dwelling elderly. Sleep 14:486-495.
11. Coleman RM, Roffwarg HP and Kennedy SJ, et al. (1982). Sleep wake disorders based on a polysomnographic diagnosis. A national cooperative study. JAMA 247:997-1003.
12. Guilleminault C (1989). Clinical features and evaluation of obstructive sleep apnea. In MH Kryger, T Roth and WC Dement, Eds, Principles and practice of sleep medicine. Philadelphia: W.B. Saunders.

13.   Bliwise DL, Feldman DE, Bliwise NG, Carskadon MA, Kraemer HC, North CS, Petta DE, Seidel WF, Dement WC (1987). Risk factors for sleep-disordered breathing in heterogeneous geriatric populations. J Am Geriatric Soc 35:132-141.
14.   American Sleep Disorders Association (1990). International Classification of Sleep Disorders. Rochester, MN: American Sleep Disorders Association.
15.   Krieger J (1990). Obstructive sleep apnea: clinical manifestations and patho-physiology. In MJ Thorpy, Ed, Handbook of sleep disorders. New York: Marcel Dekker.
16.   Guilleminault C and Stoohs R (1991). The upper airway resistance syndrome. Sleep Res 20:250.
17.   Guilleminault C, Stoohs R, Clerk A, Cetel M and Maistros P (1993). A cause of excessive daytime sleepiness: the upper airway resistance syndrome. Chest 104:781-787.
18.   Guilleminault C, Dement WC (1978). Sleep apnea syndromes and related sleep disorders. In RL Williams and I Karacan, Eds, Sleep disorders: diagnosis and treatment. New York: John Wiley.
19.   Wittig RM, Romaker A, Zorick FJ, Roehrs TA, Conway WA, Roth T (1984). Night-to-night consistency of apneas during sleep. Am Rev Respir Dis 129:244-246.
20.   Stepanski E, Lamphere J, Roehrs T, Zorick F, Roth T (1987). Experimental sleep fragmentation in normal subjects. Int J Neurosci, 33:207-214.
21.   Stepanski E, Lamphere J, Badia P, Zorick F, Roth T (1984). Sleep fragmentation and daytime sleepiness. Sleep 7:18-26.
22.   Roehrs T, Zorick F, Wittig R, Conway W, Roth T (1989). Predictors of objective level of daytime sleepiness in patients with sleep-related breathing disorders. Chest 95:1202-1206.
23.   Kribbs, NB, Getsy JE, Dinges D (1994). Investigation and management of daytime sleepiness in sleep apnea. NA Saunders, CE Sullivan, Eds, Sleep and breathing, 2/e. New York: Marcel Dekker.
24.   Guilleminault C, Billiard M, Montplasir J, Dement WC (1975). Altered states of consciousness in disorders of daytime sleepiness. J Neurol Sci 26:377-393.
25.   Carskadon, MA, Dement WC, Mitler MM, Roth T, Westbrook PR, Keenan S (1986). Guidelines for the multiple sleep latency test: a standard measure of sleepiness. Sleep 9:519-524.
26.   Roth T, Hartse KM, Zorick F, Conway W (1980). Multiple naps and the evaluation of daytime sleepiness in patients with upper airway sleep apnea. Sleep 3:425-439.
27.   Westbrook PR (1990). Sleep disorders and upper airway obstruction in adults. Otolaryngol Clin North Am 23:727-743.
28.   Findley LJ, Unverzagt ME, Suratt PM (1988). Automobile accidents involving patients with obstructive sleep apnea. Am Rev Respir Dis 138:337-340.
29.   Findley LJ, Fabrizio MJ, Knight H, Norcross BB, LaForte AJ, Suratt PM (1989). Driving simulator performance in patients with sleep apnea. Am Rev Respir Dis 140:529-530.
30.   Podszus T, Greenburg H, Scharf SM (1994). Influence of sleep state and sleep-disordered breathing on cardiovascular function. In NA Saunders and CE Sullivan, Eds, Sleep and breathing. New York: Marcel Dekker.
31.   Burack B, Pollak C, Borowiecki B, Weitzman E (1977). The hypersomnia-sleep apnea syndrome (HSA): a reversible major cardiovascular hazard. Circulation 56:111-117.

32. Millman RP, Redline S, Randall C, Carlisle CC, Levison P, Braman S (1991). The relationship between nocturnal sleep events and daytime hypertension in a population of patients with obstructive sleep apnea. Chest 99:861-866.

33. Partinen M, Jamieson A, Guilleminault C (1988). Long-term outcome for obstructive sleep apnea syndrome patients (mortality). Chest 94:1200-1204.

34. Shepard JW Jr, Garrison MW, Grither DA, Dolan GF (1985). Relationship of ventricular ectopy to oxyhemoglobin desaturation in patients with obstructive sleep apnea. Chest 88: 335-340.

35. Scharf SM, Garshick E, Brown R, Tishler PV, Tosteson T, McCarley R (1990). Screening for subclinical sleep-disordered breathing. Sleep 13:344-353.

36. Guilleminault C, Connolly S, Winkle R (1983). Cardiac arrythmia during sleep in 400 patients with sleep apnea syndrome. Am J Cardiol 52:490-494.

37. Guilleminault C, Dement WC (1988). Sleep apnea syndromes and related disorders. In RL Williams, I Karacan and C Moore, Eds, Sleep disorders: diagnosis and treatment, 2/e. New York: John Wiley.

38. He J, Kryger MH, Zorick FJ, Conway W, Roth T (1988). Mortality and apnea index in obstructive sleep apnea. Chest 94:9-14.

39. McNamara SG, Cistulli PA, Sullivan CE, Strohl KP (1994). Clinical aspects of sleep apnea. NA Saunders and CE Sullivan, Eds, Sleep and breathing, 2/e. New York: Marcel Dekker.

40. Grunstein RR, Lawrence S, Spies JM, Faaluopo P, Vermeulen W, Phillips K, Handelsman DJ, Sullivan CE (1989). Snoring in paradise—the Western Samoa sleep survey. Europ Respir J 2 (suppl 5):4015.

41. Keidar A, Zammit GK, Krespi Y (1994). The relationship between polysomnographic findings and self-reported symptoms in laser-assisted uvulopalatoplasty (LAUP) candidates. Sleep Res 23:271.

42. Pasquali R, Colella P, Cirignotta F, Mondini S, Gerardi R, Buratti P, Rinaldi-Ceroni A, Tartari F, Schiavina M, Melchionda N, Lugaresi E, Barbara L (1990). Treatment of obese patients with obstructive sleep apnea syndrome (OSAS): effect of weight loss and interference of otorhinolaryngoiatric pathology. Int J Obesity 14:207-217.

43. Rubenstein I, Colapinto N, Rotstein LE, Brown IG, Hoffstein, V (1988). Improvement in upper airway function after weight loss in patients with obstructive sleep apnea. Am Rev Respir Dis 138:1192-1195.

44. Smith PL, Gold AV, Meyrs DA, Haponik EF, Bleecker ER (1985). Weight loss in mildly to moderately obese patients with obstructive sleep apnea. Ann Intern Med 103:850-855.

45. Suratt PM, McTier RF, Findley LJ, Pohl SL, Wilhoit SC (1987). Changes in breathing and the pharynx after weight loss in obstructive sleep apnea. Chest 92:631-637.

46. Browman CP, Sampson MG, Yolles SF, Gujavarty KS, Weiler SJ, Walsleben JA, Hahn PM, Mitler MM (1984). Obstructive sleep apnea and body weight. Chest 85:435-436.

47. Guilleminault HC, Tilkian A, Dement WC (1976). The sleep apnea syndromes. Ann Rev Med 27:465-484.

48. Gastrointestinal Surgery for Severe Obesity. NIH Consensus Development Conference Statement (1991). March 25-27, 9(1).

49. Sugerman HJ, Fairman RP, Sood RK, Engle K, Wolfe L, Kellum JM (1992). Long-term effects of gastric surgery for treating respiratory insufficiency of obesity. Am J Clin Nutrition 55:597S-601S.

50. Charuzi I, Fraser D, Peiser J, Ovnat A, Lavie P (1987). Sleep apnea syndrome in the morbidly obese undergoing bariatric surgery. Gastroenterol Clin North Am 16:517-519.

51. Charuzi I, Fraser D, Peiser J, Peled, R (1992). Bariatric surgery in morbidly obese sleep-apnea patients: short- and long-term follow-up. Am J Clin Nutrition 55:594S-596S.
52. Sullivan CE, Issa FG, Berthon-Jones M, et. al (1981). Reversal of obstructive sleep apnoea by continuous positive airway pressure applied through the nares. Lancet 1: 862-865.
53. Sanders M (1990). The management of sleep-disordered breathing. In RJ Martin, Ed, Cardiorespiratory disorders during sleep, 2/e. Mt. Kisco, NY: Futura.
54. Sanders MH, Moore SE, Eveslage J (1983). CPAP via nasal mask: a treatment for occlusive sleep apnea. Chest 83:144-145.
55. Issa FG, Sullivan CE (1986). The immediate effects of nasal continuous positive airway pressure treatment on sleep pattern in patients with obstructive sleep apnea syndrome. Electroencephal Clin Neurophysiol 63:10-17.
56. Lamphere J, Roehrs T, Wittig R, Zorick F, Conway WA, Roth T (1989). Recovery of alertness after CPAP in sleep apnea. Chest:96:1364-1367.
57. Sullivan CE, Grunstein RR (1994). Continuous positive airway pressure in sleep-disordered breathing. MH Kryger, T Roth and WC Dement, Eds, Principles and practice of sleep medicine. Philadelphia: W.B. Saunders.
58. Sanders MH, Gruendl CA, Rogers RM (1986). Patient compliance with nasal CPAP therapy for sleep apnea. Chest 90:330-333.
59. Krieger J, Kurtz D (1988). Objective measurement of compliance of nasal CPAP treatment for the obstructive sleep apnea syndrome. Europ Respir J 1:436-438.
60. Kribbs NB, Pack AI, Kline LR, et al. (1993). Objective measurement of patterns of nasal CPAP use by patients with obstructive sleep apnea. Am Rev Respir Dis 147:887-895.
61. Cartwright RD, Samelson CF (1982). The effects of non-surgical treatment for obstructive sleep apnea: the tongue-retaining device. JAMA 248:705-709.
62. Cartwright RD (1985). Predicting response to the tongue-retaining device for sleep apnea syndrome. Arch Otolaryngol 111:385-388.
63. Lowe AA (1994). Dental appliances for the treatment of snoring and obstructive sleep apnea. MH Kryger, T Roth and WC Dement, Eds, Principles and practice of sleep medicine. Philadelphia: W.B. Saunders.
64. Nahmias JS, Karetzky MS (1988). Treatment of the obstructive sleep apnea syndrome using a nasopharyngeal tube. Chest 94:1142-1147.
65. Ikematsu T, Fujita S, Simmons FB, et al. (1987). Uvulopalatopharyngoplasty: variations. In D Fairbanks, S Fujita, T Ikematsu and FB Simmons, Eds, Snoring and obstructive sleep apnea. New York: Raven Press.
66. Fujita S, Conway W, Zorick F, Roth T (1981). Surgical correction of anatomic abnormalities in obstructive sleep apnea syndrome: uvulopalatopharyngoplasty. Otolaryngol Head Neck Surg 89:923-934.
67. Sher AE, Thorpy MJ, Speilman AJ, et al. (1985). Predictive value of Muller maneuver in selection of patients for uvulopalatopharyngoplasty. Laryngoscope 95:1483-1487.
68. Kamami YV (1990). Laser CO_2 for snoring: preliminary results. Acta Otorhino-laryngol Belgica 44:451-456.
69. Krespi Y, Zammit G, Keidar A, Pearlman SJ, Lund S, Urioste R (1994). Laser-assisted uvulopalatoplasty in the treatment of snoring and sleep apnea. Sleep Res 23:276.
70. Bradley TD, Rutherford R, Grossman RF, et al. (1985). Role of daytime hypoxemia in the pathogenesis of right heart failure in the obstructive sleep apnea syndrome. Am Rev Respir Dis 131:835-839.

71. Lopata M, Onal E (1982). Mass loading, sleep apnea and the pathogenesis of obesity hypoventilation. Am Rev Respir Dis 126:640-645.
72. Luce JM (1980). Respiratory complications of obesity. Chest 78:626-631.
73. White DP (1994). Central sleep apnea. In MH Kryger, T Roth and WC Dement, Eds, Principles and practice of sleep medicine. Philadelphia: W.B. Saunders.
74. Hara KS, Shepard JW (1990). Sleep in critical care medicine. In RJ Martin, Ed, Cardiorespiratory disorders during sleep, 2/e (rev). Mt. Kisco, NY: Futura.
75. Stunkard AJ, Grace WJ, Wolfe HG (1955). The night eating syndrome. Am J Med 7:78-86.
76. Aronoff NJ, Zammit GK, Urioste R (1994). The incidence of night eating in an obese adult population. Sleep Res 23:219.
77. Schenck CH, Hurwitz TD, Bundlie SR, Mahowald MW (1991). Sleep-related eating disorders: polysomnographic correlates of a heterogeneous syndrome distinct from daytime eating disorders. Sleep 14:419-431.
78. Schenck CH, Hurwitz TD, O'Connor KA, Mahowald MW (1993). Additional categories of sleep-related eating disorders and the current status of treatment. Sleep 16:457-466.
79. Aronoff NJ, Geliebter A, Hashim SA, Zammit GK (1994). The relationship between daytime and nighttime food intake in an obese night eater. Obesity Res 2:145-151.
80. Mitchell J, Aronoff NJ, Urioste R, Zammit GK (1994). Case studies of obese patients with nocturnal eating syndrome. Sleep Res 23:293.
81. Guirguis WR (1986). Sleepwalking as a symptom of bulimia. Brit Med J 293:587-588.
82. McSherry J, Ashman G (1990). Bulimia and sleep disturbance. J Fam Practice 30:102-103.
83. Roper P (1989). Bulimia while sleepwalking, a rebuttal for sane automatism? Lancet 2:796.

7

Abnormal Arachidonic Acid Metabolism in Obesity

Stephen D. Phinney, MD, PhD

Human obesity is a common disorder of unknown cause, and its prevalence in the United States is increasing (Flegal et al. 1988). The propensity for obesity has a genetic component, which implies a biochemical or metabolic mechanism enhancing energy intake or the efficiency of energy storage as triglyceride. Environmental factors such as increased dietary fat and inactivity appear to enhance the propensity for obesity. The broad range of biochemical and metabolic abnormalities associated with obesity implicates a systemic abnormality rather than a single hormone or organ as etiologic. In addition, genetic obesity in humans appears to be polygenic in nature (Stunkard et al. 1990), while most animal models exist with a defect at a single gene locus (Johnson et al. 1991). This picture would suggest that human obesity is a common manifestation of numerous metabolic, behavioral and environmental factors working alone or in combination to produce excess body fat stores. Seen from this perspective, a common biochemical etiologic thread linking the majority of severely obese humans would seem unlikely, let alone linking humans with animal models of genetic obesity as well.

Seen from another perspective, however, human obesity is a surprisingly uncommon disease in the United States. The high prevalence of environmental factors (high fat intake, low physical activity) should put most of us

The author wishes to thank his wife Huong T. Bach and the following teachers, colleagues, and students for helpful discussions leading to this hypothesis: Ralph T. Holman, Ethan A.H. Sims, Steven D. Clarke, Judith S. Stern, Patricia R. Johnson, Janis S. Fisler, Craig H. Warden, William E.M. Lands, Sachiko T. St. Jeor, Anna B. Tang, Manabu T. Nakamura, Linda Magrum, Kerry Ayre, Debbie C. Thurmond, Peter G. Davis, and Rosalind S. Odin. The research was supported in part by NIH Grant DK 35747.

at risk. However, a number of studies of human overfeeding have shown wide variations in the efficiency with which adults gain weight with the provision of similar caloric excesses (Sims et al. 1973; Bouchard et al. 1990). In this light, while behavioral and environment factors may vary, it is likely that frank obesity (e.g., body mass index > 30) is most likely to occur in those genetically predisposed.

This chapter will propose that arachidonic acid (20:4ω6, a highly unsaturated fatty acid) plays an important role in the regulation of energy balance by influencing fuel partitioning, that humans vary in their regulation of the 20:4ω6 content of important tissue pools, and that those with reduced membrane arachidonic acid are predisposed to obesity. Because of the many steps involved in the production, distribution and catabolism of arachidonic acid, there are many candidate points in its metabolism that could be influenced by genetic variation. To the extent that genetic variation in the balance of fuel disposal to oxidation versus storage benefits a species, more than one involved allele alone or in combination might promote the desired diversity, and this proposed pathway would provide a convenient network of interacting factors through which this could be achieved.

ARACHIDONIC ACID METABOLISM

To understand the alterations in 20:4ω6 metabolism with obesity, a brief background is useful. Arachidonic acid is the predominant product of desaturation and elongation (i.e., anabolism) of the omega-6 essential fatty acid (EFA) precursor linoleic acid (18:2ω6). As shown in Figure 1, this occurs via three enzymatic steps, hereafter called the hepatic fatty acid anabolic pathway (HFAAP). These same enzymes participate in the anabolism of alpha-linolenic acid (18:3ω3) to eicosapentaenoic acid (20:5ω3) and on to docosahexaenoic acid (22:6ω3). That these latter steps do not occur to an appreciable extent with ω6 fatty acids (i.e., taking 20:4ω6 to 22:5ω6) indicates that specific steps in the pathway are remarkably selective of substrate, and also suggests that the product 20:4ω6 is selectively conserved and regulated. Once produced, arachidonic acid is concentrated in phospholipids (PL) and cholesteryl esters (CE) relative to triglyceride (TG) and free fatty acid (FFA). Neither the details of the regulation of the HFAAP nor the specific mechanism for the bioconcentration of 20:4ω6 in PL and CE are known. Based upon metabolic studies, there is presumed to be feedback inhibition of 20:4ω6 on delta-6 desaturase (dotted line, Figure 1).

"Classic" EFA deficiency as first described in animals in 1929 (Burr and Burr 1929) and in adult humans in 1970 (Holman 1970) involved deprivation of 20:4ω6 and its precursor 18:2ω6 to the point that the activated HFAAP produces an excess of the nonessential product 20:3ω9 (see Figure 1). When the ratio of this secondary HFAAP product 20:3ω9 (also called Mead acid after Dr. James Mead) compared to serum arachidonic acid reaches 0.4, the

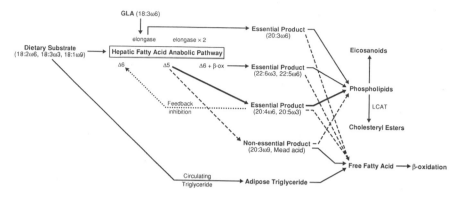

Figure 1. Pathways of essential (and nonessential) fatty acid anabolism involving omega-6, omega-3, and omega-9 families metabolized via the "hepatic fatty acid anabolic pathway" (HFAAP). All three substrate fatty acids utilize the same enzymes in common: delta-6 desaturase, elongase, and delta-5 desaturase. Only the omega-3 family fatty acids undergo substantial further anabolism to yield 22-carbon product with a double bond in the delta-4 position (produced by a pair of elongations, delta-6 desaturation and a 2-carbon beta-oxidation). Solid lines indicate major pathways, dashed lines are secondary pathways, and the dotted line indicates feedback inhibition. GLA=gamma-linolenic acid.

threshold of EFA deficiency has been reached (Holman 1970). In enterally fed animals and humans, this occurs with chronic intakes of omega-6 fatty acids at less than 0.5 to 1.0 percent of total energy. In humans, this rarely occurs except with parenteral feeding or with chemically defined enteral feeding. An additional factor forestalling EFA deficiency in humans is the relatively large adipose TG reserve. In adults eating a typical North American diet, human adipose TG contains 10 to 20 percent 18:2ω6 (or more than 1 to 2 kg for even normal-weight adults), so this will cover even long periods of privation at the projected minimum need for linoleic acid at 1 to 2 g per day.

While this minimum requirement for 18:2ω6 is fairly well established, the daily human requirement for arachidonic acid is not. The efficiency with which the minimum intake of linoleic acid can be conserved and moved through the HFAAP to arachidonic acid is also unknown. That is, under conditions of 18:2ω6 restriction, what percent of mobilized 18:2ω6 is converted to 20:4ω6 as opposed to that lost to beta-oxidation? Thus the range for daily production and catabolism of arachidonic acid via all routes of disposal (i.e., the rate of net arachidonic acid catabolic flux) in normal humans remains to be determined.

An indirect approach to this issue can be found in studies of human vegetarians, as the only appreciable dietary sources of arachidonic acid are found in animal flesh and animal fats. Thus vegetarians are dependent upon the HFAAP to provide all of their daily 20:4ω6 needs. Both vegans and semi-vegetarians have lower proportions of arachidonic acid in their serum phospholipids and cholesteryl esters (Phinney et al.1990), indicating that dietary 20:4ω6 is a significant source of this fatty acid in the omnivores. A conservative estimate is that an omnivorous human consumes up to 500 mg of arachidonic acid daily (Garg and Grundy 1988; Phinney et al. 1990). As this appears to enhance the circulating 20:4ω6 pool, this observation implies that an intake of 500 mg of arachidonic acid represents a significant proportion of an adult human's daily need.

Also of interest in this study was the observation that the vegan vegetarians also had significant elevations in the proportion of Mead acid in the serum PL and free fatty acid fractions. While still only a minor fraction and well below the level indicative of overt EFA deficiency, this observation implies that the fatty acid anabolic pathway yields 20:3ω9 as a secondary product. In other words, the relative proportion of 20:3ω9 in serum (or liver) PL could function as a marker of HFAAP flux (see Figure 1). The significance of this observation to obesity will be established below.

ARACHIDONIC ACID IN METABOLIC REGULATION

Since the discovery that most prostaglandins and leukotrienes are the products of arachidonic acid, there has been a burgeoning array of agents and actions through which 20:4ω6 and its metabolites exert regulatory effects on cellular and organ function (Hartl and Wolfe 1990). Of interest to the topic of obesity is the strong correlation between muscle PL arachidonic acid and insulin sensitivity (Borkman et al. 1993), and the reduction of hepatic lipogenesis by 20:4ω6 in vitro (Odin et al. 1987) and in vivo (Williams et al. 1990). Considering just these functions alone, a paucity of arachidonic acid in phospholipids would increase peripheral insulin resistance and accelerate hepatic lipogenesis at the expense of skeletal muscle glycogen (reduced due to impaired muscle glucose uptake) and hepatic glycogen.

Another emerging function of arachidonic acid is its participation in the release of insulin by the pancreatic beta cell (Turk et al. 1992). To perform this function, 20:4ω6 is released from phosphatidyl inositol (PI) on the inner lamella of the membrane. If the membrane PI were relatively deficient in arachidonic acid, then insulin release might be impaired. In another scenario, however, if there were an inappropriately accelerated release of 20:4ω6 from the membrane, then basal insulin release might be enhanced by the increased flux of arachidonic acid into the cytosol. Assuming that regeneration of PI 20:4ω6 does not fully compensate, however, then membrane 20:4ω6 would be reduced, and the membrane response to maximal insulin stimulation would be impaired.

ABNORMAL ARACHIDONIC ACID IN OBESITY

Schouten and co-workers (1981) reported a rise in serum PL arachidonic acid when obese patients lost weight. As there were no normals for comparison in this study, it was unclear if the patients started low and rose to normal, or if their serum PL arachidonic acid had risen to supranormal during the diet. In addition, this study did not report repeat measures of serum PL 20:4ω6 when the patients were weight-stable following weight loss.

To address this issue, a human study was undertaken to obtain serum samples before, during, and after weight loss by very low-calorie dieting (VLCD) (Phinney et al. 1991). Compared to values derived from a population of healthy, normal weight adults (Phinney et al. 1990), the obese patients had significantly depressed serum PL 20:4ω6 before weight loss. During the VLCD, their serum PL arachidonic acid rose to normal, but it fell back to the pre-weight loss depressed value when they were weight stable following (and despite) major weight loss. Concurrent with these shifts in their PL 20:4ω6, these patients' CE 20:4ω6 rose from normal to supranormal, but returned to normal after the weight loss. These data suggest that our dieting subjects started with an abnormal distribution of arachidonic acid prior to weight loss, and this abnormality persisted in the post-dieting phase despite substantial correction of their obesity. Clearly this was not simply a systemic deficiency of 20:4ω6, as the CE arachidonic acid content remained at or above normal values throughout the weight loss phase. In addition, Mead acid, the marker of EFA deficiency (Holman 1970), declined during the VLCD; and adipose tissue release of the omega-6 precursor linoleic acid was copious (> 20 g/d) during the diet (Phinney et al. 1990).

In parallel with these observations in humans, there is evidence for abnormal arachidonic acid metabolism in the obese Zucker rat as well. There are two reports of low proportions of 20:4ω6 in liver PL of obese Zucker rats compared to lean (Blond et al. 1989; Guesnet et al. 1990). Both of these papers concluded that the obese animals had impaired arachidonic acid production, but the latter reported a relative elevation in hepatic PL 20:5ω3 in the obese animals. As endogenous production of 20:5ω3 utilizes the same fatty acid anabolic pathway (see Figure 1) as 20:4ω6, this observation suggested either a loss in specificity for omega-6 substrate by the HFAAP, or an accelerated systemic catabolism of arachidonic acid necessitating increased pathway flux. If the latter were the case, then one would expect an increased level of the ω6 intermediate 20:3ω6, along with secondary pathway products such as 20:5ω3 and 20:3ω9.

To address this question of the distribution of 20:4ω6 and the secondary HFAAP products 20:3ω9 and 20:5ω3, lean and obese Zucker rats were given free access to a defined diet for 60 days and gavaged daily with 0.1 ml of soybean oil (Phinney et al. 1993). While this study confirmed the previous finding of low arachidonic acid in liver PL from obese animals, liver and serum CE 20:4ω6 were significantly elevated, as were the secondary products 20:3ω9 and 20:5ω3 in multiple liver and serum fractions. In addition, the arachidonic acid precursor 18:2ω6 was depressed in all fractions, while its intermediate 20:3ω6 was elevated in all fractions. These results indicate accelerated HFAAP activity, possibly in an attempt to compensate for either increased catabolism or maldistribution of arachidonic acid in the obese animals.

In assessing the metabolic differences between lean and obese Zucker rats, the nonessential HFAAP product 20:3ω9 deserves specific attention. Despite its low proportion in the lipid fractions assayed (0.05 to 0.5 percent), fastidious sample handling and gas chromatography technique allow its accurate determination (Phinney et al. 1990). The implications of our observations noted above are that Mead acid is produced as a minor product of HFAAP, but in more or less constant proportion with arachidonate. As the latter is subject to bioconcentration and catabolism in other tissues, hepatic (and possibly serum) PL 20:3ω9 may serve as a surrogate marker of hepatic 20:4ω6 production.

GAMMA-LINOLENIC ACID FEEDING OF ZUCKER RATS

To further enhance arachidonic acid production in this animal model of obesity, identical groups of lean and obese Zucker rats in this study were gavaged with 0.1 ml of black currant oil methyl ester concentrate (70 percent gamma-linolenic acid [GLA, 18:3ω6]) (Phinney 1993). As shown in Figure 1, the 18:3ω6 bypasses the rate-limiting enzyme (delta-6 desaturase) in the HFAAP. The GLA-gavaged lean animals were unaffected in weight gain, food intake, body composition, and liver PL 20:4ω6 compared to soy-gavaged lean animals. With the GLA obese animals, however, there was reduced food intake, reduced weight gain, and reduced percent body fat compared to soy-gavaged obese controls. Concurrently, the GLA gavage achieved its goal of increasing the liver PL 20:4ω6 to normal; and simultaneously the PL 20:3ω9 was significantly reduced.

While the GLA gavage did not create a phenotypically lean animal from an obese genotype, it did reduce total weight and adiposity, and it markedly reduced food intake. This latter effect was confirmed in a follow-up study using a graded dose of GLA adjusted to increasing body weight (Thurmond et al. 1993). In the last 20 days of the 60-day gavage period, the GLA obese animals spontaneously ate the same amount of food as the lean controls gavaged with soy. As with the prior GLA study, however, this study also did not produce a genetically obese animal with a normal (lean) body composition. Thus the GLA gavage had its most pronounced effect on food intake, achieved only a modest reduction in percent body fat, and did not bring lean body mass up to normal. This result is not unlike that achieved with enforced calorie restriction in the obese Zucker rat (Cleary 1980), but the critical differences were that the GLA-induced reduction in food intake was "voluntary," and the GLA effect on food intake and growth was specific only to the obese genotype.

These effects of manipulating arachidonic acid production in the liver of the obese Zucker rat suggest that the reduced proportion of 20:4ω6 in hepatic PL (or some closely related fraction) is causally linked to the hyperphagia of this animal model, possibly through enhanced lipogenesis via the mechanism described above. However, correcting the hepatic PL 20:4ω6 deficit by enhanced production (GLA gavage) did not appear to resolve other metabolic problems outside of the liver. These observations are compatible with the hypothesis that there is a systemic problem with arachidonic acid conservation, and that further enhancing its flux out of the liver does not cure the systemic problem. In other words, perhaps the enhanced systemic use of arachidonic acid is the primary metabolic defect in this model of genetic obesity. In this case, the hepatic PL 20:4ω6 deficit is a secondary defect when arachidonic acid production via the HFAAP cannot keep pace; and this in turn allows increased hepatic lipogenesis which further compounds the obesity problem by shifting carbohydrate calories into the lipid pool (Figure 2, enhanced fatty acid synthase [FAS] in liver).

POTENTIAL CAUSES AND CONSEQUENCES OF INCREASED 20:4ω6 FLUX

In a small pilot study, the arachidonic acid content of phosphatidyl inositol was assessed in liver from lean and obese Zucker rats (Phinney 1992). Whereas the total liver PL (containing phosphatidyl choline, phosphatidyl serine, phosphatidyl ethanolamine, sphingolipids, and cardiolipin) showed a 20:4ω6 decrement of 14 percent in obese compared to lean, its decrement in liver PI was 31 percent. This surprising result indicates that one of the most important pools of regulatory substrate (PI) (Kinsella 1990) has experienced a more pronounced loss of arachidonic acid than the mixed PL pool. This result needs to be confirmed, as the analysis is very delicate and the number of animals was small. However, especially if confirmed in tissues outside the liver, it would indicate an abnormality in cellular regulation affecting all tissues utilizing PI for membrane signal transduction.

The most interesting possibility suggested by our data would be that the release of arachidonic acid from PI itself is the problem, with the metabolic consequences being due as much to the poorly restrained release of PI products (inositol triphosphate [IP$_3$], diacylglycerol [DAG], and free 20:4ω6) as from the paucity of arachidonic acid remaining in the PI. A potential sign that this is occurring is the observation of increased intracel-

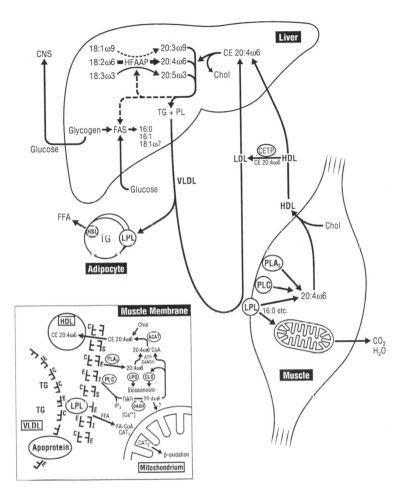

Figure 2. A hypothetical diagram for the arachidonic acid cycle, indicating the exchange of 20:4ω6 between liver and the periphery (e.g., muscle). In this scheme, the recycling of 20:4ω6 to the liver is accomplished via cholesteryl ester (CE).

Definitions: HFAAP=hepatic fatty acid anabolic pathway (see Figure 1); TG= triglyceride; PL=phospholipid; FA=fatty acid synthase; CN= central nervous system; VLDL=very low-density lipoprotein; LPL=lipoprotein lipase; HSL=hormone sensitive lipase; FFA=free fatty acid or nonesterified fatty acid; LDL=low-density lipoprotein; HDL=high-density lipoprotein; CET=cholesteryl ester transfer protein; Chol=free cholesterol; PLC=phospholipase C; PLA₂=phospholipase A₂.

In the muscle enlargement: ACAT=acyl cholesterol acyl transferase; LPO= lipoxygenase CLO=cyclooxygenase; IP₃=inositol triphosphate; DA=diacylglycerol; DAGH= diacylglycerol hydrolase; CAT=carnitine acyl transferase; [Ca⁺⁺]= intracellular free calcium concentration. The letters C, E, I and S refer respectively to the phospholipid polar head groups choline, ethanolamine, inositol and serine.

lular calcium in hepatocytes from obese Zucker rats (Zemel 1990). This could be the consequence of IP_3 release, which releases calcium from the Golgi apparatus and via calcium channels. Increased intracellular calcium has also been noted to characterize erythrocytes from obese humans (Resnick et al. 1992), suggesting the commonality of this finding in the syndromes of obesity across species.

DISTURBED OMEGA-6 METABOLISM
IN MULTIGENIC MOUSE OBESITY

In addition to the above information on disturbed EFA metabolism in the Zucker rat and in human obesity, there is also evidence for a similar problem in the multigenic mouse model of obesity as well (Phinney et al. 1993). The backcross progeny of (C57BL/6J x *Mus spretus*) x C57BL/6J have been characterized by Fisler and co-workers (1993) as ranging in carcass fat from 1 to 50 percent, while both parents are relatively lean. Arachidonic acid was not reduced in liver PL of the obese animals; however, both PL 20:3ω6 and 20:3ω9 were increased in this tissue. In addition, liver PL 20:3ω6 and 20:5ω3 both correlated with percent carcass fat ($p < 0.0001$ and 0.005, respectively). These results are compatible with accelerated hepatic arachidonic acid production (as indicated by increased PL content of its intermediate and two secondary products); but unlike the obese Zucker rat, these mice were able to compensate by increasing the HFAAP to the degree that hepatic PL 20:4ω6 remained normal.

The linear relationship between carcass fat and both 20:3ω6 and 20:5ω3 in hepatic PL in this mouse model implies a multiple-step, graded disturbance in fatty acid metabolism. This in turn implies the interaction of two or more genes affecting the metabolism of arachidonic acid. As noted in the introduction, with multiple genes potentially affecting the same pathway, a wide range of variation in peripheral 20:4ω6 flux could explain the diversity of body composition responses seen in this animal model, and possibly in humans as well.

This concept is reinforced by the relationship between serum insulin and hepatic fatty acids in this animal (Phinney et al. 1993). Hepatic PL 20:3ω9, 20:3ω6, and 22:6ω3 were all positively correlated ($p < 0.01$) with fasting serum insulin in these mice; whereas hepatic PL 20:4ω6 had no significant correlation with serum insulin. This is not in conflict with the negative correlation recently reported between muscle PL 20:4ω6 and serum insulin (Borkman et al. 1993), as the liver is the metabolic "donor" for arachidonic acid, and thus would not necessarily show parallel effects if the problem in 20:4ω6 metabolism originated in the periphery. Thus our observations strongly support a link between increased HFAAP activity and insulin resistance, and extends the conclusions of Borkman (1993) to the concept that increased arachidonic acid flux in the periphery (rather than a reduced static level in muscle PL) is a functional correlate to insulin resistance.

CE 20:4ω6 AS SURROGATE MEASURE OF ITS PERIPHERAL FLUX

If the above argument holds and there is indeed accelerated release of arachidonic acid from PL (PI) into the cytosol, what is its fate? If allowed to remain as nonesterified 20:4ω6, it would be a potential substrate for eicosanoid synthesis via lipoxygenase or cyclooxygenase pathways, it could be peroxidized, or it could be recovered intact. This latter option might allow regeneration of PL in situ. Another means of recovery might be via esterification to cholesterol, yielding cholesteryl arachidonate (CE 20:4ω6). This cholesteryl ester could be returned to the liver via HDL particles, which are typically very rich in CE.

While hepatic recovery and recycling of 20:4ω6 from the periphery has not been previously described, it helps explain a number of observations in the above studies of fatty acid metabolism in obese animals and humans (see Figure 2). The obese Zucker rat has an increased proportion of arachidonic acid in both the serum and hepatic CE fractions (Phinney et al. 1993). Of the two fractions, however, the serum CE has the greater 20:4ω6 enrichment (in both lean and obese genotypes), suggesting that the periphery rather than the liver is the source of the enriched CE 20:4ω6. In the polygenic mouse model of obesity, the liver CE of the obese contains more arachidonic acid than does that of the lean animals (Phinney et al. 1993). This is compatible with the concept that arachidonic acid is processed into PL and/or TG in the liver, exported to membranes in the periphery by VLDL, released into the cytosol in the process of signal transduction, recovered by esterification to cholesterol as CE 20:4ω6, and returned to the liver as HDL. In other words, there is a cycle between liver and the periphery involving 20:4ω6 used in signal transduction that employs lipoproteins as vehicles of transport.

In obese humans, serum CE has either the same proportion of 20:4ω6 as leans when the serum PL is deficient (Phinney et al. 1991), or it is increased when the serum PL 20:4ω6 is normal (Phinney, Tang et al. 1992). While indirect evidence, these observations are nonetheless compatible with an increase in the return of free arachidonic acid from the periphery. Taken in the context of the indications for increased HFAAP activity noted above, the overall picture is consistent with this hypothesis.

Assuming that this is the case, however, it is clear that the peripheral recovery and hepatic recycling of 20:4ω6 via HDL transport is less than quantitative. If it were, then the HFAAP would not be enhanced in obesity. Thus there must be at least some catabolic loss of arachidonic acid in the periphery, making the "arachidonic acid cycle" far less than 100 percent efficient. This should be observed as increased eicosanoid products or peroxidation products, or alternatively as increased clearance of carbon from 20:4ω6 as CO_2 as a result of beta-oxidation (see Figure 2).

POTENTIAL FOR VARYING END-ORGAN EFFECTS ASSOCIATED WITH OBESITY

As there are many potential steps involved in the insertion, release, and recovery of arachidonic acid from membranes, there are enough independently coded proteins to allow for the polygenic expression of obesity in the multigenic mouse model (and also in humans) to occur via variations in the same common pathway. In addition, there may be differences in the expression of the enzymatic abnormality between organs, and in the same person over time (Fabsitz et al. 1992), thus allowing for the obvious heterogeneity of the syndromes of obesity while remaining consistent with this unifying hypothesis. This heterogeneity, especially between organs, could also help to explain the variations in the health risks of obesity associated with insulin resistance, such as hypertension and type II diabetes (Reaven 1988).

One important gap in this picture is the potential role for arachidonate in the regulation of adipocyte proliferation and function. It is possible that the adipocyte proliferation is a primary participant in the 20:4ω6-mediated events, as there is at least one report of arachidonic acid metabolites participating in the differentiation of adipocytes (Serrero et al. 1992). If this were not the case, however, there are still the regulatory effects of 20:4ω6 on hepatic lipogenesis and its effect on insulin-mediated glucose disposal in the periphery. Both would contribute to a shift of glucose from direct use as energy-yielding substrate toward its use as substrate for lipogenesis.

CLINICAL IMPLICATIONS OF ABNORMAL OMEGA-6 METABOLISM IN OBESITY

This new perspective on EFA metabolism in obesity has little immediate clinical utility. The gamma-linolenate treatment that reduced food intake in the obese Zucker rat is unlikely to be effective in humans, as this animal has an extreme form of fatty acid metabolic disturbance resulting in frank depletion of liver PL 20:4ω6. This was not seen in the multigenic mouse model, and may not occur in humans as well. In addition, the 18:3ω6 treatment did not produce a lean animal, indicating that the hyperphagia can be uncoupled from the abnormal partitioning of substrate in the periphery. This in turn supports the possibility that a peripheral metabolic abnormality is primary. Assuming that this involves arachidonic acid release from PL in the periphery, then enhancing its production in the liver would not solve the problem. To the extent that 18:3ω6 treatment might increase peripheral 20:4ω6 release, it might in fact cause harm by amplifying responses to incidental inflammatory or thrombogenic stimuli.

One potential early use of our observations would be in the diagnosis and classification of syndromes of obesity. While our initial results from small groups of severely obese humans (Phinney et al. 1991; Phinney et al. 1992) show fairly uniform abnormalities in PUFA metabolism, casting a wider net may allow us to differentiate between two moderately obese adults, one with an aberrant omega-6 fatty acid pattern but with weight held partially in check by diet restriction, while another person might have a more normal fatty acid pattern with weight excess secondary to behaviorally induced overeating. The information yielded by a serum fatty acid profile might allow more effective triage for therapeutic intervention, and would strongly indicate that the person with the biochemical abnormality receive treatment appropriate for a chronic disease with a metabolic etiology.

SUMMARY

This chapter has presented data from humans, Zucker rats, and mice which indicates that obesity is associated with a disturbance in omega-6 fatty acid metabolism. While others have interpreted this observation in rats as an impairment in arachidonic acid production, more careful examination supports the concept of accelerated systemic 20:4ω6 flux with obesity in all three species. These observations suggest a normal cycle of arachidonic acid export from the liver to membranes in the periphery, its release into the cytosol and recovery as cholesteryl arachidonate, and return to the liver via LDL/HDL. This cycle appears to be increased in both rodent models of obesity and in humans. An increase in arachidonic acid release from membranes could overstimulate some metabolic regulatory pathways, while reducing substrate availability to others, resulting in a wide range of organ effects and tissue manifestations of the disease. As it must be assumed that this common disturbance in arachidonic acid metabolism is the result of a number of different genetic lesions within and between species, the metabolic manifestations and end-organ effects of obesity could differ as well. This hypothesis offers a new perspective on the normal metabolism of arachidonic acid, a unifying hypothesis for the etiology of genetic obesity, and an explanation for some of the diverse manifestations commonly associated with obesity.

REFERENCES

Blond J-P, Henchiri C, Bezzard J (1989). Delta-6 and delta-5 desaturase activities in liver from obese Zucker rats at different ages. Lipids 24:389-395.
Borkman M, Storlien LH, Pan DA, Jenkins AB, Chisholm DJ, Campbell LV (1993). The relation between insulin sensitivity and the fatty acid composition of skeletal muscle phospholipids. N Engl J Med 328:238-244.
Bouchard C, Tremblay A, Despres J-P, Nadeau A, Lupien P-G, Theriault G, Dussault J, Moorjani S, Pinault S, Fournier G (1990). The response to long-term overfeeding in identical twins. N Engl J Med 322:1477-1482.

Burr GO, Burr MM (1929). A new deficiency disease produced by the rigid exclusion of fat from the diet. J Biol Chem 82:345-367.

Cleary MP, Vasselli JR, Greenwood MRC (1980). Development of obesity in Zucker obese (fa/fa) rat in absence of hyperphagia. Am J Physiol 238:E284-E292.

Fabsitz RR, Carmelli D, Hewitt JK (1992). Evidence for independent genetic influences on obesity in middle age. Int J Obesity 16:657-666.

Fisler JS, Warden CH, Pace MJ, Aldons JL (1993). BSB: a new mouse model of multigenic obesity. Obesity Res 1 1:271-280.

Flegal KM, Harlan WR, Landis JR (1988). Secular trends in body mass index and skinfold thickness with socioeconomic factors in young adult women. Am J Clin Nutrition 48:535-543.

Garg A, Bonanome A, Grundy SM, Zhang ZJ, Unger RH (1988). Comparison of a high carbohydrate diet with a high monounsaturated-fat diet in patients with non-insulin-dependent diabetes mellitus. N Engl J Med 319:829-834.

Guesnet P, Boune J-M, Pascal G, Durand G (1990). Tissue phospholipid fatty acid composition in genetically lean and obese Zucker female rats on the same diet. Lipids 25:517-522.

Hartl WH, Wolfe RR (1990). The phospholipid/arachidonic acid second messenger system: its possible role in physiology and pathophysiology of metabolism. J Parenteral Enteral Nutrition 14:416-427.

Holman RT (1971). Essential fatty acid deficiency. Prog Chem Fats Other Lipids 9:275-348.

Johnson PR, Greenwood MRC, Horwitz BA, Stern JS (1991). Animal models of obesity: genetic aspects. Ann Rev Nutrition 11:325-353.

Kinsella JE (1990). Lipids, membrane receptors, and enzymes; effects of dietary fatty acids. J Parenteral Enteral Nutrition 14:2005-2175.

Odin RS, Finke BA, Blake WL, Phinney SD, Clarke SD (1987). Modification of fatty acid composition of membrane phospholipid in hepatocyte monolayer with n-3, n-6, and n-9 fatty acids and its relationship to triacylglycerol production. Biochim Biophys Acta 921:378-391.

Phinney SD, Odin RS, Johnson SB, Holman RT (1990). Reduced arachidonate in serum phospholipids and cholesteryl esters associated with vegetarian diets in humans. Am J Clin Nutrition 51:385-392.

Phinney SD, Tang AB, Johnson SB, Holman RT (1990). Reduced adipose 18:3ω3 with weight loss by very low calorie dieting. Lipids 25:798-806.

Phinney SD, Davis PG, Johnson SB, Holman RT (1991). Obesity and weight loss alter polyunsaturated lipid metabolism in humans. Am J Clin Nutrition 51:831-838.

Phinney SD, Tang AB, St Jeor ST (1992). Obesity but not waist-hip ratio associated with abnormal essential fatty acid metabolism. Am J Clin Nutrition 56:771.

Phinney SD, Tang AB, Thurmond DC, Stern JS (1992). Correction of deficient liver phospholipid arachidonate in obese Zucker rats with reduced food intake and weight gain. J Cellular Biochem Abstract Suppl 16B:265.

Phinney SD, Fisler JS, Tang AB, Warden CH (1993). Liver fatty acid composition correlates with body fat and gender in a multigenic mouse model of obesity. FASEB J 7:A281.

Phinney SD, Fisler JS, Tang AB, Warden CH (1993). Fatty acid markers of hepatic arachidonic flux correlate with serum insulin and glucose in a multigenic mouse model of obesity. Obesity Res 2:77S.

Phinney SD, Tang AB, Thurmond DC, Nakamura MT, Stern JS (1993). Abnormal polyunsaturated lipid metabolism in the obese Zucker rat with partial metabolic correction with gamma-linolenic acid. Metabolism 42:1127-1140.

Reaven GM (1988). Banting lecture 1988: role of insulin resistance in human disease. Diabetes 37:1595-1607.

Resnick LM, Gupta RK, Bhargava KK, Gruenspan H, Alderman MH, Laragh JH (1991). Cellular ions in hypertension, diabetes, and obesity. Hypertension 17:951-975.

Schouten JA, van Gent CM, Popp-Snijders CM, van der Veen EA, van der Voot HA (1981). The influence of low-calorie (240 kcal/day) protein-carbohydrate diet on serum lipid levels in obese subjects. Int J Obesity 5:333-339.

Serrero G, Lepak NM, Goodrich SP (1992). Paracrine regulation of adipose differentiation by arachidonate metabolites: prostaglandin F$_2\alpha$ inhibits early and late markers of differentiation in the adipogenic cell line 1246. Endocrinology 131:2545-2551.

Sims EAH, Danforth E Jr, Horton ES, Bray GA, Glennon TA, Salans LB (1973). Endocrine and metabolic effects of experimental obesity in man. Recent Prog Horm Res 29:457-496.

Stunkard AJ, Harris JR, Pedersen NL, McClearn GE (1990). The body-mass index of twins who have been reared apart. N Engl J Med 322:1483-1487.

Thurmond DT, Tang AB, Nakamura MT, Stern JS, Phinney SD (1993). Time-dependent effects of progressive gamma-linolenate feeding on hyperphagia, weight gain, and erythrocyte fatty acid composition during growth of Zucker obese rats. Obesity Res 1:118-125.

Turk J, Gross RW, Ramanadham S (1993). Amplification of insulin secretion by lipid messengers. Diabetes 42:367-374.

Williams MA, Tinoco J, Tang Y-T, Bird MI, Hincenbergs I (1989). Feeding pure docosahexaenoate or arachidonate decreases plasma triacylglycerol secretion in rats. Lipids 24:753-758.

Zemel MB, Sowers JR, Shehin S, Walsh MF, Levy J (1990). Impaired calcium metabolism associated with hypertension in Zucker obese rats. Metabolism 39:704-708.

8

Obesity and the Endocrine System

Walter Futterweit, MD

A thorough and elegant historical perspective of obesity reflecting the cultural and scientific values of the observers has been compiled by Bray. From sloth and gluttony to disobedience to nature, the afflicted obese person had not only to confront his own affliction, but also the moral judgment of those around him.[1]

It is of historical importance that much interest was generated by Frolich's report in 1901 of a 14-year-old boy with severe headaches, rapid weight gain and diminution of vision who was found to be very obese and short and who also had gynecomastia with small testes.[2] His penis was normal but embedded in pubic fat. His pubic hair was minimal and no axillary hair was present. An intracranial tumor was suspected and at surgery, a tumor—probably a cystic craniopharyngioma—was found and the cystic contents were removed.

This case and later publications suggested that the obesity was related to the hypothalamus and this syndrome was termed Frohlich's syndrome. Further studies later determined that gonadotropins were reduced or absent and some factor from the hypothalamus was lacking in stimulating pituitary secretion of gonadotropins. The resulting adiposogenital syndrome could be replicated experimentally with stereotactic techniques by inducing specific hypothalamic lesions with resulting hyperphagia and obesity. A number of lesions and etiologies were associated with Frohlich's syndrome, including inflammatory diseases of the midbrain, as well as hypothalamic and pituitary tumors and granulomatous diseases. The clinical concept of Frohlich's syndrome has been misapplied over the years and the eponym has been loosely applied to obese boys and girls whose sexual

The author is grateful for the technical assistance of Richard A. Weiss in the preparation of this chapter. The helpful comments of Dr. Jeffrey I. Mechanick are also appreciated.

maturity was delayed. Associated hypothalamic involvement was frequently cited, namely, diabetes insipidus, hypothermia and evidence of some pathological intracranial process.

The common misconception that obesity is often an endocrine aberration must be strongly disclaimed. Yet it is of more than casual interest that virtually all obese subjects manifest endocrine abnormalities secondary to the obese state. In view of the potentially serious metabolic and endocrine complications of obesity these manifestations should be sought and intervention applied early in the course of the disease.

The next several sections are presented to guide the involved physician to potential, albeit rare, causes of obesity. These involve considerable time and patience, but they may offer insight as to the pathogenesis of the obesity.

HISTORY AND PHYSICAL EXAMINATION

The following components should be included in the patient's history:

1. Age of onset of obesity; duration of obesity; if recent how much distribution
2. Eating habits; sociocultural factors
3. Sedentary occupation; degree of exercise; aging; inactivity
4. Drug ingestion or administration; systemic and topical glucocorticoids, estrogens, androgens, progestins, insulin, sulfonylurea, sodium valproate, cyproheptadine, phenothiazines (chlorpromazine, thioridazine, mesoridazine), tricyclic antidepressants (amitriptyline, imipramine and nortriptyline), lithium
5. Ethnicity and socioeconomic factors
6. Mental state, emotional conflicts, self-image and other psychiatric factors; onset of the above
7. Nicotine withdrawal
8. Alcohol abuse
9. Family history of obesity and fat distribution
10. History of medical illnesses
11. Onset of menarche and puberal changes, change in menses, skin texture, tendency to easy bruisability, hirsutism, galactorrhea, polydypsia, polyuria, visual disturbances, mood swings, gynecologic history of previous procedures (laparotomy, removal of cysts), infertility, seizure disorder, gynecomastia, hypertension, diabetes mellitus, headaches, somnolence, facial puffiness or rounding, husky voice, lethargy, symptoms of hypoglycemia (tremulousness, sweats, confusion, impaired mentation, craving for sweets and the response to food), anosmia, thermal dysregulation

The following components should be part of the physical examination:

1. Body mass index (BMI) measurement (weight in kg/height in square meters): normal = 20 to 25, moderate risk = BMI 30 to 40; height, weight, distribution of fat (pelvic fat girdle), generalized or central obesity
2. Waist:hip ratio
3. Cushingoid features, facial plethora, cervicodorsal and supraclavicular fat pad, facial mooning, central obesity with relatively thin extremity fat, violaceous striae, muscle tone, proximal muscle wasting, thin skin
4. Hypothyroidism
5. Hypogonadism, genitalia, eunuchoidism, anosmia, cryptorchidism
6. Hirsutism (terminal coarse hairs), acne, alopecia, pubic hair distribution, oiliness of facial skin, seborrhea
7. Acanthosis nigricans (nape of neck, axillae, groin)
8. Type of escutcheon (male or female)
9. Achrocordions, skin tags
10. Gynecomastia, galactorrhea
11. Eyes: fundi (retinitis pigmentosa, papilledema, gross testing of visual fields)
12. Macroglossia
13. Thyromegaly
14. Skin coarseness, or fine texture of skin
15. Pallid skin color, lemony palms and facies color
16. Ecchymoses
17. Brawny pretibial edema
18. Blood pressure reading
19. Pelvic exam
20. Mental status
21. Achilles tendon reflex—check for normal or delayed relaxation phase
22. Lipomatosis
23. Short, stubby hands with shortened metacarpals (dimpling of the 4th metacarpal head)

Examination of the patient must include assessment of fat distribution, including central (android, upper-body) or peripheral (gynoid, lower-body), as well as assessment of abnormal body fat distribution (e.g., pelvic) in male hypogonadism.

The waist:hip ratio (WHR) also is important in defining the type of fat distribution. This is obtained by measuring the minimal waist circumference by the maximal hip circumference. A WHR in the male greater than 0.9 and in the female greater than 0.8 is associated with the presence of central accumulation of fat cells and is a prognostic risk factor for diabetes mellitus, hypertension, stroke, atherosclerosis and hyperlipidemia.

In any obese hypertensive patient the possibility of Cushing's syndrome must be considered. Thorough examination for this serious but potentially curable disorder as well as a reversible form of obesity is necessary, as well as laboratory evaluation of the etiology of the Cushing's syndrome.

Similarly, an obese woman who is hirsute and oligomenorrheic with signs of hyperandrogenism which may include resistant acne, acanthosis nigricans, seborrhea or male pattern scalp hair loss should have a thorough general and pelvic examination and laboratory studies to define the source of the hyperandrogenism.

Although hypogonadism is not always associated with obesity, there are patients who often do have associated weight gain. These patients may be sought out by assessing their gender habitus and body characteristics, as well as by noting the genitalia and size of testes and ovaries. The presence or absence of gynecomastia should be noted and in both men and women the presence of galactorrhea. A prepuberal etiology of hypogonadism may be established by noting the presence of eunuchoidal proportions (i.e., an arm span 2 inches or greater than the height and pubic arch to floor: crown to pubic arch ratio also increased by at least 2 inches). These changes will not be noted in instances of panhypopituitarism where growth hormone is reduced. Evidence of eunuchoidism, anosmia and frequent presence of cryptorchidism may be seen in patients with Kallmann's syndrome. Patients with Klinefelter's syndrome often display no abnormality of the arm span:height measurement, but often demonstrate an increase in the pubic arch to floor: crown to pubic arch ratio (lower segment) measurement.

Hypothalamic dysfunction on examination may be noted with abnormal visual findings and neurologic signs. Additional findings may include symptoms referable to impaired release of pituitary hormones leading to impairment of growth, hypogonadism, hypothyroidism, diabetes insipidus and galactorrhea. Further diagnostic testing should define the entity.

BASIC LABORATORY TESTS IN EVALUATION OF OBESITY

To a clinician confronted with an obese patient the most pertinent laboratory data should not only relate to the rare endocrine or systemic entities that are associated with or may indeed cause the obesity, but to the potential complications of the obese state. Thus after one performs a 24-hour urine for urine free cortisol (corrected for total creatinine) one may test the patient with an overnight 1.0 mg dexamethasone suppression study if clinically indicated (a normal response would be a serum cortisol less than $5\mu g/dL$). Standard thyroid function studies are also indicated, including serum thyroxine (T_4), thyroid-stimulating hormone (TSH), triiodothyronine (T_3), thyroid-binding globulin (TBG), and the T_4:TBG ratio which corrects for the altered TBG often seen in obesity with a TBG rise possibly reflecting that seen in obese patients with a fatty liver. Alterations of sex hormones should be looked for particularly if symptoms reflect impairment of the hypothalamic-pituitary-gonadal axis. Furthermore, other studies (including those reflecting glucose intolerance, hyperinsulinism and serum lipids) should be evaluated. These include a fasting measurement of blood glucose and insulin and a glucose tolerance test with measurement of serum insulin. Many of the sophisticated endocrine studies listed below under the various endocrine categories involved in obesity are not indicated in routine evaluation of simple obesity, but are reviewed so as to give a broad outline of the immense endocrine and metabolic consequences of obesity.

OBESITY IN ENDOCRINE DISEASES

Endocrine or systemic causes of obesity are very rare with estimates ranging from 1 to 2 percent or less. Most obese patients have obesity which is apparently unrelated to an underlying endocrine etiology. Obesity may be an associated sign in certain metabolic, endocrine and genetic disorders. The fact, however, that endocrine disease can be associated with obesity and may be a major symptom does make it important that an endocrinopathy be excluded. Many diseases are associated with obesity and some systemic diseases involve major endocrine organs causing endocrinopathies which then may lead to increased weight, hyperphagia or abnormal fat distribution. Of major importance is the fact that simple obesity most often is associated with development of endocrine dysfunction which may cause a number of potentially serious complications. The fact that approximately 20 to 30 percent of the American adult population is overweight (namely, 20 percent or more over the ideal weight) makes it imperative that the physician treating such a patient always bears in mind a possible primary or associated endocrine or systemic disease.

The following endocrine and systemic disease categories have been associated with obesity, with a major emphasis on the endocrine disorders that may be associated with obesity:

1.   Hypothalamic Syndromes and Pituitary Diseases
     a. Infiltrative lesions: granulomas—sarcoidosis, histiocytosis X; tumors—craniopharyngioma, astrocytoma, pituitary adenomas, gliomas, chordomas, meningiomas, metastases; inflammatory—meningitis, tuberculosis, syphilis, postviral encephalopathies; metabolic—hemochromatosis (hemosiderin-laden macrophages)
     b. Trauma
     c. Postpartum pituitary necrosis (Sheehan's syndrome)
     d. Hypothalamic surgery
     e. Hypothalamic-pituitary irradiation

      f. Gonadotrophin-releasing hormone deficiency (Kallmann's syndrome)

      g. Panhypopituitarism

      h. Growth hormone failure

      i. Laron dwarfism

      j. Cushing's disease (pituitary-dependent)

      k. Hydrocephalus

      l. Primary empty sella syndrome

2. Thyroid

      a. Hypothyroidism—autoimmune (Hashimoto's thyroiditis)

      b. Secondary hypothyroidism

      c. Hypothalamic-pituitary dysfunction

      d. Postablation with radioactive iodine treatment associated with autoimmune sufficiency

      e. polyglandular (thyroid, adrenal)

3. Adrenal Cortex

      a. Cushing's syndrome secondary to adrenal tumor

4. Ovarian

      a. Polycystic ovary syndrome

      b. Hyperthecosis

      c. Functional sex steroid-producing tumor (masculinizing, feminizing)

5. Testicular

      a. Primary hypogonadism (Anorchia, Klinefelter's syndrome)

      b. Defects in testicular steroidogenesis

      c. Postinfectious (mumps, gonorrhea)

      d. Castration

      e. Myotonia dystrophica

6. Pancreatic

      a. Insulinoma

      b. Hyperinsulinism

7. Genetic

      a. Prader-Willi syndrome

      b. Laurence-Moon-Biedl syndrome

      c. Alstrom's syndrome

      d. Carpenter syndrome

      e. Cohen syndrome

8. Miscellaneous Systemic Diseases

      a. Down's syndrome

      b. Partial lipodystrophy

      c. Multiple lipomatosis

      d. Pseudohypoparathyroidism

      e. Cushing's syndrome secondary to ectopic ACTH or CRF secretion (frequently carcinoma of lung and bronchial carcinoid)

   f. Pseudo-Cushing's disease (secondary to alcohol abuse)
   g. Lipid storage disease

ENDOCRINE AND METABOLIC ABNORMALITIES IN OBESITY

Although the frequency of endocrine disorders causing obesity is small, the metabolic and hormonal consequences of obesity are frequently present. The more severe the degree of obesity the more likely it is that endocrine consequences will ensue. The latter may be a causative factor in some of the more serious complications of obesity. The present consensus is that the alterations in metabolic and endocrine function in obesity are secondary rather than primary. Although the underlying causes of obesity are poorly understood, there are frequent metabolic and endocrine sequelae which should be looked for and evaluated. Furthermore, there are a variety of abnormalities that are demonstrable on endocrine testing. These include abnormalities of the hypothalamic-pituitary, hypothalamic-pituitary-gonadal axes and others, as well as very important changes in insulin dynamics. It is of the utmost importance to the treating physician to be aware of these changes in view of the potential for complications as well as misinterpretation of some of the tests of endocrine function found in the obese individual. The following summarize some of the alterations of endocrine function seen in obesity.

Pancreas: Insulin Resistance

The most important parameter and metabolic disturbance of obesity is the association with hyperinsulinemia. The basal levels as well as responses to glucose loads, tolbutamide, arginine, leucine and glucagon are exaggerated. Enhanced secretion of C-peptide insulin also follows administration of glucose.The finding of abnormalities of pancreatic beta cells in obesity lends further support. Administration of insulin by various techniques reveals a subnormal drop in blood glucose. Most investigators conclude that the insulin resistance (IR) seen in the obese patient results from a post-receptor defect of insulin action in target tissue. Women with a BMI greater than 26.8 may be defined as obese and at this level of BMI have associated IR, while those under 26.8 are not.[3]

The definition of IR is that of a metabolic state wherein physiologic insulin concentrations produce a less than normal biologic response.[4] In simple terms, since the fasting blood glucose level reflects to a great extent the rate of hepatic glucose release which is regulated by the insulin concentration, one has an opportunity to assess IR by noting the fasting blood glucose:insulin level ratio. The higher the insulin level the more insulin resistant the individual. A glucose (mg/dL):insulin (μU/mL) ratio less than 6 is characteristic of obese patients and of impaired glucose tolerance and syndrome X.[4] This ratio has certain pitfalls but is a fair estimate of IR. One may assume quite accurately that all obese patients have some degree of IR. The IR contributes to further hyperinsulinemia and the resulting effects of insulin which contribute to hypertension, hypertriglyceridemia, decreased HDL cholesterol and increased LDL cholesterol. The fact that insulin enhances renal absorption of sodium and water[5] and the effects on vascular smooth muscle increasing endothelial proliferation are possible sequelae of hyperinsulinemia. Insulin may thus be considered a "secret killer"[6] leading to the great morbidity associated with obesity. The question as to why some nonobese individuals develop IR is intriguing and studies of patients with Syndrome X[7] (resistance to insulin-stimulated glucose uptake, impaired glucose tolerance, hyperinsulinemia, increased levels of VLDL and triglycerides, decreased levels of LDL cholesterol and hypertension) do not as yet indicate the prime etiology. It is possible that IR is not sufficient to account for Syndrome X and that possible genetic defects may be important.

There are also biologic factors including disorders of energy metabolism whereby there is a decrease in caloric needs in obese patients lower than those found in the nonobese.[8] Data indicate that there is an increased metabolic rate which is directly related to increased body weight.[9] This metabolic adaptation in obesity is an important key in the understanding of the pathogenesis and perpetuation of the obese state.

IR should also be sought in nonobese subjects with polycystic ovary syndrome,[10] diabetes mellitus, lupus erythematosus and some other autoimmune entities characterized by antibodies to the insulin receptor.[11]

After weight reduction insulin clearance, production and sensitivity normalize.[12] Data of Jimenez and co-workers[12] suggest that the reduction of hyperinsulinemia in massively obese patients after weight loss reflects an early increased insulin clearance rather than a decrease in insulin production. The latter occurs later during the weight reduction. The initial increased insulin clearance lowers the serum insulin and C-peptide levels. Thus the changes that follow weight reduction often follow a reversible pattern.[12]

Hypothalamic-Pituitary Axis

Obesity results in reduced growth hormone (GH) secretion and an impaired response to growth hormone-releasing hormone (GHRH).[13-17] The impaired response to GHRH excludes a GHRH deficiency as being responsible for the reduced GH found in obese subjects. An attenuated GH response also occurs following other provocative stimuli such as L-dopa, glucagon, arginine, fasting, insulin-induced hypoglycemia, exercise, opioids, sleep and nicotinic acid.[14] Reversibility of defects following weight reduction[18] suggests that the impairment of pituitary GH response to GHRH and other stimuli is a result rather than a cause of the obesity. The attenuation of GH response following insulin-induced hypoglycemia may reflect impaired GHRH release as the pathophysiologic mechanism resulting in the impaired GH response.[14]

It should be stressed that the regulation of pituitary GH secretion is the stimulatory effect of GHRH and the negative regulatory effect of somatostatin. In considering hypothalamic control of GH the data are speculative.[19] Impairment of pituitary responses of prolactin (PRL) and thyrotropin to thyrotropin-releasing hormone (TRH) as well as chlorpromazine have been demonstrated in obesity.[20-22] Divergent results on PRL secretion, however, have been reported by others.[23] Basal levels of serum prolactin are usually normal in the obese nonhirsute as well as hirsute women when compared to nonobese women.[24]

GH secretion reduction in the obese is associated with a decreased GH half-life with increased metabolic clearance of GH.[15] The reduction of GH has important clinical implications which may perpetuate the obesity. Decreased GH secretion results in a decrease of lean body mass and an increased percentage of body fat.[14] It is of interest that despite reduced GH levels in obesity, the concentrations of plasma IGF-I (insulin-like growth factor, somatomedin-C), which is synthesized by the liver in response to GH and other factors, are normal or increased.[15,16] Increased IGF-I levels may directly suppress GH secretion via a negative feedback mechanism.[16] The suppression of GH via IGF-I appears to involve somatostatin release. The increased hypothalamic release of somatostatin thus may be an integral part of the impaired GH release in obesity. The interplay of mechanisms which may result in decreased GH release such as a putatively increased somatostatinergic tone[19,23,25] or possible feedback on GH via increased IGF-I may be important mechanisms in the pathophysiologic events associated with obesity in man. One may thus consider the direct stimulation of somatostatin by insulin or via IGF-I as being responsible for impaired pituitary GH responses.[26] Studies by Cordido and co-workers[19,23] of suppression of endogenous somatostatin lend support to the hypothesis that an enhanced somatostatinergic tone is a distinct event in obesity. Direct stimulation of IGF-I by insulin has been hypothesized.[25,27,28] The mechanisms for alterations of IGF-I and GH in obesity are yet to be fully elucidated and it may be that abnormalities in tissue levels, binding and inhibitors of IGF-I may play an important role in the reduction of GH secretion in obesity. Thus although a number of defects have been associated and may possibly result in a reduced GH secretion, the precise mechanism is yet to be fully defined.

Hypothalamic-Pituitary-Ovarian Axis

A number of endocrine abnormalities may be present in women with obesity. These can include oligomenorrhea, amenorrhea, infertility, dysfunctional bleeding, luteal phase insufficiency, hirsutism, acne, seborrhea and male pattern alopecia.[29] Some obese girls may have early onset of menarche (Frisch-Revelle hypothesis)[30,31] wherein body weight achieves 48 kg or approximately 22 percent of body fat. A number of obese women may experience menses to their mid-50s. Some patients with premature menopause have also been described. Enhanced peripheral conversion of androgens, mainly androstenedione to estrone, may account for the increased incidence of endometrial carcinoma in the morbidly obese and even in moderately obese women. In the morbidly obese woman there is a sixfold enhanced conversion of the androstenedione to estrogen (15 percent as opposed to 2 percent in nonobese women), much of this due to the enhanced aromatization conversion by the stromal portion of increased adipose cells.[33] Adipose tissue contains the aromatase enzyme which utilizes some of the androgen precursors and converts them to estrogens.[34,35] In addition fat tissue contains 17b-hydroxysteroid dehydrogenase which converts estradiol to estrone.[34] Thus fat tissue is an important reservoir of sex steroids and forms significant amounts of circulating estrogens.[34]

Abnormalities of androgens are frequently seen in obese women. It has been hypothesized that the decrease of SHBG may result as a direct effect of insulin on its hepatic production.[36] The degree of reduction of SHBG appears to be directly proportional to the degree of obesity. The consequences of reduced SHBG are those of elevated levels of free estrogens[37] as well as non-SHBG-bound (presumably free and biologically active) testosterone.[38] Decreased SHBG also results in increased metabolic clearance rates (MCRs) of testosterone and other androgens for which there is high binding affinity. Thus, despite normal androgen plasma levels in some women with obesity, the enhanced turnover of androgens leads to increased tissue exposure.[39,40] Some but not all obese women demonstrate elevated androgen levels of androstenedione, testosterone and dehydroepiandrosterone sulfate (DHEAS).[41] The hyperandrogenemia appears to be more common in obese women with an increase of the WHR.[42] Some of these effects are seen in the gynecologic and pilosebaceous manifestations of obesity which clinically are not that different from those found in the polycystic ovary syndrome (PCO).[43]

The effects of a decreased SHBG and an increase in free testosterone may be different in men and in pre- and postmenopausal women.[44] Since reduction in SHBG is associated with hyperinsulinemia and insulin resistance, the possible relationship and risk factor for later development of noninsulin-dependent diabetes mellitus (NIDDM) was studied by Haffner and co-workers.[44] The investigators found that increased androgenicity as evaluated by a decreased SHBG was an important independent risk factor for NIDDM in pre- and postmenopausal women. No such relationship was found in men where they are already maximally androgenized. This confirms previous data by Lindstedt and associates[45] who demonstrated that low SHBG predicted the incidence of NIDDM in a 12-year follow-up study of both pre- and postmenopausal women in Sweden.

Many of the endocrine changes resulting from obesity are reversible, resulting in conversion of the anovulatory cycles to normal cycles as well as reducing hyperandrogenemia[46-49] and the elevation of LH levels.[48,49] Obese infertile women who lost 15 percent of body weight conceive easier without any other treatment and the increased levels of testosterone and androstenedione decline significantly by weight reduction alone.[47] It may be possible that obesity by itself is the inciting factor in the pathogenesis of PCO.

It should be noted that not all obese women develop anovulation or menstrual dysfunction and, conversely, that not all women with PCO are obese (less than 40 to 50 percent).[50,51] Most obese women maintain normal menses with variable serum LH. Although some studies demonstrate normal LH levels and pulsatility in obese women,[52] others have demonstrated reduced LH and amplitude of pulse levels as well as pulsatility.[24]

Why is it that some obese women develop menstrual dysfunction including amenorrhea and others do not?[53] Regularly cycling obese women had a 30 percent reduction of mean SHBG and a 70 percent increase of free non-SHBG-bound (physiologically free) testosterone compared to non-obese women. Studies of the amenorrheic obese women demonstrated a significant reduction of SHBG and an increase in total testosterone and androstenedione compared to the ovulatory obese women. The increased free estrogens may create a positive feedback on LH secretion leading to increased pituitary sensitivity to gonadotropin-releasing hormone (GnRH), which in turn augments ovarian androgen production as in PCO. Unlike patients with PCO where normoprolactinemia or hyperprolactinemia may be found,[51,54] some obese women may have low PRL and attenuated PRL responses to TRH.[20] Obesity may aggravate an already present defect in some women resulting in anovulation and amenorrhea.[47,55]

Studies of insulin response to oral glucose load in obese eumenorrheic women with and without hirsutism and women with PCO (mean BMI 35 kg/m^2) demonstrate that the rate of increase in insulin as a function of the BMI was twofold greater in women with PCO than the other two obese groups.[56] Thus it appears that women with PCO differ from most obese women who do not have anovulation in that the degree of IR is more pronounced with increasing weight.

Hyperandrogenemia may be facilitated by a direct effect of insulin on the ovaries via IGF-I receptors[57,58] mediating LH binding with augmented ovarian androgen response to LH.[49]

Body weight influences the direction of estrogen metabolism to more or less potent forms. While thin women have an increase of the 2-hydroxylated form of estradiol, obese women have less of the latter and more of other potent estrogens.[59] The stromal portion of the adipocyte is primarily involved in the extraglandular aromatization of androstenedione to estrone and is therefore of great importance in the peripheral conversion of this androgen to estrone.[60] Some investigators[61,62] describe increased 17-alpha oxidation of estradiol in obese women and speculate that susceptibility to certain hormone-dependent cancers may result as a consequence of the derangements of estradiol metabolism.[63]

Hypothalamic-Pituitary-Testicular Axis

Although the serum testosterone is decreased in markedly obese male subjects,[27,64] clinically there is no decreased libido or potentia and testicular size and spermatogenesis generally remain unaltered.[41] The low total serum testosterone represents the biologically bound and inactive form while the free or unbound testosterone remains in the normal or slightly increased range. This is due to a reduction of SHBG.[65] However, in massively obese men (more than 200 to 250 percent of ideal body weight) there is a decrease in testosterone and free testosterone as well, resulting in hypogonadism.[66-68] This results from increased peripheral conversion of testosterone to estradiol, which is directly related to the extent of obesity.[69]

Other androgens are normal in male obesity, including serum androstenedione and DHT.[67,70] There are some obese men who demonstrate elevated levels of serum estradiol and/or estrone due to increased production rates.[69] The latter result from enhanced peripheral conversion of androstenedione to estrogens largely as a result of the increase in adipose tissue.[64,69] This correlates with the weight gain and declines after weight reduction.[66,69-72]

Serum LH and FSH levels are usually in the normal range in obese men with normal responses to GnRH or clomiphene citrate.[22,65,69] Some suppression of serum FSH may also occur in some obese males as a result of enhanced aromatization of androgens to estrogens by the increased body fat cells.[67] Leydig cell response to human chorionic gonadotropin is also normal, indicating a normal Leydig cell reserve in obesity.[65] Although massively obese men may occasionally demonstrate reduced serum LH and FSH, the changes revert to normal following weight reduction.[66,67]

Hypothalamic-Pituitary-Adrenal Axis

In view of the importance of excluding Cushing's syndrome in any patient presenting with progressive obesity, sometimes of several years' duration, it is of utmost importance to be aware of the impact of obesity itself on the parameters that reflect the hypothalamic-pituitary-adrenal (HPA) axis.

Discrepancies in the studies of the hypothalamic-pituitary-adrenal axis in obesity have been cited in the literature.[73] These include cortisol production rates leading to increased production rate of cortisol, responses of plasma cortisol to insulin-induced hypoglycemia, and the response of ACTH to the hypothalamic corticotropin-releasing factor (CRF). The elegant study of Pasquali and co-workers[73] with obese women related the activity of the HPA axis to varying patterns of body fat distribution. The findings of this group demonstrated (1) an elevated urine free cortisol excretion rate in obese women with an abdominal fat distribution and (2) higher ACTH and cortisol responses to CRF stimulation in the latter more than those found in women with peripheral body fat distribution as well as normal weight women. It is thus hypothesized that obese women with abdominal fat distribution may have a hyperactive HPA axis. This may be due to increased sensitivity of CRF at the pituitary level resulting in ACTH hypersecretion.[73] These studies are an extension of a previous study by Marin and associates,[74] who demonstrated an increased secretion of urine free cortisol and an enhanced serum cortisol response to ACTH in obese women with abdominal body fat distribution as compared to obese women with a peripheral body fat distribution and nonobese women.

The fact that the morning cortisol in the women with abdominal fat distribution is normal or even slightly reduced implies the theoretical possibility of cortisol resistance.[75] Basal cortisol and ACTH levels are similar in nonobese and the two different types of body fat distribution in women.[73]

The above studies[74,75] warrant attention in that they may explain the varying data that have appeared in the literature regarding the effects of obesity on the HPA axis. Impairment of insulin-induced hypoglycemic response of cortisol in the morbidly obese[20] does not negate the fact that the vast majority of obese women have normal response of serum cortisol to a hypoglycemic stimulus. A rapid decline in cortisol secretion rate and urinary 17-hydroxycorticoids may follow a brief 9-day fast, which is well prior to a major change in body fat, weight, or lean body mass.[76]

The normal plasma cortisol, overnight 1 mg dexamethasone test and the normal diurnal variation of cortisol in obesity[74] differentiate obesity from Cushing's syndrome. The increase in urinary 17-hydroxycorticoids in obese patients is related to body weight and if measured and calculated per kilogram of body weight, the value would be in the normal range.

It appears that the female adrenal cortex is more responsive to ACTH than the male in terms of glucocorticoid production. Thus equivalent cortisol secretion rates are obtained in men at the expense of higher ACTH release.[77] Although cortisol secretion rates do not differ between men and women, the increased ACTH levels and pulse frequency found in men as well as the increased 24-hour production rate for ACTH in men as opposed to women indicate increased adrenocortical responsiveness in women to ACTH.

Increased production rates (PR) of androstenedione and dehydroepiandrosterone (DHEA) in obese women are associated with and result from increased metabolic clearance rates (MCR) of adrenal androgens.[78] Thus there may be normal levels of these androgens in obese women despite an increased production rate. In view of the strong correlation between BMI and the MCRs and PRs of androstenedione and DHEA, the hyperandrogenism in obese women should decline as the BMI declines with dieting.

Previous data on relating DHEA and DHEAS levels in human obesity to reduced incidence of cardiovascular disease in men and lipid changes have been hampered by absence of studies relating these changes to body fat distribution.[79] Circulating DHEAS levels in 96 women were correlated with trunk and skinfold thicknesses and total and regional body fat from dual x-ray absorptiometry (DXA). The study of Williams and co-workers demonstrated that truncal fat as determined by DXA was associated with increased serum DHEAS levels in normally menstruating Caucasian women.[79] Circumference ratios such as the WHR are not as sensitive indicators of fat distribution as skin:skinfold thickness ratios or DXA results. The waist:hip ratio was not significantly correlated to the DHEAS or DHEA level.[79,80] The association between increased truncal fat and DHEAS with reduced total leg fat reported by Williams in normally menstruating women lends greater emphasis to the association between truncal obesity and cardiovascular risk factors in these women. No relationship was found between total body fat or age.

Hypothalamic-Pituitary-Thyroidal Axis

Although there are data indicating abnormalities of thyroid indices in obesity, there is no strong evidence for any clinically apparent defect in the hypothalamic-pituitary-thyroidal axis.The basal serum T_4, free T_4, TSH level and response of TSH to TRH is normal in obese subjects.[81] It has been demonstrated that overfeeding results in a rise in serum triiodothyronine (T_3) and an infrequent decline of reverse T_3 (rT_3). These results occur both in short-term and long-term feeding experiments.[82] These results are opposite to those seen in patients who are fasting,[83-85] where an increase of rT_3 and a decline of T_3 are noted. The T_3 levels change in view of an effect of nutrition on the peripheral conversion of T_4 to T_3, as well as on the metabolic clearance of T_3. Thus in chronic overfeeding there is accelerated production of T_3 from T_4 (thyroxine) as well as an increased metabolic clearance of T_3, while these are reduced markedly in fasting states. Nutritional states do not alter the production of T_4. Thus the evidence favors a major role of nutrition (mainly alterations in carbohydrate intake) rather than body weight in determining thyroidal adaptation to food intake.[86]

There has been controversy regarding possible thyroid hormone resistance in obesity. Decreased cellular levels of thyroid hormone receptors have been demonstrated in obesity.[87,88] Clinically, however, this concept has not been verified in view of the absence of large doses of triiodothyronine to reduce adipose tissue. The effect of T_3 administration appears to reduce lean body mass rather than fat tissue.[89]

Parathyroid, Vitamin D and Calcium

Elevated parathyroid levels have been found in patients with obesity,[41,90] and this decreases with weight loss. This is associated with increased urinary cyclic AMP as well as serum 1,25-dihydroxyvitamin D.[90] Obese subjects have normal or reduced serum ionizable calcium, indicating secondary hyperparathyroidism as an attempt to compensate for their reduction in serum calcium.[41] The latter may result as a consequence of a reduction of 25-hydroxyvitamin D,[90,91] or a result of the form in which calcium is transported in the blood.[41,92] The result of any reduction of effective serum calcium can give osteomalacia which has been found on bone biopsies in some obese patients.[91] Certainly the role of parathyroid hormone regulation and dysfunction in obesity requires further study.

Gastrointestinal (GI) Hormones

Since ingestion of food contributes largely to the development of obesity, the mechanism of preabsorptive "satiety signals" from the GI tract is essential in the understanding of the mechanism that controls the size and frequency of meals.[93]

Cholecystokinin

Cholecystokinin (CCK) is a small intestinal peptide that is released after ingestion of food and exerts a negative feedback signal to limit food size as well as other GI effects.[94] Intravenous administration of the octapeptide of CCK has reduced food intake in human studies[95] and the effect is rapid, dose-related and transient. Administration of CCK receptor antagonists increases food intake in humans.[96] The peripheral satiety of CCK is in part mediated by specific effects on the pyloric stomach sphincter as well as via afferent vagus nerve fibers going to not yet fully defined areas of the brain containing CCK receptors. Thus the processing of the satiety signal carried by the vagal afferents to the brain is as yet unclarified. There are some data implicating the dorsal hindbrain as an important area in integrating visceral information.

Glucagon

Administration of the pancreatic hormone glucagon to humans induces variable reduction in satiety.[93] Recent data indicate that glucoreceptor cells in the liver are necessary for the satiety effect. The glycogenolytic effect is not a factor in the satiety effect of glucagon. A physiologic role for glucagon in regulating food intake is suggestive. Variable data are present indicating an elevation of glucagon in human obesity.[97-100]

Bombesin

Bombesin (BBS) and BBS-like peptides are found in the GI tract and brain. Neural disconnection of gut fibers prevents the BBS-induced satiety.[101] More data are needed to assess the importance of these substances in the regulation of food in humans.

Other Peptides

Somatostatin from the pancreas, GI tract and brain may also inhibit food intake. Subdiaphragmatic vagotomy blocks the satiety effect of somatostatin.

Pancreatic polypeptide increases postprandially and data on its effect in regulation of appetite are not yet convincing. Reduced basal and postprandial secretion of pancreatic polypeptide (especially after protein-rich meals) has been reported in obesity when compared to normal subjects,[102] while another group demonstrated no difference between obese and normal subjects.[103] Evidence that it exerts a physiologic curb on appetite is not convincing.

No effect has been shown to date of secretin and gastrin on experimental food intake in animals.

High basal and an exaggerated stimulated immunoreactive gastric inhibitory peptide (GIP)[104,105] has been hypothesized to play a role in the pathogenesis of the hyperinsulinemia of obesity and early noninsulin-dependent diabetes mellitus (NIDDM).[104] Different observers have found variable evidence for a hypothesis that GI factors may overstimulate the pancreas, leading to hyperinsulinemia of obesity and early NIDDM. GIP responses to nutrients have varied according to different studies[104-106] and at this time there are no definitive data supporting the role of GIP in the pathogenesis of hyperinsulinemia of obesity.[105]

The levels of vasoactive intestinal polypeptide appear to be increased in obesity.[107,108] Its precise role, as well as that of the other previously mentioned GI hormones, if any, has to be further clarified.

Miscellaneous Endocrine Alterations in Obesity

Obese patients, particularly those who are massively so, have increased salt and water retention,[86] which is enhanced by carbohydrate intake. Fasting and weight loss results in urinary sodium loss. The latter is reduced with refeeding, resulting in sodium retention and a rise in aldosterone secretion. Spironolactone can block this rise by reducing the effect of aldosterone on the renal tubule.[109] A role of insulin in the regulation of sodium reabsorption during fasting and refeeding has been established.[110] Insulin appears to decrease sodium excretion by a direct effect on the renal tubule.[110] Glucagon has been demonstrated to enhance natriuresis in starvation[111] via a direct renal tubular effect. Thus the initial effects of starvation or semi-starvation in weight loss may be due to natriuresis related to changes in insulin and glucagon.[112,113] Parenthetically, plasma renin and aldosterone levels are normal in obesity.

The fact that insulin enhances renal absorption of sodium and water (antinatriuretic effect)[5,112] and the ill effects on vascular smooth muscle (increasing endothelial proliferation) are serious sequelae of insulin resistance. Insulin may thus be considered a "secret killer,"[6] leading to the great morbidity associated with obesity.

Vasopressin (AVP, ADH) concentration is normal in obesity, but its suppression after a water load and its stimulation with insulin-induced hypoglycemia are attenuated.[63,114,115] The latter normalizes after weight reduction. The majority of obese patients do not have clinically important dysfunction of salt and water metabolism.[41]

Beta-endorphin levels are elevated in obesity and do not normalize after weight reduction.[116,117] The hyperendorphinemia and absence of circadian cyclicity are present in association with a normal serum cortisol.[93] The presence of beta-endorphin in other organs such as the pancreas, testes and ovary has been demonstrated.[116,118] These may play a role in the hyperendorphinemia of obesity.

Insulin has been shown to increase plasma norepinephrine levels.[119] Jung and co-workers[120] noted that the obese patients who had an impaired prolactin response to insulin-induced hypoglycemia also had no rise of plasma norepinephrine to hypoglycemia, while the plasma adrenaline response was normal. This suggests that hypothalamic alterations in obesity may be present as well as those of the sympathetic nervous system.[52] This may involve serotoninergic pathways involving prolactin secretion as well as noradrenergic fibers in the brain. The synthesis of neurotransmitters may also be affected by dietary change, thereby influencing a reduction of sympathetic activity and noradrenaline turnover.[52] Whether this is a primary or secondary defect in obesity is uncertain.

Thus there have been conflicting reports relating to changes in catecholamine concentrations in obese subjects.[121,122] Responses to pharmacologic intervention suggest that perhaps subtle defects in adrenergic tone may be present in some patients with obesity.[86]

Neuroendocrine-Clinical Hypothalamic Syndromes

Hypothalamic dysfunction and lesions can produce obesity. The obesity resulting from experimentally produced lesions of the ventromedial nuclei has been known for many years. Other regions of the hypothalamus are also involved and surgically produced lesions can also produce obesity.[123] These are associated with heterogeneous derangements which manifest themselves clinically other than as increased food intake. Hyperinsulinemia and hyperphagia result from obesity of the ventromedial hypothalamus (VMH) as well as the paraventricular hypothalamus (PVH). The hyperinsulinemia does increase appetite, contributing to the hyperphagia, but is not the only mechanism. Of importance is the participation of the autonomic nervous system in the formation of hyperinsulinism in VMH lesions. Hyperactivity of vagal tone as well as hypoactivity of the sympathetic nervous system have been reported as being associated with the hyperinsulism of VMH-lesioned rats.[124]

A number of hypothalamic entities may produce obesity in man.[125,126] The different etiologies include tumors, inflammatory diseases, trauma, surgery and other diseases which may involve the VMH or surrounding areas of the hypothalamus.[125] Clinically, the features associated with hypothalamic obesity may include sequelae of papilledema (headaches and impaired vision), endocrine dysfunction of the hypothalamic-pituitary axis (reproductive dysfunction, diabetes insipidus, hypothyroidism and hypoadrenalism, as well as impaired growth). Miscellaneous neurologic and physiologic abnormalities may include coma, seizures, somnolence, personality changes, as well as hypo- and hyperthermia.[125,126]

Genetic Syndromes Associated with Obesity

Genetic factors in obesity are well known and have been summarized in excellent reviews.[127-129] Another causative factor is endocrine disorders which, although rare, are distinctly associated with obesity. They are characterized by distinct dysmorphic features and include the Prader-Willi syndrome, Laurence-Moon and Bardet-Biedl syndromes, Alstrom-Hallgren syndrome, Cohen syndrome and Carpenter syndrome. These are summarized in detail by Bray.[125,130]

The disorder that is most frequently cited is the Prader-Willi syndrome. Deletions or translocations on the short arm of chromosome 15 are often present. These patients present with obesity, hypotonic musculature, mental retardation, hypogonadism, short stature and small hands and feet. The syndrome often shows up in siblings.[131] Morphology of the brain has been found to be normal.

The Bardet-Biedl syndrome is suggested by the association of obesity with retinitis pigmentosa and polydactylism.[132] Hypogonadism is frequently present in these genetic syndromes.

Hyperlipidemia

The reader is referred to excellent reviews of hyperlipidemia and risk factors for atherosclerosis in obesity.[133,134]

Tumor Necrosis Factor Alpha

Cytokines are low-molecular proteins produced by many cell types which include T-cells. Some of their functions include the regulation of immune and inflammatory responses, paracrine or autocrine activity at low concentrations, as well as interactions with high-affinity receptors on cell surfaces. Recent experiments have demonstrated that cytokines may be involved in obesity as well as cachexia.[135,136]

Since adipose tissue is the major site of action for energy storage as well as mobilization, studies of adipocyte physiology and metabolism have demonstrated significant effects of tumor necrosis factor alpha (TNFα), one of the cytokines, in leading to suppression of adipose-specific genes, including enzymes involved in lipogenesis. Administration of TNFα leads to hypertriglyceridemia and an increase in very-low-density lipoproteins in rats and humans, as well as an effect on appetite and gastrointestinal function.[135] There are data which indicate that TNFα may be a mediator of insulin resistance. It is interesting to speculate on a possible independent role for TNFα despite its well-established link with cachexia. It appears that the concentration of the cytokine TNFα is crucial. The concentrations that are produced in obese rodents as well as those that produce insulin resistance when administered exogenously are far lower than those which induce other symptoms such as cachexia. Further studies are necessary to establish whether TNFα expression in fat is an important association of human obesity.[135,136]

CONCLUSION

The metabolic consequences of obesity, although serious, are but a pale reflection of the mental anguish, self-doubt and reduced productivity of patients afflicted with this serious disorder. The role of the physician and ancillary disciplines must be to have an awareness of the occult manifestations of the condition and to direct appropriate help to the patient. The morbidity and later complications are serious and demand early diagnosis and therapeutic intervention.

The hyperinsulinism and attendant consequences of insulin resistance must be evaluated fully. The metabolic alterations of gonadal function, particularly in the female, may lead to endocrine-dependent neoplasia. The numerous endocrine abnormalities seen in the obese patient make it essential that the treating physician look for metabolic abnormalities already present or any potentially reversible pathophysiologic state prior to providing the patient with appropriate dietary and other support. Although rare, there are endocrinopathies that do manifest themselves as obesity and it is the responsibility of the treating physician to exclude them. To that end it is hoped that this review has served its purpose.

NOTES

1. Bray GA (1992). Obesity: historical development of scientific and cultural ideas. In P Bjorntorp and BN Brodoff, Eds, Obesity. Philadelphia: JB Lippincott.

2. Frohlich A (1901). Ein fall von tumor der hypophysis cerebri ohne akromegalie. Wien Klin Reindsch 15:883, 906.

3. Campbell PJ, Gerich JE (1990). Impact of obesity on insulin action in volunteers with normal glucose tolerance: demonstration of a threshold for the adverse effect of obesity. J Clin Endocrinol Metab 70:1114-1118.

4. Cara JF (1991). Insulin resistance in obese and nonobese men. J Clin Endocrinol Metab 73:691-695.

5. DeFronzo RA (1981). The effect of insulin on renal sodium metabolism: a review with clinical implications. Diabetologia 21:165-171.

6. Foster DW (1989). Insulin resistance—a secret killer? N Engl J Med 320:733-734.

7. Reaven GM (1988). Banting Lecture 1988. Role of insulin resistance in human disease. Diabetes 37:1595-1607.

8. Hirsh J, Leibel RL (1991). A biological basis for human obesity. J Clin Endocrinol Metab 73:1153-1157.

9. James WPT, Davies HL, Bailes J, et al. (1978). Elevated metabolic rates in obesity. Lancet 1:1122-1125.

10. Dunaif A, Segal KR, Futterweit W, et al. (1989). Profound peripheral insulin resistance, independent of obesity, in polycystic ovary syndrome. Diabetes 38:1165-1174.

11. Kahn CR (1980). Role of insulin receptors in insulin-resistant states. Metabolism 29:455-466.

12. Jimenez J, Zuniga-Guajardo S, Zinman S, et al. (1987). Effect of weight loss in massive obesity on insulin and C-peptide dynamics: sequential changes in insulin production, clearance and sensitivity. J Clin Endocrinol Metab 64:661-668.

13. Williams T, Berelowitz M, Joffe SN, et al. (1984). Impaired growth hormone responses to growth hormone-releasing factor in obesity. N Engl J Med 311:1403-1407.

14. Iranmanesh A, Veldhuis JD (1992). Clinical pathophysiology of the somatotropic (GH) axis in adults. Endocrinol Metab Clin North Am 21:783-816.

15. Veldhuis JD, Iranmanesh A, Ho KKY, et al. (1991). Dual defects in pulsatile growth hormone secretion and clearance subserve the hyposomatotropism of obesity in man. J Clin Endocrinol Metab 72:51-59.

16. Loche S, Cappa M, Borrelli P, et al. (1987). Reduced growth hormone response to growth hormone-releasing hormone in children with simple obesity: evidence for somatomedin-C mediated inhibition. Clin Endocrinol (Oxf) 27:145-153.

17. Dieguez C, Page MD, Scanlon MF (1988). Growth hormone neuroregulation and its alterations in disease states. Clin Endocrinol (Oxf) 28:109-143.

18. Ball MF, El-Khodary AZ, Canary JJ (1972). Growth hormone response in the thinned obese. J Clin Endocrinol Metab 34:498-511.

19. Cordido F, Penalva A, Dieguez C, et al. (1993). Massive growth hormone (GH) discharge in obese subjects after the combined administration of GH-releasing hormone and GHRP-6: evidence for a marked somatotroph secretory capability in obesity. J Clin Endocrinol Metab 76:819-823.

20.   Kopelman PG, White N, Pilkington TRE, et al. (1979). Impaired hypothalamic control of prolactin secretion in massive obesity. Lancet 1:747-750.
21.   Cavagnini F, Maraschini C, Pinto M, et al. (1981). Impaired prolactin secretion in obese patients. J Endocrinol Invest 4:149-153.
22.   Amatruda JM, Hochstein M, Hsu TH, et al. (1982). Hypothalamic and pituitary dysfunction in obese males. Int J Obesity 6:183-189.
23.   Cordido F, Dieguez C, Casanueva FF (1990). Effect of central neurotransmission enhancement by pyrodostigmine on the growth hormone secretion elicited by clonidine, arginine, or hypoglycemia in normal and obese subjects. J Clin Endocrinol Metab 70:1361-1370.
24.   Grenman S, Ronnemaa T, Irjala K, et al. (1986). Sex steroid, gonadotropin, cortisol and prolactin levels in healthy, massively obese women: correlation with abdominal fat cell size and effect of weight reduction. J Clin Endocrinol Metab 63:1257-1261.
25.   Kopelman PG, Noonan K (1986). Growth hormone response to low dose intravenous injections of growth hormone-releasing factor in obese and normal weight women. Clin Endocrinol (Oxf) 24:157-164.
26.   Berelowitz M, Szabo M, Frohman LA, et al. (1981). Somatomedin-C mediates growth hormone negative feedback by effects on both the hypothalamus and the pituitary. Science 212:1281.
27.   Glass AR, Burman KD, Dahms WT, et al. (1981). Endocrine function in human obesity. Metabolism 30:89-104.
28.   Komorowski JM, Pawlikowski M (1979). Relationship between insulin and somatotropin in obesity. Endokrinol 73:209-213.
29.   Hartz AJ, Barboriak PN, Wong A, et al. (1979). The association of obesity with infertility and related menstrual abnormalities in women. Int J Obesity 3:57-73.
30.   Frisch RE, McArthur JW (1974). Menstrual cycles: fatness as a determinant of minimum weight for height necessary for their maintenance or onset. Science 185:949-951.
31.   Crawford JD, Osler DC (1975). Body composition at menarche: the Frisch-Revelle hypothesis revisited. Pediatrics 56:449-458.
32.   Bray GA (1985). Complications of obesity. Ann Intern Med 103:1052-1062.
33.   Siiteri PK (1987). Adipose tissue as a source of hormones. Am J Clin Nutrition 45:277-282.
34.   Deslypere JP, Verdonck L, Vermeulen A (1985). Fat tissue: a steroid reservoir and site of steroid metabolism. J Clin Endocrinol Metab 61:564-570.
35.   Pasquali R, Casimirri F (1993). The impact of obesity on hyperandrogenism and polycystic ovary syndrome in premenopausal women. Clin Endocrinol (Oxf) 39:1-16.
36.   Plymate SR, Matej LA, Jones RE, et al. (1988). Inhibition of sex hormone-binding globulin production in the human hepatoma (Hep G2) cell line by insulin and prolactin. J Clin Endocrinol Metab 67:460-463.
37.   Apter D, Bolton NJ, Hammong GL, et al. (1984). Serum sex hormone-binding globulin during puberty in girls and in different types of adolescent menstrual cycles. Acta Endocrinol (Kbh) 107:413-419.
38.   Vermeulen A, Ando S (1979). Metabolic clearance rate and interconversion of androgens and the influence of the free androgen fraction. J Clin Endocrinol Metab 48:320-326.
39.   Evans DJ, Hoffman RG, Kalkhoff RK, et al. (1983). Relationship of androgenic activity to body fat topography, fat cell morphology and metabolic aberrations in premenopausal women. J Clin Endocrinol Metab 57:304-310.

40. Rosenfield RL (1975). Studies of the relation of plasma androgen levels to androgen action in women. J Steroid Biochem 6:695-702.
41. Glass A (1989). Endocrine aspects of obesity. Med Clin North Am 73:139-160.
42. Kirschner MA, Samojlik E, Drejka M, et al. (1990). Androgen-estrogen metabolism in women with upper-body versus lower-body obesity. J Clin Endocrinol Metab 70:473-479.
43. Futterweit W (1984). Pathophysiology of polycystic ovarian disease. In W Futterweit, Polycystic ovarian disease. New York: Springer-Verlag.
44. Haffner SM, Valdez RA, Morales PA, et al. (1993). Decreased sex hormone-binding globulin predicts noninsulin-dependent diabetes mellitus in women but not in men. J Clin Endocrinol Metab 77:56-60.
45. Lindstedt G, Lundberg PA, Lapidus L, et al. (1990). Low sex hormone-binding globulin concentration as independent risk factor for development of NIDDM: 12-year follow-up of population study of women in Gothenburg, Sweden. Diabetes 40:123-128.
46. Mitchell GW, Rogers J (1953). The influence of weight reduction on amenorrhea in obese women. N Engl J Med 249:835-836.
47. Bates GW, Whitworth NS (1982). Effect of body weight reduction on plasma androgens in obese, infertile women. Fertil Steril 38:406-409.
48. Harlass FE, Plymate SR, Fariss BL, et al. (1984). Weight loss is associated with correction of gonadotropin and sex steroid abnormalities in the obese anovulatory female. Fertil Steril 42:649-652.
49. Pasquali R, Antenucci D, Casimirri F, et al. (1989). Clinical and hormonal characteristics of obese amenorrheic hyperandrogenic women before and after weight loss. J Clin Endocrinol Metab 68:173-179.
50. Futterweit W (1984). Clinical features of polycystic ovarian disease. In W Futterweit, Polycystic ovarian disease. New York: Springer-Verlag.
51. Goldzieher JW (1981). Polycystic ovarian disease. Fertil Steril 35:371-394.
52. Jung R (1984). Endocrinological aspects of obesity. J Clin Endocrinol Metab 13:597-612.
53. Zhang YW, Stern B, Rebar RW (1984). Endocrine comparison of obese menstruating and amenorrheic women. J Clin Endocrinol Metab 58:1077-1083.
54. Futterweit W (1984). Hyperprolactinemia. In W Futterweit, Polycystic ovarian disease. New York: Springer-Verlag.
55. Plymate SR, Fariss BL, Bassett ML, et al. (1981). Obesity and its role in polycystic ovary syndrome. J Clin Endocrinol Metab 52:1246-1248.
56. Rittmaster RS, Deshwal N, Lehman L (1993). The role of adrenal hyperandrogenism, insulin resistance and obesity in the pathogenesis of polycystic ovarian syndrome. J Clin Endocrinol Metab 76:1295-1300.
57. Cara JF, Fan J, Azzarello A, et al. (1990). Insulin-like factor I enhances luteinizing hormone binding to rat ovarian theca-interstitial cells. J Clin Invest 86:560-565.
58. Adashi EY, Resnick CE, D'Ercole AJ, et al. (1986). Insulin-like growth factors as intraovarian regulators of granulosa cell growth and function. Endocrinol Rev 6:400-420.
59. Fishman J, Boyar RM, Hellman L (1975). Influence of body weight on estradiol metabolism in young women. J Clin Endocrinol Metab 41:989-991.
60. Casey ML, MacDonald PC (1983). Origin of estrogen and regulation of its formation in postmenopausal women. In HJ Buchsbaum, Ed, The menopause. New York: Springer-Verlag.
61. Schneider J, Bradlow HL, Strain G, et al. (1983). Effects of obesity on estradiol metabolism: decreased formation to nonuterotropic metabolites. J Clin Endocrinol Metab 56:973-978.

62. Klinga K, von Holst T, Runnebaum B (1983). Influence of severe obesity on peripheral hormone concentration in pre- and post-menopausal women. Europ J Obstet Gynecol Reprod Biol 14:103-112.

63. Foster DW (1992). Eating disorders: obesity, anorexia nervosa and bulimia nervosa. In JD Wilson and DW Foster, Eds, Williams textbook of endocrinology, 8/e. Philadelphia: WB Saunders.

64. Kley HK, Edelman P, Kruskemper HL (1980). Relationships of plasma sex hormones to different parameters of obesity in male subjects. Metabolism 29:1041-1045.

65. Glass AR, Swerdlof RS, Bray GA, et al. (1977). Low serum testosterone and sex hormone-binding globulin in massively obese men. J Clin Endocrinol Metab 45:1211-1219.

66. Kley HK, Deselaers T, Peerenboom H (1981). Evidence of hypogonadism in massively obese males due to decreased free testosterone. Horm Metab Res 13:639-641.

67. Strain GW, Zumoff B, Kream J, et al. (1982). Mild hypogonadotropic hypogonadism in obese men. Metabolism 31:871-875.

68. Givens JR (1991). Reproductive and hormonal alterations in obesity. In P Bjorntorp and BN Brodoff, Eds, Obesity. Philadelphia: JB Lippincott.

69. Schneider G, Kirschner MA, Berkovitz A, et al. (1979). Increased estrogen production in obese men. J Clin Endocrinol Metab 48:633-638.

70. Stanik S, Dornfeld LP, Maxwell MH, et al. (1981). The effect of weight loss on reproductive hormones in obese men. J Clin Endocrinol Metab 53:828-832.

71. Kley HK, Deselaers T, Peerenboom H, et al. (1980). Enhanced conversion of androstenedione to estrogens in obese males. J Clin Endocrinol Metab 51:1128-1132.

72. Zumoff B, Strain GW, Kream J, et al. (1981). Obese young men have elevated plasma estrogen levels but obese premenopausal women do not. Metabolism 30:1011-1014.

73. Pasquali R, Cantobelli S, Casimirri F, et al. (1993). The hypothalamic-pituitary-adrenal axis in obese women with different patterns of body fat distribution. J Clin Endocrinol Metab 77:341-346.

74. Marin P, Darin N, Amemiya T, et al. (1992). Cortisol secretion in relation to body fat distribution in obese premenopausal woman. Metabolism 41:882-886.

75. Streeten DHP (1993). Editorial: is hypothalamic-pituitary-adrenal hyperactivity important in the pathogenesis of excessive abdominal fat distribution? J Clin Endocrinol Metab 77:339-340.

76. Garces LY, Kenny FM, Drash A, et al. (1968). Cortisol secretion rate during fasting of obese adolescent subjects. J Clin Endocrinol Metab 28:1843-1847.

77. Roelfsema F, Van Den Berg G, Frolich M, et al. (1993). Sex-dependent alteration in cortisol response to endogenous adrenocorticotropin. J Clin Endocrinol Metab 77:234-240.

78. Kurtz BR, Givens JR, Komindrs S, et al. (1987). Maintenance of normal circulating levels of androstenedione and dehydroepiandrosterone in simple obesity despite increased metabolic clearance rates: evidence for a servo-control mechanism. J Clin Endocrinol Metab 64:1261-1267.

79. Williams DP, Boyden TW, Pamenter RW, et al. (1993). Relationship of body fat percentage and fat distribution with dehydroepiandrosterone sulfate in premenopausal females. J Clin Endocrinol Metab 77:80-85.

80. DePergola G, Giagulli VA, Garuti G, et al. (1991). Low dehydroepiandrosterone circulating levels in premenopausal obese women with very high body mass index. Metabolism 40:187-190.

81. Azizi F (1978). The effect of dietary composition on fasting-induced changes in serum thyroid hormones and thyrotropin. Metabolism 27:935-942.

82. Danforth E, Horton ES, O'Connell L, et al. (1979). Dietary-induced alterations in thyroid hormone metabolism during overnutrition. J Clin Invest 64:1336-1347.

83. Vagenakis AG, Burger A, Portnay GI, et al. (1975). Divergence of peripheral thyroxine metabolism from activating to inactivating pathways during complete fasting. J Clin Endocrinol Metab 41:191-194.

84. Jung RT, Shetty PS, James WPT (1980). Nutritional effects on thyroid and catecholamine metabolism. Clin Science 58:97-108.

85. Carlson HE, Drenick EJ, Chopra IJ, et al. (1977). Alterations in basal and TRH-stimulated serum levels of thyrotropin, prolactin and thyroid hormones in starved obese men. J Clin Endocrinol Metab 45:707-713.

86. Bray GA (1989). Obesity: an endocrine perspective. In LJ DeGroot, Ed, Endocrinology, 2/e. Philadelphia: WB Saunders.

87. Burman KD, Latham KR, Djuh YY (1980). Solubilized nuclear thyroid hormone receptors in circulating human mononuclear cells. J Clin Endocrinol Metab 51:106-116.

88. Kvetny J (1985). Nuclear thyroxine receptors and cellular metabolism in obese subjects before and after fasting. Horm Metab Res 21:60-65.

89. Bray GA, Melvin KEW, Chopra IJ (1973). Effect of triiodothyronine on some metabolic responses of obese patients. Am J Clin Nutrition 26:715-721.

90. Bell NH, Epstein S, Greene A, et al. (1985). Evidence for alteration of the vitamin-D endocrine system in obese subjects. J Clin Invest 76:370-373.

91. Compston JE, Vedi S, Ledger JE, et al. (1981). Vitamin D status and bone histomorphometry in gross obesity. Am J Clin Nutrition 34:2359-2363.

92. Andersen T, McNair P, Fogh-Andersen N, et al. (1986). Increased parathyroid hormone as a consequence of changed complex binding of plasma calcium in morbid obesity. Metabolism 35:147-151.

93. Gibbs J, Smith GP (1992). Effect of brain-gut peptides on satiety. In P Bjorntorp and BN Brodoff, Eds, Obesity. Philadelphia: JB Lippincott.

94. Smith GP, Gibbs J, Jerome C, et al. (1981). The satiety effect of cholecystokinin: a progress report. Peptides 2(Suppl 2):57-59.

95. Smith GP, Gibbs J (1987). The effect of gut peptides on hunger,satiety and food intake in humans. Ann NY Acad Sci 499:132-136.

96. Wolkowitz OM, Gertz B, Weingartner H, et al. (1990). Hunger in humans induced by MK-329, a specific peripheral-type cholecystokinin-receptor antagonist. Biol Psychiatry 28:169-173.

97. Gossain VV, Srivasta L, Rovner DR, et al. (1983). Plasma glucagon in simple obesity: effect of exercise. Am J Med Sci 286:4-10.

98. Starke AAR, Erhardt G, Berger M, et al. (1984). Elevated pancreatic glucagon in obesity. Diabetes 33:277-280.

99. Meryn S, Stein D, Straus EW (1986). Pancreatic polypeptide, pancreatic glucagon and enteroglucagon in morbid obesity and following gastric bypass operation. Int J Obesity 10:37-42.

100. Vasquez B, Nagulesparan M, Unger RH (1983). Fasting and postprandial plasma glucagon and glucagon-immunoreactivity are normal in obese Pima Indians. Horm Metab Res 15:218-220.

101. Stuckey JA, Gibbs J, Smith GP (1985). Neural disconnection of gut from brain blocks bombesin-induced satiety. Peptides 6:1249-1252.

102. Marco J, Zulueta MA, Correas I, et al. (1980). Reduced pancreatic polypeptide secretion in obese subjects. J Clin Endocrinol Metab 50:744-747.

103. Wahl TO, Schimke RN, Kyner JL, et al. (1979). Human pancreatic polypeptide (HPP) in obese adults. Diabetes 28(Suppl 2):436.
104. Mazzaferri EL, Starich GH, Lardinois CK, et al. (1985). Gastric inhibitory polypeptide responses to nutrients in Caucasians and American Indians with obesity and noninsulin-dependent diabetes mellitus. J Clin Endocrinol Metab 61:313-321.
105. Service FC, Rizza RA, Westland RE, et al. (1984). Gastric inhibitory polypeptide in obesity and diabetes mellitus. J Clin Endocrinol Metab 58:1133-1140.
106. Salera M, Giacomoni P, Pironi L, et al. (1982). Gastric inhibitory polypeptide release after oral glucose: relationship to glucose intolerance, diabetes mellitus and obesity. J Clin Endocrinol Metab 55:329-336.
107. Tomkin GH, Ardill J, Lafferty H, et al. (1983). Vasoactive intestinal polypeptide in obesity. Int J Obesity 7:153-160.
108. Andrews WJ, Henry RW, Alberti KGMM, et al. (1981). The gastro-entero-pancreatic hormone response to fasting in obesity. Diabetologia 21:440-445.
109. Boulter PR, Hoffman RS, Arky RA (1973). Pattern of sodium excretion accompanying starvation. Metabolism 22:675-683.
110. DeFronzo RA (1982). Insulin secretion, insulin resistance and obesity. Int J Obesity 6:73-82.
111. Saudek CD, Boulter PR, Arky RA (1973). The natriuretic effect of glucagon and its role in starvation. J Clin Endocrinol Metab 36:761-765.
112. Kolanowski J (1981). Influence of insulin and glucagon on sodium balance in obese subjects during fasting and refeeding. Int J Obesity 2(Suppl 1):105-114.
113. Kolanowski J, Salvador G, Desnecht P, et al. (1977). Influence of glucagon on natriuresis and glucose-induced sodium retention in the fasting obese subject. Europ J Clin Invest 7:167-175.
114. Coiro V, Chiodera P (1987). Effect of obesity and weight loss on the arginine vasopressin response to insulin-induced hypoglycemia. Clin Endocrinol (Oxf) 27:253-258.
115. Drenick EJ, Carlson HE, Robertson GL, et al. (1977). The role of vasopressin and prolactin in abnormal salt and water metabolism of obese patients before and after fasting and during refeeding. Metabolism 26:309-317.
116. Genazzani AR, Fachinetti F, Petraglia F, et al. (1986). Hyperendorphinemia in obese children and adolescents. J Clin Endocrinol Metab 62:36-40.
117. Giovannini C, Fachinetti F, Ciucci E, et al. (1987). Diet-induced weight loss doesn't correct hyperendorphinemia in obese patients. J Endocrinol Invest 10(Suppl 3):1987-1993.
118. Bruni JF, Watkins WB, Yen SSC (1979). Beta-endorphin in the human pancreas. J Clin Endocrinol Metab 49:649-651.
119. Welle S, Lilaviv U, Campbell G (1981). Thermic effect of feeding in man: increased plasma norepinephrine levels following glucose but not protein or fat consumption. Metabolism 30:953-958.
120. Jung RT, Campbell RG, James WPT, et al. (1982). Altered hypothalamic and sympathetic responses to hypoglycemia in familial obesity. Lancet 1:1043-1046.
121. Kjeldsen SE, Eide I, Aakesson I, et al. (1983). Influence of body weight on plasma catecholamine patterns in middle-aged, normotensive men. Scand J Clin Lab Invest 43:339-342.
122. Gustafson AB, Kalkhoff RK (1982). Influence of sex and obesity on plasma catecholamine response to isometric exercise. J Clin Endocrinol Metab 55:703-708.
123. Inoue S (1992). Animal models of obesity: hypothalamic lesions. In P Bjorntorp and BN Brodoff, Eds, Obesity. Philadelphia: JB Lippincott.

124. Inoue S, Mullen YS, Bray GA (1983). Hyperinsulinemia in rats with hypothalamic obesity: effects of autonomic drugs and glucose. Am J Physiol 245:R372-R378.
125. Bray GA (1989). Classification and evaluation of the obesities. Med Clin North Am 73:161-184.
126. Bray GA (1992). An approach to the classification and evaluation of obesity. In P Bjorntorp and BN Brodoff, Eds, Obesity. Philadelphia: JB Lippincott.
127. Bouchard C (1989). Genetic factors in obesity. Med Clin North Am 73:67-81.
128. Bouchard C (1992). Genetic aspects of human obesity. In P Bjorntorp and BN Brodoff, Eds, Obesity. Philadelphia: JB Lippincott.
129. York DA (1992). Genetic models of animal obesity. In P Bjorntorp and BN Brodoff, Eds, Obesity. Philadelphia: JB Lippincott.
130. Bray GA (1984). Syndromes of hypothalamic obesity in man. Pediatric Ann 13:525-536.
131. Bray GA, Dahms WT, Swerdloff RS, et al. (1983). The Prader-Willi syndrome: a study of 40 patients and a review of the literature. Medicine 62:59-80.
132. Klein D, Ammann F (1969). The syndrome of Laurence-Moon-Bardet-Biedl and allied diseases in Switzerland. Clinical, genetic and epidemiological studies. J Neurol Sci 9:479-513.
133. Assmann G, Schulte H (1992). Obesity and hyperlipidemia: results from the prospective cardiovascular Munster (PROCAM) study. In P Bjorntorp and BN Brodoff, Eds, Obesity. Philadelphia: JB Lippincott.
134. Bierman EL, Brunzell JD (1992). Obesity and atherosclerosis. In P Bjorntorp and BN Brodoff, Eds, Obesity. Philadelphia: JB Lippincott.
135. Hotamisligil GS, Shargill NS, Spiegelman BM (1993). Adipose expression of tumor necrosis factor : direct role in obesity-linked insulin resistance. Science 259:87-91.
136. Spiegelman BM, Hotamisligil GS (1993). Through thick and thin: wasting, obesity and TNF. Cell 73:625-627.

9

Methodological Issues in Obesity Research: Examples from Biometrical Genetics

David B. Allison, PhD

Scientists are frequently interested in discovering causal relations among variables. The great physicist Max Planck once said, "The law of causality is...in my opinion, our most valuable signpost—to help us find our bearings in a bewildering maze of occurrences and to show us the direction in which scientific research must advance in order to achieve fertile results" (Planck 1958, p. 387).

Much of the practice of modern scientific research can be characterized as an iterative process whereby one (1) specifies a causal model that one believes may account for some observations; (2) makes a prediction about data based on the model; (3) collects some data; (4) compares the data collected in step 3 to the data expected in step 2 via an appropriate statistical analysis; and (5) returns to step 1, modifying the model as necessary to account for discrepancies between the observed and expected data. These steps are prototypic, but things do not always proceed in such a rigidly sequential manner. Generally, a somewhat freer flow occurs among these steps.

Biometrical genetics is fundamentally the study of the causes of phenotypic variation. Thus the field of biometrical genetics represents a good vantage point from which to examine some common problems in the implementation of the iterative scientific process described above. In this chapter, I will describe four common problems in the implementation of this process. Although my examples will be drawn from biometrical genetic

The author is grateful to Michael C. Neale of the Department of Psychiatric Genetics at the Medical College of Virginia whose tutelage inspired much of this chapter.

studies of human obesity, the issues are not unique to either biometrical genetics or obesity research.

ISSUE 1: THE NEED TO CONSIDER MEASUREMENT ERROR

Many researchers fail to consider measurement error when collecting, analyzing and interpreting their data. This issue primarily involves steps 3 and 4 above. Before proceeding further, a definition is in order. By measurement error I refer to the random component of measurements. In other words, that aspect of a measurement that is normally distributed with a mean of zero and is uncorrelated with the construct being measured. This is to be distinguished from *bias* which implies some systematic error (Nunnally 1978).

The most important thing to understand about measurement error is that it attenuates effects. Equation 1 is a classic formula from measurement theory,

$$r_o = r_t\sqrt{r_{xx}r_{yy}}$$ (1)

where r_o is the observed correlation between X and Y, r_t is the true correlation between X and Y, and r_{xx} and r_{yy} are the reliabilities of X and Y, respectively. What this means is that, other things being equal, to the extent that the measurements of X and Y are unreliable (prone to error), the observed relation between X and Y will be an underestimate of their true relation.

Although ideally one would like to eliminate measurement error, this is generally believed to be impossible. This is because our measurements are always imperfect manifestations of the latent constructs we are interested in—or, more eloquently, "Imagine the condition of men living in a sort of cavernous chamber underground... Like ourselves...prisoners so confined would have seen nothing of themselves or of one another, except the shadows thrown by the fire-light on the wall of the cave facing them" (Plato 1958 ed., pp. 227-228). That is, we see shadows and must infer reality. Thus there are two ways to handle measurement error (besides ignoring it). The first is to minimize it. The second is to be aware of, measure and model it. Unfortunately, measurement error is often simply ignored. Consider the following example.

Krondl and co-workers (1983) studied the heritability[1] of food preferences using the standard twin design. They asked twins to rate their preferences for each of 25 foods on a five-point scale. The heritability of each food was analyzed separately. For several foods (e.g., Brussels sprouts) the monozygotic (MZ) intra-pair variance exceeded the dizygotic (DZ) intra-pair variance. Although Krondl correctly points out that "when the MZ intra-pair mean square exceeds the DZ intra-pair mean square estimation of heritability is inappropriate," one must wonder how this could occur. If one takes these values seriously, one can imagine a scenario in which, at an early age, MZ twins are very similar in their preference for Brussels sprouts. Thus MZ twins who intensely like Brussels sprouts simultaneously reach for the sprouts when they are placed on the dinner table. This results in a fierce battle. By chance, one twin wins the fight, is rewarded by getting the sprouts and has his liking further increased. The other twin, having been mauled, develops a phobia of Brussels sprouts. Thus, MZ twins turn out to be dissimilar in their preferences for Brussels sprouts relative to DZ twins.

Since this scenario is clearly absurd, one would do better to look at methodological reasons for this anomalous result. Asking people about single foods is like asking them a single question of a questionnaire. Single items measuring certain traits are often unreliable. Thus Krondl's anomalous result is probably nothing more than the random fluctuation of sample statistics accentuated by unreliable measurement. One way to minimize this problem is through aggregation (Allen and Yen 1979). When several indicators (e.g., questionnaire items) of the same construct are added together, the "true" variance accumulates more rapidly than the error variance and a reliable measure results.

This strategy of aggregation was successfully applied by Rozin and Millman (1987) when measuring preferences for variety in ice cream among twins. They asked subjects to respond to a number of items and combined the responses into a single index. Rozin and Millman estimated the reliability (test-retest) of their measurements to be .88. Thus a fairly reliable measurement was obtained yielding observed correlations for ice cream variety preference of .72 for MZ twins and .41 for DZ twins. Using the formula $h^2 = 2(r_{mz} - r_{dz})$, a heritability estimate of .62 is reached. However, we can use Equation 1 to correct the observed correlations for attenuation and solve for r_t by using .88 as an estimate of r_{xx} and r_{yy} (the reliability is presumed to be the same for both twins). This yields correlations of .82 for MZ twins and .47 for DZ twins, suggesting that a more accurate heritability estimate is .70. Thus by minimizing and measuring their measurement error, Rozin and Millman allow it to be modeled and more reasonable answers are thereby attained.

The next three problems all relate to step 1, the specification of the model.

ISSUE 2: THE NEED TO MAKE THE
UNDERLYING MODEL EXPLICIT

Researchers often seem to be operating as though they have some causal model in mind but fail to make the model explicit. Since the model should influence the data analysis strategy, if the model is not made explicit, one cannot evaluate the adequacy of the data analysis and the conclusions thereby reached. Worse yet, the researchers themselves may conduct an analysis that is not consistent with their model.

One of the most common examples of this error is "over-control." Over-control occurs when one controls for a variable that is an integral link in the causal chain one is interested in. Controlling for things seems to be scientifically *en vogue*. The more things one controls for, the "tighter" one's study appears to be. Sir Ronald Fisher, perhaps the preeminent statistician of the twentieth century, stated, "In no case, however, can we judge whether or not it is profitable to eliminate a certain variate unless we know, or are willing to assume, a qualitative scheme of causation" (Fisher 1958, pp. 190-191).

Consider the left panel of Figure 1. This model postulates that both X_1 and X_2 may influence Y and that X_1 and X_2 may be correlated, but do not directly cause one another. If one wanted to test a model in which X_1 has a causal influence on Y, it would be important to control for X_2. Now consider the right panel of Figure 1. Here X_1 is postulated to have a causal influence on Y, but this is mediated through X_2. In this case, controlling for X_2 breaks the causal chain between X_1 and Y. If one wanted to test whether X_1 had a causal influence on Y, controlling for X_2 would be an example of over-control. In fact, as Papineau (1989) points out, due to the infinitely contin-

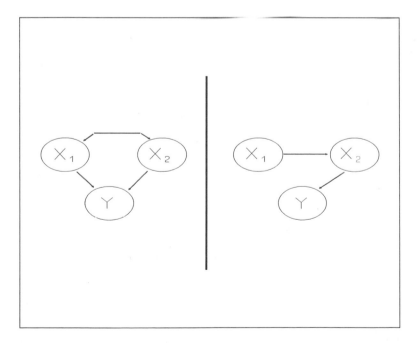

Figure 1. Two biometrical genetic models.

uous nature of time, this type of analysis, if taken to an extreme, ensures that causality will never be demonstrated.

A germane example of this can be found in a twin study reported by Austin and co-workers (1987). Using the traditional formula $h^2 = 2(r_{mz}-r_{dz})$, they estimated the heritability (h^2) of body mass index (BMI) to be .89. However, they note that monozygotic (MZ) twins were more similar to each other than were dizygotic twins (DZ) with respect to certain behaviors, including aspects of eating behavior. Austin therefore controlled for these variables and re-estimated the heritability of BMI to be .73. While I do not intend to imply that .89 is a more reasonable heritability estimate than .73, it seems that this analysis represents a probable example of over-control. It is well known that many behaviors are genetically influenced (Eaves et al. 1989; Plomin et al. 1989) and eating behavior appears to be no exception (De Castro 1993). It is quite possible that one way the genotype influences BMI is through food intake (Allison et al. 1993). If this is the case, Austin's group has controlled away part of the very thing they are interested in studying (i.e., over-control). Perhaps an explicit statement of their underlying causal model would have clarified the situation.

ISSUE 3: THE NEED TO CONSIDER THE IMPLICATIONS OF THE MODEL

There is an old joke: a university freshman wants to know what 2 plus 2 equals. The student asks a math professor who replies, "Exactly 2 plus exactly 2 is exactly 4." The student then goes to the engineering department and asks an engineering professor who replies, "Approximately 2 plus approximately 2 is approximately 4." Finally, the student asks a statistics professor. The statistics professor looks around surreptitiously, leans forward and whispers, "How much do you want it to be?"

There is probably some truth to the common perception that a good statistician can "torture the data until they confess," that is, get any answer desired. However, along the way to getting that answer, decisions and choices will have to be made. Often these decisions become integral parts of the model. If the model is made explicit, its implications can be considered and one can judge the reasonableness of the conclusions thereby reached.

An example of a situation in which the implications of chosen models have perhaps been insufficiently considered concerns the heritability of BMI. Figure 2 summarizes the results of biometrical genetic studies of BMI from two different authors. It is striking that Bouchard and co-workers (1988) obtain a heritability of .05, while Stunkard's group (1990) obtains a heritability of .69 (for women). Although several explanations for this discrepancy can be proposed (e.g., different types of relatives studied, age-specific genetic effects, sampling differences, etc., see Meyer and

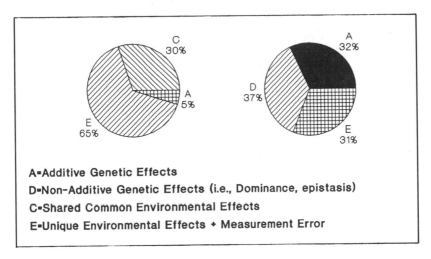

Figure 2. How heritable is obesity? Results of biometrical genetic studies of body mass index from two different authors. (Adapted with permission from C Bouchard et al, Inheritance of the amount and distribution of human body fat, Int J Obesity 12:205-215, 1988; and from AJ Stunkard et al, The body mass index of twins who have been reared apart, N Engl J Med 322:14301437, 1990.)

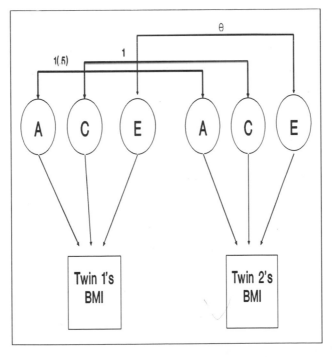

Figure 3. ACE model of the inheritance of body mass index.

Stunkard [1993] for further detail), one point that has not been explicitly discussed is differences in the models' fit to the data.

In biometrical genetics an ACE model is one in which the phenotype is believed to result from the causal influence of A (alleles acting *Additively*), C (the shared *Common* environment), and E (unique *Environmental* experiences) (Neale and Cardon 1992). The model fit by Bouchard (1988) is essentially a variant of an ACE model. Although the Stunkard team (1990) eventually settled on an ADE model (D represents alleles acting multiplicatively, e.g. Dominance), they began by trying and rejecting an ACE model. Figure 3 pictorially represents an ACE model.

By and large, the major difference between the way Stunkard and Bouchard model the data concerns the parameter labeled *e* in Figure 3. Typically, *e* (the correlation between twins' unique and random influences) is taken to 0.0 for all twins. In other words, unique environmental experiences and measurement error, which comprise *e*, are by definition uncorrelated. Stunkard's group maintains this convention. However, Bouchard's group frees *e* and allows it to take on a different value for siblings, DZ twins and MZ twins. In their analysis of BMI, this parameter is estimated at .16 for DZ twins and .96 for MZ twins. These values are quite close to the theoretical correlations for nonadditive genetic influences *(D)* of .25 for DZ twins and 1.00 for MZ twins. Thus Bouchard (1988) does with *e* what Stunkard (1990) does with *D*. Bouchard's analysis essentially says "I'm more willing to believe in a violation of the equal environments assumption[2] than in dominant/recessive genes for BMI." To this point, such a position must be seen as a viable alternative. However, what are the implications of this model and the specific parameter estimates obtained?

The *e* of .96 for MZ twins is remarkably close to the upper limit of 1.00. What it implies is that MZ twins share almost all their experiences (at least those that influence BMI) in common. In fact, when Bouchard (1988) applied this same model to measures of fat mass and percent body fat, *e* did reach 1.00. This model implies that MZ twins *never* have a single experience that influences their BMI that their co-twin does not also have. Moreover, it implies that either there is no measurement error (anyone who has ever tried to measure body fat *in vivo* will immediately recognize the improbability of this event) or that measurement error is perfectly correlated across MZ twins but not DZ. The latter outcome is inconsistent with the nature of measurement error (i.e., its randomness).

Thus the implications of the model that estimates the heritability of BMI to be .05 appear to be untenable. By carefully examining these implications, we are able to choose between two otherwise anomalously discrepant results reported in the literature.

ISSUE 4: THE NEED TO CONSIDER ALTERNATIVE
OR COMPETING MODELS

Demonstrating that a particular model fits the data well is only one criterion by which we may judge the validity of a model. To the greatest extent possible, it is also important to rule out competing models that might fit the data equally well. The use of commingling analysis to detect the action of major genes for obesity presents a good example of this.

Commingling occurs when two or more component distributions are mixed into one larger distribution. Commingling results when one cause has a much larger effect on a trait than the many other smaller factors influencing the trait and is generally taken as a sign of major gene action. That is to say, the rift between the component distributions is assumed to originate from the effect of a major gene.

Understanding the rationale behind commingling analysis requires an appreciation of the "null" model. The null model assumes that the phenotype (e.g., adiposity) is the result of numerous independent small causes (i.e., many genes and many environmental influences). When many independent effects of roughly equivalent magnitude are added up, the resulting phenotypic frequency distribution tends to be normally distributed (by the central limit theorem). However, if one cause (e.g., one gene) has a much larger impact, the resulting distribution would not be normal but would instead look like a skewed, or in extreme cases, multimodal distribution. This is because the total distribution is now a mixture of several smaller component distributions that have been commingled.

Typically, commingling analyses proceed as follows. One begins with the null model, which assumes that the frequency distribution is normal. A normal distribution can be fully characterized by three things: the mean (μ), the variance (σ^2) and the probability density function for a normal distribution.[3] Given the above, the probability (or "likelihood") that the observed data come from a multivariate normal distribution with mean and variance s^2 is calculated. Next, a more complex model is proposed in which the observed data are hypothesized to come from k normal distributions each with its own μ and σ^2. Values for μ and σ^2 are selected to maximize the likelihood of the model and the likelihood is calculated. A model with k normal distributions can be compared to a model with k–1 multivariate normal distributions via a likelihood-ratio test. The quantity $-2\ln(L_{k-1}/L_k)$ is assumed to be approximately distributed as χ^2 where L_{k-1} is the likelihood of obtaining the observed data with k–1 distributions and L_k is the likelihood of obtaining the observed data with k distributions. If the χ^2 is statistically significant, the more complex model with k distributions fits the data significantly better than the simpler model with k–1 distributions which is then rejected and major gene action is presumed.

Several studies have used the above approach with obesity-related variables (e.g., Allison et al. 1993; Borecki et al. 1991; Price et al. 1989, 1991; Price and Stunkard 1989). While the methodology is always faithfully implemented, only the "null" model of a single normal distribution is considered as an alternative to commingling. An equally plausible alternative might be a truncated distribution since biology imposes a "floor" on one's possible BMI.

Figure 4 shows a histogram with overlaying density function for a sample of simulated BMI values. Initially, 5000 cases were simulated from a normal distribution with a mean of 21 and a standard deviation of 10. However, since people with BMIs below 12.0 are unlikely to live, I "killed" (deleted) all subjects with BMIs below 12. Had these data been subjected to commingling analysis as described above, there would undoubtedly have been sufficient evidence to prefer a model of commingled distributions over one normal distribution. However, this would miss the true process gener-

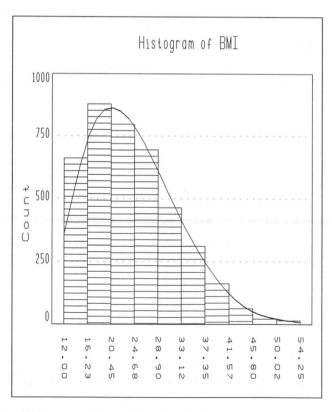

Figure 4.   Histogram with overlying density function for a sample of simulated body mass index values.

ating the observed data. Schork and co-workers (1990) have described methods for incorporating truncation models into commingling analyses. If future research considers these alternative or competing models against commingling and finds that the commingling model provides a better fit to the data, we can have far greater confidence in the conclusion of major gene action.

NOTES

1. Heritability (h^2) can be defined as that proportion of the between-person variance in the phenotype that is attributable to between-person variance in the genotype.
2. The equal environments assumption is critical to use of the standard twin design. The equal environments assumption states that MZ twins are no more likely to be concordant for exposure to the phenotype-relevant environment than are DZ twins.
3. The probability density function for the univariate normal distribution is given by:

$$f = \frac{1}{\sqrt{2\pi\sigma^2}} \exp\left[\frac{-(X-\mu)^2}{2\sigma^2}\right]$$

REFERENCES

Allen MJ, Yen WM (1979). Introduction to measurement theory. Monterey, CA: Brooks/Cole.

Allison DB, Heshka S, Gorman BS, Heymsfield SB (1993). Evidence of commingling in human eating behavior. Obesity Res 1:339-344.

Austin MA, King MC, Bawol RD, Hulley SB, Friedman GD (1987). Risk factors for coronary heart disease in adult female twins. Am J Epidemiol 125:308-318.

Borecki IB, Rice T, Bouchard C, Rao DC (1991). Commingling analysis of generalized body mass and composition measures: the Quebec family study. Int J Obesity 15:763-773.

Bouchard C, Perusse L, Leblanc C, Tremblay A, Theriault G (1988). Inheritance of the amount and distribution of human body fat. Int J Obesity 12:205-215.

De Castro JM (1993). Genetic influences on daily intake and meal patterns of humans. Physiol Behav 53:777-782.

Eaves LJ, Eysenck HJ, Martin NG (1989). Genes, culture and personality: an empirical approach. New York: Academic Press.

Fisher RA (1958). Statistical methods for research workers. New York: Hafner.

Krondl M, Coleman P, Wade J, Milner J (1983). A twin study examining the genetic influence on food selection. Human Nutrition 34A:189-198.

Meyer JM, Stunkard AJ (1993). Genetics and human obesity. In AJ Stunkard and TA Wadden, Eds, Obesity: theory and therapy. New York: Raven Press.

Neale MC, Cardon LR (1992). Methodology for genetic studies of twins and families. Dordrecht, Netherlands: Kluwer.

Nunnally JC (1978). Psychometric theory. New York: McGraw-Hill.

Papineau D (1989). Pure, mixed and spurious probabilities and their significance for a reductionist theory of causation. In P Kitcher and WC Salmon, Eds, Scientific explanation. Minneapolis: University of Minnesota Press.

Planck M (1958). The concept of causality in physics. In HJ Koren, Ed, Readings in the philosophy of nature. Westminster, MD: Newman Press.

Plato (1958). The republic. New York: Oxford University Press.

Plomin R, DeFries JC, McClearn GE (1989). Behavioral genetics, 2/e. New York: WH Freeman.

Price RA, Ness R, Sorenson TIA (1991). Changes in commingled body mass index distributions associated with secular trends in overweight among Danish young men. Am J Epidemiol 133:501-510.

Price RA, Stunkard AJ (1989). Commingling analysis of obesity in twins. Human Heredity 39:121-135.

Price RA, Sorenson TIA, Stunkard AJ (1989). Component distributions of body mass index defining moderate and extreme overweight in Danish men and women. Am J Epidemiol 130:193-201.

Schork NJ, Weder AB, Schork MA (1990). On the asymmetry of biological frequency distributions. Genetic Epidemiol 7:427-446.

Stunkard AJ, Harris JR, Pederson NL, McClearn GE (1990). The body mass index of twins who have been reared apart. N Engl J Med 322:1430-1437.

10

Therapeutic Weight Loss: A Serious Need for Guiding Principles Grounded in Physiology

Theodore B. VanItallie, MD

It is no secret that obesity is most commonly treated by therapeutic energy restriction; that is, by means of a diet that provides fewer calories than the obese patient expends. Although almost everybody knows such a diet induces weight loss, that seems to be about all many people do know about the subject. Indeed, it is disquieting that despite all the attention given to the problem of obesity by the U.S. government and voluntary health agencies and despite the proliferation of numerous commercial weight-loss programs—some supervised by physicians and dietitians and others by lay "counselors" —there is as yet no consensus concerning (1) the principles that should guide therapeutic weight reduction; (2) the minimum professional qualifications that should be required of those who undertake to treat obesity; and (3) the gaps in knowledge that must be closed if obesity is to be treated with optimal safety and effectiveness.

The unfortunate fact is that, for the most part, therapeutic caloric restriction is not carried out in any systematic way or with adequate consideration of the available scientific information about the physiology of weight loss. Compare, for example, the current dietary treatment of obesity with the current pharmacologic treatment of hypertension. The treatment of hypertension is at least systematic, being based on a large body of experimental

This chapter is adapted from TB VanItallie, The dietary treatment of severe obesity, in JE Hamner, ed, The 1988 distinguished professorship lectures (Memphis: University of Tennessee Press, 1989); and from MU Yang and TB VanItallie, Effect of energy restriction on body composition and nitrogen balance in obese individuals. In TA Wadden and TB VanItallie, eds, Treatment of the seriously obese patient (New York: Guilford Press, 1992).

133

information about the disorder and about the agents used to manage it. There is substantial agreement among most experts on how to treat hypertension—and this is no accident. Many scientific gatherings have been convened in an effort to arrive at a consensus about treatment. Treatment of hypertension is the responsibility of physicians who are, for the most part, well informed about the physiology and pharmacology of the subject.

In sad contrast, therapeutic weight reduction remains in a comparatively primitive state. Many weight-reduction programs—even those operated by physicians—still prescribe the same reducing diet to virtually all of their clients, regardless of their size, age, sex, or level of physical activity. Many of those who treat obese patients do not appear to comprehend the potential hazards of too rapid weight loss. Indeed, the physiologic effects on the body of therapeutic energy restriction and the adverse health consequences of these effects are insufficiently understood by many of those who now assume responsibility for the care of obese patients. Sometimes the results of this ignorance can be catastrophic for the patient.

In this chapter, I attempt to make two major points. The first is that the therapeutic induction of substantial weight loss in an obese individual is a serious matter. It should not be undertaken by unqualified people or by those who are not knowledgeable about obesity and its treatment. On the other hand, I would not want to interfere with the right of overweight individuals to "go on a diet" or voluntarily increase the level of their physical activity. In the present context, I refer to organized programs designed to treat, usually for a prolonged period, individuals with serious obesity who are unable to help themselves.

The second point is that the induction of therapeutic weight loss does not have to be a haphazard procedure performed under the supervision of persons who know little or nothing about the physiologic effects of their regimens. As I shall attempt to demonstrate, there is sufficient scientific information of acceptable quality available about the way in which the human body responds to caloric restriction to permit the formulation of reasonable principles of weight reduction treatment.

The overriding concern in the dietary treatment of obesity is surely the safety of the patient. When the safety of weight loss is considered, two factors must be given attention. First, one must be certain to provide the obese patient with a weight-reduction diet that is nutritionally adequate and appropriate, except for its energy content. Second, the calorically restricted diet should not induce excessive losses of body protein. The latter consideration is emphasized in this discussion.

WEIGHT LOSS: QUALITY VERSUS QUANTITY

It is important to distinguish between the quality of weight less and its quantity. It is all too common these days to encounter print advertisements and TV commercials promoting diets and other kinds of treatments whose focus is on quantity of weight loss. Such emphasis on rapid weight loss is both irrational and irresponsible; yet, not surprisingly, it has great appeal to many frustrated overweight persons.

What is weight loss of good quality? At our present stage of knowledge, the best way to answer this question is to consider the composition of the "excess weight" carried about by obese persons. Webster and co-workers (1984) addressed this issue by analyzing measurements of body composition made on 104 women who ranged in age from 14 to 61 and whose fat content varied from 6 to 60 percent of body weight. They found that differences in weight between women of similar height (uncorrected for frame size) can be attributed to a mixture of components that is about 75 percent fat and 25 percent fat-free mass (FFM). This observation has been confirmed in 111 obese patients (43 men and 68 women) by Vaswani and associates (1993). On the basis of such findings, Garrow (1993) has concluded that in the treatment of obese patients, it is desirable that no more than 25 percent of the weight loss be FFM.

If this recommendation is taken as a standard by which the long-term safety of a low-calorie diet can be judged, it is possible to derive tentative guidelines for designing optimal calorie-restricted diets for the treatment of obesity.

In developing appropriate guidelines, the first step one might take is to look at the energy value of 1 pound of "lost weight" of acceptable composition; that is, no more than 25 percent FFM and no less that 75 percent fat. The relevant calculations, as shown in Figure 1, indicate that 1 pound (454.5 g) of lost weight of acceptable composition corresponds to an energy deficit of about 3200 kcal. Thus, at a deficit of 1000 kcal per day, assuming water equilibrium, it should take 3.2 days to lose 1 pound of weight of acceptable composition. This corresponds to about 0.3 pound (136 g) per day.

If the rate of weight loss remains greater than 0.3 pound per 1000 kcal deficit, then the quality of the loss becomes increasingly poor. As shown in Figure 2, at an energy deficit of 1000 kcal per day and a rate of weight loss of 0.77 pound per day, an obese patient on a calorically restricted diet is actually losing more FFM than fat. If an excessive rate of weight loss continues for a prolonged period, the body will become increasingly protein-depleted, with all the attendant adverse consequences.

Factors Affecting Composition of Therapeutic Weight Loss

There are at least three important factors that determine the quality of weight loss during therapeutic weight reduction: the first is the energy content of the diet; the second is the macronutrient composition of the diet; and the third is the patient's body composition—namely, the degree of severity of the patient's obesity.

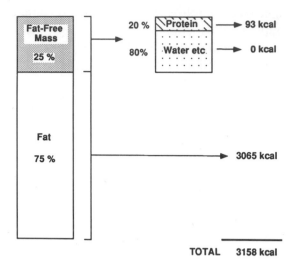

Figure 1.   Energy value of 1 pound of "lost weight" of acceptable composition (25 percent fat-free mass and 75 percent fat). At a deficit of 1000 kcal/day, it will take 3.2 days to lose 1 pound. Thus, to maintain a weight loss of acceptable composition, the rate of loss should not exceed an average of pound/day. (Reproduced with permission from MU Yang and TB VanItallie, Effect of energy restriction on body composition and nitrogen balance in obese individuals. In TA Wadden and TB VanItallie, eds, Treatment of the seriously obese patient. New York: Guilford Press, 1992.)

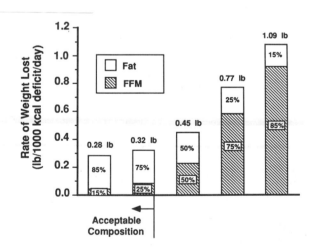

Figure 2.   Composition of weight at different rates of weight reduction (assuming water equilibrium). Values are normalized to pounds per 1000-kcal/day deficit. (Reproduced with permission from MU Yang and TB VanItallie, Effect of energy restriction on body composition and nitrogen balance in obese individuals. In TA Wadden and TB VanItallie, eds, Treatment of the seriously obese patient. New York: Guilford Press, 1992.)

Let us first consider the role of the diet's energy content. This role is indicated in Figure 3, which summarizes several reports taken from the literature. The figure clearly shows the inverse relationship between calorie intake and cumulative nitrogen deficit.

Second, let us look briefly at the contribution to the quality of weight loss of the diet's composition. In this regard, Boozer and co-workers (1993) have shown that rats fed energy-restricted high-fat diets retained more body fat than rats fed isocaloric low-fat diets. (The contribution of dietary protein will be considered later in the chapter.)

Finally, let us examine the relationship between the degree of obesity of a patient and the quality of weight loss during energy restriction. Figure 4 (left panel) shows that total starvation is far better tolerated by obese than by nonobese persons. These studies (VanItallie and Yang 1977) and others (e.g., Garrow 1993) indicate that the body composition of the obese patient at any given time during caloric restriction plays an important role in determining the composition of the weight that is lost.

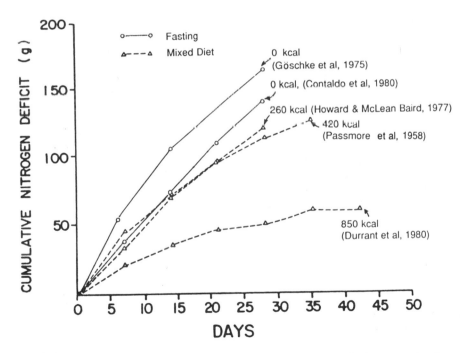

Figure 3. Cumulative nitrogen deficits in obese women on daily energy intakes ranging from 0 to 850 kcal. (Adapted from TB VanItallie and A Abraham, Some hazards of obesity and its treatment. In J Hirsch and TB VanItallie, eds, Recent advances in obesity research IV. Proceedings of the Fourth International Congress on Obesity. London: John Libbey, 1985.)

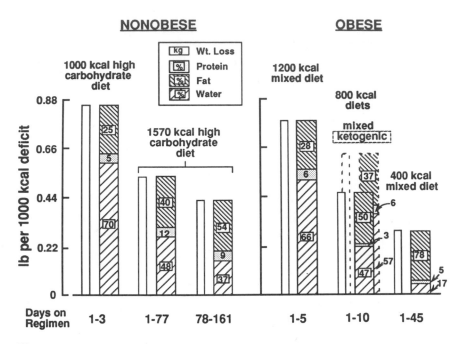

Figure 4. Effect of energy intake and duration during caolric restriction on rate and composition of weight loss in onobese and obese subjects. All values have been normalized to pounds per 100-kcal deficit. (Adapted from T. VanItallie and MU Yang, Current concepts in nutrition: diets and weight loss. N Engl J Med 297:1158-1161, 1977. Adapted by permission of The New England Journal of Medicine.)

IMPORTANCE OF CONSERVING BODY PROTEIN

Obviously, the body can only lose so much protein or FFM without getting into serious trouble. The precise danger range is not yet known, but it needs to be emphasized that the amount of intracellular protein normally present in the body is less than one might imagine. Some estimates have placed it at 5 to 6 kg (see Figure 5). It seems clear when the fat-free mass index falls to a certain point (say 50 to 20 percent below the 5th percentile), death is almost inevitable (VanItallie et al. 1990). Unfortunately, we know very little about what happens to intracellular protein in patients who remain on very-low-calorie diets for prolonged periods.

It is conceivable that some of the side effects of severe restriction of dietary energy can be explained by the resulting development of a protein-catabolic state, accompanied by various metabolic adaptations designed to conserve protein. Eventually, actual intracellular protein depletion could develop with resulting adverse functional and morphologic changes. Some of the side effects listed below may not be related to protein privation but

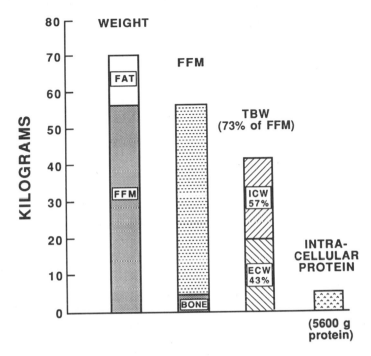

Figure 5. Body composition of a 70-kg reference man. Values are derived from the International Commission on Radiological Protection, 1984. (Reproduced with permission from MU Yang and TB VanItallie, Effect of energy restriction on body composition and nitrogen balance in obese individuals. In TA Wadden and TB VanItallie, eds, Treatment of the seriously obese patient. New York: Guilford Press, 1992.)

could reflect other physiologic responses to the "therapeutic" creation of an acute and chronic energy deficit:

Gastrointestinal disturbances such as nausea, vomiting, diarrhea and constipation

Fatigue

Orthostatic dizziness (occasional syncope)

Cold intolerance

Skin dryness

Brittle nails

Hair loss

Muscle cramps

Amenorrhea

Decrease in libido

Euphoria

Insomnia

Anxiety, irritability, depression

Less commonly reported side effects include:

Occult arrhythmias

Gallstone formation with biliary colic

Pancreatitis early in refeeding

Disorientation with regard to self-identity and body image

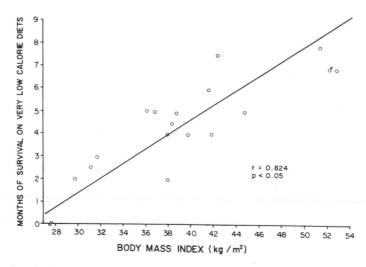

Figure 6.   Relationship of duration of survival of 17 obese dieters on very-low-calorie diets to prediet BMI, showing regression of duration of survival (in months) on BMI for 17 obese persons who died during or shortly agter completing prolonged adherence to 300- to 500-kcal diets. The diets usally derived all their energy from typtophan-supplemented collagen or gelatin hydrolysates. In general, the most obese subjects (as inferred from BMI) survived the longest. (Reproduced with permission from TB VanItallie and MU Yang, Cardiac dysfunction in obese dieters: a potentially lethal complication of rapid, massive weight loss. Am J Clin Nutrition 39:695-702, 1984.)

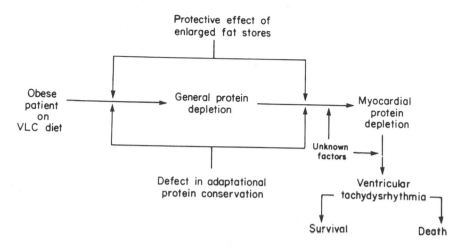

Figure 7. Postulated sequence of events linking prolonged use of very-low-calorie diets to prolonged periods experience rapid, massive weight loss accompanied by varying degrees of depletion of body and, specicifically, myocardial protein. Rate of protein loss is modulated by the size of the fat depot and the ability of the vofy to call forth adaptational processes that favor protein conservations in plasma and tissue. Other factors, some as yet unknown, also may affect the heart's vulnerability to ventricular arrthythmias. (Reproduced with permission from TB VanItallie and MU Yang, Cardiac dysfunction in obese dieters: a potentially lethal complication of rapid, massive weight loss. Am J Clin Nutrition 39:695-702, 1984.)

Apart from its other adverse effects, progressive protein deficit appears capable of promoting cardiac dysfunction. One manifestation of such dysfunction is prolongation of the QTc interval during rapid massive weight loss. This change in the ventricular repolarization process renders the dieting patient vulnerable to the occurrence of a lethal ventricular arrhythmia. In this regard, the correlation reported in 1984 by VanItallie and Yang between the prediet body mass indexes of a group of 17 liquid protein diet victims and their duration of life on the liquid protein seems relevant (Figure 6). We have calculated that these avid dieters died after they had lost approximately 15 kg of FFM—namely, about 3 kg of intracellular protein. By the time of death, the most obese subjects in this group had lost in excess of 30 percent, while the least obese had lost 10 to 15 percent of their initial weight. Our formulation of the possible mechanism responsible for the deaths, which attributes the QTc interval prolongation to protein malnutrition of the heart, is shown in Figure 7.

In 1985, Rassmussen and Andersen published a report from Copenhagen on the relationship between QT changes and nutritional status during weight loss after gastroplasty. The authors analyzed electrocardiograms, serum electrolytes, plasma concentration of prealbumin and retinol-binding protein (RBP), and dietary intakes in 22 women during weight loss after gastroplasty for morbid obesity. The QT interval corrected for heart rate (QTc) was prolonged (.44 sec) in 32 percent of subjects on one or more occasions. The occurrence of QTc prolongation was significantly associated with protein intakes well below the recommended amounts of 44 g per day —namely, below 34 g per day. These low protein intakes were associated with low concentrations in plasma of prealbumin. QTc prolongation was not associated with inadequate mineral intake, and occurred in spite of normal serum levels of calcium, magnesium, potassium, and sodium. The authors concluded that, because QTc prolongation may precede fatal arrhythmia, adequate protein intake is essential during weight reduction.

Several points need to be emphasized in connection with the Copenhagen study. First, the study confirms that QTc prolongation can occur in the absence of electrolyte derangement. Second, supplementing the diet with recommended doses of vitamins and minerals did not prevent QTc prolongation.

SUGGESTED TREATMENT GUIDELINES

Can any of the information or ideas touched on in this discussion be used to develop more rational guidelines to assure safe and effective weight loss? The answer is a qualified "yes." Regrettably, the supply of reliable scientific information that can be used to help us develop guidelines is sparse. Nevertheless, there is enough to make a beginning.

First, weight reduction diets should be tailored to the individual needs of the patient. As discussed earlier, several principles have to be kept in mind when a calorie-reducing regimen is prescribed. First and foremost, we have to remember that the ability of overweight individuals to tolerate calorie restriction (that is, to conserve body protein during weight loss) depends in considerable part on the degree of severity of their obesity. Thus, morbidly obese individuals generally can tolerate very-low-calorie diets (providing 400 to 800 kcal per day) far better than moderately obese persons can. As patients lose more and more fat during treatment, their ability to protect their protein stores during caloric restriction appears to be increasingly compromised. Thus, during therapeutic weight loss, the percent energy deficit that is prescribed should be periodically adjusted to the changes that have occurred in quantity of body fat or in the body mass index (BMI).

Percent energy deficit is the percent reduction from maintenance energy intake brought about by a prescribed low-calorie diet. Thus, if the daily energy intake needed to maintain the weight of an obese patient is 2400 kcal, a 600 kcal weight-reduction diet would create a 75 percent energy deficit. A 300-calorie diet would create an 87.5 percent deficit. In most clinical settings, the energy intake required to maintain weight (in effect, the spontaneous daily

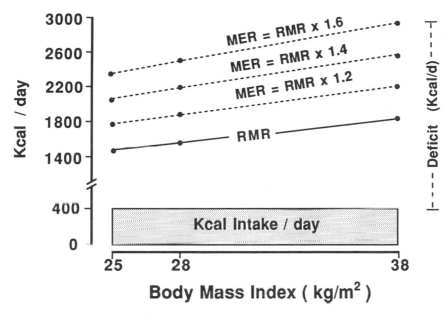

Figure 8. A 400-kcal/day diet will induce diverse energy deficits depending on factors such as sex, age, body size, and physical activity level. The values shown are for three females, 40 years old and 67 inches in height, with different body mass indices. Energy deficit is determined by subtracting the appropriate maintenance energy requirements (MER) from the daily calorie intake, and MER is estimated from resting metabolic rate (RMR) and daily level of physical activity. (Reproduced with permission from MU Yang and TB VanItallie, Effect of energy restriction on body composition and nitrogen balance in obese individuals. In TA Wadden and TB VanItallie, eds, Treatment of the seriously obese patient. New York: Guilford Press, 1992.)

energy expenditure) must be determined from the estimated resting energy expenditure and the estimated level of physical activity.

The rationale for prescribing a "percent calorie deficit," rather than some arbitrary energy intake, arises from the simple fact that people often differ widely in their daily maintenance energy requirement (MER). A 900-kcal diet will produce a far greater nutritional stress in a large, physically active man whose daily MER is 3200 kcal than it will in a small, physically inactive woman whose MER is 1800 kcal. In addition, the MER progressively decreases as more and more weight is lost.

As indicated in Figure 8, the MER of individuals of similar age and stature will differ materially depending on such factors as BMI and habitual level of physical activity. Thus, a 400 kcal/day diet will induce diverse energy deficits depending on factors such as sex, age, body size, and physical activity level. The values shown in the figure are for three females,

40 years old and 67 inches in height, with different BMIs and levels of physical activity.

MER is calculated by multiplying the resting metabolic rate by a coefficient that reflects the contribution to total energy expenditure of the daily level of physical activity. Energy deficit is determined by subtracting the appropriate MER from the daily calorie intake.

Because the severity of a calorically restricted diet is best expressed in terms of percent energy deficit, it is reasonable to characterize weight reduction diets in this fashion. Thus, as shown in Table 1, the most severely obese patients are permitted the most drastic caloric restriction. (As a patient's BMI decreases with successful weight loss, the allowable percent caloric deficit should be adjusted downward, as indicated in the table.)

For less severe obesity, the percent energy deficit permitted is correspondingly smaller. It seems prudent to set a limit below which energy intake should not be further reduced. The treatment method described herein sets that limit at 800 kcal per day. In this regard, the patient needs to have at least a rough understanding and acceptance of the physiologic rationale for keeping rate of weight loss in check.

It is important to emphasize that the foregoing system for prescribing a calorie-reduced diet is only a guide designed to help the patient lose weight at a rate compatible with a composition of loss of acceptable quality—namely, a weight loss that on average is at least 75 percent fat and no more than 25 percent FFM. Whether this goal is actually achieved in any given case can only be reliably ascertained if the body composition of the obese patient is monitored during weight loss. If weight loss is too rapid or if body composition measurements show that the proportion of weight lost as FFM is consistently too high, an upward adjustment of the energy content of the diet is mandatory.

Table 1. Adjustment of Energy Deficit — Actual Intake Minus the Maintenance Requirement (MER) — to the Concurrent Body Mass Index (BMI)

BMI (kg/m²)	Prescribed Energy Deficit (as % of MER)
25.0 - 27.9	40
28.0 - 31.9	50
32.0 - 35.9	60
36.0 - 39.9	65
40.0 - 43.9	70

To calculate the appropriate calorie prescription, use the following equation:
Prescribed kcal = MER − (% energy deficit × MER)

DIETARY FORMATS

Optimizing the Protein Content of Low-Calorie Diets

The optimal level of protein intake for obese individuals who continue to adhere faithfully to a low-calorie diet is not clearly known. There appears to be a limit on how much protein one can add to a low-calorie diets and still obtain an increasingly beneficial effect on nitrogen balance. In this regard Yang and VanItallie (1984) studied a series of obese individuals maintained for 64 days on either of two low-calorie diets (600 to 800 kcal/day as determined by bomb calorimetry), consisting of protein alone at 1.5 per kilogram of optimal weight (kg_{opt}) per day or an equal mixture of protein and carbohydrate (each at 0.75 g kg_{opt}/day). On the average, the diet that consisted almost entirely of protein did not spare body protein better or induce a greater rate of weight loss than did the 50/50 mixture of protein and carbohydrate.

Although a case could therefore be made for limiting the protein content of a low-energy diet to a point where it provides no more than half of its calories as protein (i.e., 75 g in a 600-kcal diet), no one seems to know just how far the protein content of an energy-restricted diet can be reduced without the production of undesirable metabolic and clinical effects. As mentioned earlier, Rassmussen and Andersen (1985) found that post-gastroplasty patients who consistently consumed less than 34 g of protein per day exhibited adverse changes in rapidly turning over plasma proteins (pre-albumin and RBP), and were at considerable risk of developing QTc interval prolongation and ventricular arrhythmia. Accordingly, when a weight reduction diet is prescribed, it is prudent to provide a generous amount of high-quality protein (perhaps an excessive amount) rather than risk inducing protein depletion with a hypocaloric diet that is too low in protein content.

SUMMARY

In this chapter I have tried to call attention to an anomalous situation that still obtains in the field of obesity therapy—namely, that weight reduction treatment continues to be undertaken by physicians and nonphysicians with little or no understanding of, or attention to, the effect of energy restriction on body composition and, more particularly, on the body's fat-free mass and intracellular protein status. As a consequence of neglect of the scientific information available about the physiologic consequences of caloric restriction, low-calorie diets are routinely prescribed without consideration of the maintenance energy needs of the patient or the possible adverse effects of too-rapid weight loss. It seems entirely feasible that guidelines can be developed to help make the prescription of low-calorie diets a more rational and systematic procedure—one based on the available scientific knowledge about the effect of energy restriction and diet composition on the rate and composition of weight loss. Specifically, it is suggested that, rather than prescribe a low-calorie diet with an arbitrarily fixed energy content, it makes better sense to prescribe an energy deficit that is geared to the changing maintenance energy needs of the obese patient and the gradually diminishing severity of the obesity during successful treatment.

It is also suggested that rates of weight loss be restrained by the physician so that they do not exceed 0.3 pound (136 g) per 1000 kcal deficit. If this guideline rate of weight loss is adhered to during prolonged weight reduction, fat-free mass will be better preserved and fewer adverse side effects are likely to occur. In addition, the use of a calorie-reduced diet in treatment of the obese patient will be medically more sound and rational, in contrast to the haphazard, unscientific, and occasionally unsafe approaches that are so widely used at the present time.

REFERENCES

Boozer CN, Brasseur A, Atkinson RL (1993). Dietary fat affects weight loss and adiposity during energy restriction in rats. Am J Clin Nutrition 58:846-852

Garrow JS (1993). Composition of weight loss during therapeutic dietary restriction. In JG Kral and TB VanItallie, eds, Recent developments in body composition analysis: methods and applications. London: Smith-Gordon.

Rassmussen LH, Andersen T (1985). The relationship between QTc changes and nutrition during weight loss after gastroplasaty. Acta Med Scan 217:271-275.

VanItallie, TB (1989). The dietary treatment of severe obesity. In JE Hamner, III, ed, The 1988 distinguished visiting professorship lectures. Memphis: University of Tennessee.

VanItallie TB, Abraham S (1985). Some hazards of obesity and its treatment. In J Hirsch and TB VanItallie, eds, Recent advances in obesity research IV. Proceedings of the Fourth International Congress on Obesity: London: John Libbey.

VanItallie, TB, Yang MU (1977). Current concepts in nutrition: diets and weight loss. N Engl J Med 297:1158-1161.

VanItallie TB, Yang MU (1984). Cardiac dysfunction in obese dieters: a potentially lethal complication of rapid, massive weight loss. Am J Clin Nutrition 39:695-702.

VanItallie TB, Yang MU, Heymsfield SB, Funk RC, Boileau RA (1990). Height-normalized indices of the body's fat-free mass and fat mass: potentially useful indicators of nutritional status. Am J Clin Nutrition.

Vanswani AN, Gamble MV, VanItallie TB (1993). Body composition changes in obese patients during weight reduction: estimation by electromagnetic scanning technology. In JG Kral and TB VanItallie, eds, Recent developments in body composition analysis: methods and applications. London: Smith-Gordon.

Webster JD, Hesp R, Garrow JS (1984). The composition of excess weight in obese women estimatied by body density, total body water, and total body potassium. Hum Nutr Clin Nutr 38C:299-306.

Yang MU, VanItallie TB (1984). Variability in body protein loss during protracted, severe caloric restriction. Role of triiodothyronine and other possible determinants. Am J Clin Nutrition 40:611-622.

Yang MU, VanItallie TB (1992). Effect of energy restriction on body composition and nitrogen balance in obese individuals. In TA Wadden and TB VanItallie, eds, Treatment of the seriously obese patient. New York: Guilford Press.

11

Rational Nutrition Component of Comprehensive Weight Management

Jane M. Rees, MS, RD

Current scientific knowledge about the problem of obesity mandates new approaches to weight management. The most relevant research conclusions are: the prominence of genetics plus weight gain and loss history in determining an individual body's response to its energy supply, both internal stored energy and newly consumed energy, the ineffectiveness of short interventions and semi-starvation and the potency of gratification as a determinant of behavior (National Institutes of Health 1992; Sears 1951). While these conclusions are relevant to all aspects of a multidisciplinary weight management protocol, they are especially important to consider in designing the nutritional component.

PROPOSED PRINCIPLES

The following principles are proposed as guides for nutritional therapy in comprehensive weight management because they integrate factors that can no longer be overlooked in intervention strategies applied to human obesity.

1. *Historical and initial knowledge, attitudes and behavior, as well as physical characteristics, will be assessed and changes monitored.* Human problems with a biopsychosocial etiology, such as eating disorders, require intervention in the knowledge base, the attitudes and the behaviors of the people affected (Bruch 1973; Crisp 1980). The intellectual, affective, behavioral and physical aspects of each obese patient's present and life-long situation will be

Research for this chapter was supported by Grant MCJ-000970 from the Maternal and Child Health Bureau of the U.S. Department of Health and Human Services and the Nielsen Family Grant.

evaluated initially, a fitting intervention developed and changes monitored (Rees 1993). Patients can control increases in knowledge and improvement in attitudes and behaviors, meaning that it is appropriate to focus on improvement in these areas when measuring success. Because of physiologic variation, changes brought about in the body by changes in behavior are not predictable or controllable and therefore not appropriate as the focus of measures of success (Rees 1990). Physical changes will be monitored to help the patient and the therapeutic team know more about an individual's physiologic makeup and response to the environment.

2. *Information about nutrients in food and how the body uses them will be provided in a manner that enables patients to acquire a working knowledge of nutrition.* In an age when information about traditional foods is no longer passed down through generations, nor generally applicable when it is, knowledge about the role of the six basic nutrients is essential. To live normally, patients who are vulnerable to excess fat storage need to be able to assess the food content and choose a balance of nutrients, under any circumstance, among newly developed foods, "diet" products and snack foods, for example. Furthermore, they must believe this skill is important to them and that they are in control of their food consumption (Rees and Trahms 1989). They must understand and act on the understanding that food intake is a matter of survival rather than an element of life that they can allow to be influenced by fashion or advertising claims about energy (positive) or calories (negative). Interventions must help them overcome messages that larger people do not need food. Specifically they must know that nutrients are the chemicals that, along with oxygen, keep a person alive; calories are a measure of energy, not of food volume or "fat"; and the word diet is not just a verb that implies restriction.

3. *Patients will be helped to develop positive attitudes about themselves and their abilities to gain knowledge and change behaviors.* Self-efficacy is one of the few factors consistently associated with success in changing food-related behaviors. The psychosocial component of a multifaceted weight management program will address this core issue (Rodin, Schank and Striegel-Moore 1989). The nutrition component must also incorporate messages about a positive concept of the self, empowering patients to take appropriate steps in learning and changing behavior. Sophisticated counseling techniques developed in the social sciences are needed to convey nutrition messages effectively (Hackney and Cormier 1979). Simplistic behavior modification strategies and group education are useful adjuncts, but as the sole methods for facilitating change by seriously affected patients, they are not adequate (Boxer and Miller 1987).

Along with improving self-concept and support for patients undertaking the difficult task of managing their weight, the psychosocial component of a multidisciplinary program will address personality and family dysfunction in counseling (Epstein, Valoski, Wing and McCurley 1990;

Harkaway 1987; Mellon, Slinkard and Irwin 1987). The medical specialist will rule out genetic, metabolic and endocrinologic syndromes, assess growth and sexual maturity in young patients and biochemical status (Arden 1992), as well as participating in setting goals, planning action and motivating patients, spouses and families.

4. *Patients will be helped to normalize eating and exercise behaviors and to nurture themselves.* Learning to eat an amount of food appropriate for their height, age and gender and to exercise at the optimum level compatible with their physical makeup are skills patients can maintain for life in their efforts to control their weight. Extremes are unhealthy in the long and even short term. Just as the body cannot be deprived of air or water, it cannot be deprived of food without negative consequences (Keys, Brozek, Hanschel, Mickelsen and Taylor 1950).

Patients will need to be taught to incorporate pleasures that are deemphasized in our culture in comparison with the consumption of food (Ornstein and Sobel 1989). Replacing unhealthy behaviors, often practiced to achieve immediate gratification and sensory input, with healthy behaviors to achieve the same ends is effective compared to solely relying on prohibitions.

5. *Patients will be guided in establishing realistic goals for change and accepting physiologic consequences.* Examples in learning to play musical instruments and improve interpersonal relationships teach that change in human endeavors is achieved in a series of small increments, except in the instance of people with an exceptional talent in a particular area. Realistically, patients can manage to achieve a series of small changes in their habits. They need guidance to establish reasonable goals (Hackney and Cormier 1979) because the traditional messages about changing their situation have emphasized speed and unrealistic achievement. For example, replacing a glass of whole milk daily with a glass half filled with 2 percent and the rest whole milk is probably an accomplishable task and an appropriate goal, compared to changing multiple foods in the habitual diet all at once.

In the same way, patients need help understanding that whatever changes they permanently make are indeed positive but will not lead to a predictable body reaction. They will need to accept their bodies as they are determined genetically and by their history up to seeking treatment, not as they would like them to be (National Institutes of Health 1992). They will need to learn to reject negative, uninformed messages about body shape and size and to fight discrimination that will continue to be directed toward themselves, even if they are in as complete control possible (Allon 1979; Tobias and Gordon 1980). They will probably have to go through a grieving process for the body society describes as "normal."

Physical alterations resulting from realistic changes in energy intake and output will generally be less dramatic than people have been led to expect. The rate of fat gain may stabilize or decrease first. Fat stores may eventually stabilize and over time, as the reversible factors maintaining fat stores are reversed, total fat can decrease. When a variety of biochemical, anthropometric and other physical parameters are monitored in detail (Rees 1993), there is a greater chance that some positive change will be detected than when only gross weight is measured.

6. *Appropriate rewards for progress will be built in.* Patients need to be taught about rewards because in many instances society has taught them to reward themselves with food or miraculous promises of weight loss. Each small increment of increased knowledge or change in attitude or behavior is an opportunity for reward (Sears 1951) with appropriate substitutes for traditional "biological reinforcers," now known to be counterproductive because they have unpredictable results. The nutritional therapist teaches patients to reward themselves by:

a. Providing tangible and social rewards
b. Planning rewards jointly (therapist and patient)
c. Guiding patients to reward themselves
d. Observing patients to spontaneously reward themselves

NEW PRINCIPLES TO ELIMINATE THE NEGATIVE CHARACTERISTICS OF TRADITIONAL NUTRITION MANAGEMENT

The proposed principles will replace the following characteristics of the nutrition component in past obesity research and treatment, which have been shown at best to be ineffective and at worst detrimental:

1. Ignoring genetic and life-long body type.
2. Relying on superficial, "cookbook" training without teaching facts and processes, leaving patients dependent on external strategies and unable to deal with their own long-term problems.
3. Taking a punitive or strictly disciplinary approach that fosters a judgmental attitude toward oneself and a defensive and inflexible attitude toward change.
4. Coupling dietary restriction with excessive exercise while ignoring the need for physical and psychological nurturing of the self.
5. Having unrealistic expectations for change increments and resulting body alterations.

The principles proposed here can be defended on scientific grounds and, following revisions made through informed debate, they can become the guiding principles for the nutrition components of comprehensive research and treatment protocols.

REFERENCES

Allon N (1979). Self-perceptions of the stigma of overweight in relationship to weight-losing patterns. Am J Clin Nutrition 32:470-480.

Arden MR (1992). Adolescent obesity. In L McAnarney, Ed, Textbook of adolescent medicine. Philadelphia: WB Saunders.

Boxer GH, Miller BD (1987). Treatment of a 7-year-old boy with obesity hypoventilation (pickwickian syndrome) on a psychosomatic inpatient unit. J Am Acad Child Adol Psychiatry 26:798-805.

Bruch H (1973). Eating disorders. New York: Basic Books.

Crisp AH (1980). Anorexia nervosa: let me be. New York: Grune & Stratton.

Epstein LH, Valoski A, Wing RR, McCurley J (1990). Ten-year follow-up of behavioral, family-based treatment for obese children. JAMA 264:2519-2523.

Hackney H, Cormier LS (1979). Counseling strategies and objectives. Englewood Cliffs, NJ: Prentice Hall.

Harkaway JE (1987). Family intervention in the treatment of childhood and adolescent obesity. In JC Hansen and JE Harkaway, Eds, Eating disorders. Rockville, MD: Aspen.

Keys A, Brozek J, Henschel A, Mickelsen O, Taylor HL (1950). The biology of human starvation (2 vols). Minneapolis: University of Minnesota Press.

Mellon LM, Slinkard LA, Irwin CE (1987). Adolescent obesity intervention: validation of the SHAPEDOWN program. J Am Diet Assoc 87:333-338.

National Institutes of Health (1992). National Institutes of Health technology assessment conference statement, March 30—April 1, 1992: Methods for voluntary weight loss and control. Bethesda, MD: U.S. Department of Health and Human Services.

Ornstein R, Sobel D (1989). Healthy pleasures. Reading, MA: Addison-Wesley.

Rees JM (1993). A comprehensive protocol for assessment of obese adolescents and evaluation of their progress in managing weight. Ann NY Acad Sci 699:280-286.

Rees JM (1990). Management of obesity in adolescence. Med Clin North Am 74:1275-1289.

Rees JM, Trahms CM (1989). Nutritional influences on physical growth and behavior in adolescence. In GR Adams, R Montemayor and TP Gullotta, Eds, Biology of adolescent behavior and development. Newbury Park, CA: Sage.

Rodin J, Schank D, Striegel-Moore R (1989). Psychological features of obesity. Med Clin North Am 73:47-66.

Sears RR (1951). A theoretical framework for personality and social behavior. Am Psychol 6:476.

Tobias A, Gordon JB (1980). Social consequences of obesity. J Am Diet Assoc 76:338-342.

12

Food Control Training as a Successor to Dieting: A New Model for Weight Management

Stephen Pernice Gullo, PhD
with the assistance of
Michael E. Swiander, MA

Obesity is a medical condition that is notoriously resistant to treatment (Bjorval and Rossner 1986; Jeffery and Forster 1987; National Institutes of Health [NIH] 1985, 1992; Sash 1977; Stunkard 1984; Wooley and Wooley 1979). Very low caloric diets, behavior modification, drugs, gastric and intestinal surgery, and most commercial weight loss programs have produced varying degrees of short-term success, but research indicates that very few individuals who go through these programs achieve and maintain normal weights (Wolfe 1992; Fatis et al. 1989; Anderson et al. 1988; Rodin et al. 1988; Cairella 1987; Bjorval and Rossner 1986; Kramer et al. 1986; Wadden et al. 1985; Stuart 1978). If the goal of treatment for obesity is to be defined as permanent or long-term maintenance of weight loss, current statistics indicate that existing therapeutic measures are not effective in achieving this goal (NIH 1985, 1992).

Although behavioral treatments have established themselves as the prevalent short-term successful nonsurgical therapy, weight loss is more often associated with cognitive change than with behavioral change (Kalodner and DeLucia 1991; Wilson and Brownell 1980; Jeffrey et al. 1978). Salivation, appetite and food intake are all strongly influenced by beliefs and expectations, especially for restrained eaters (Jansen and Van Den Hout 1991; Woody et al. 1981; Rolls et al. 1976; Mahoney 1975; Pudel 1975). Pretreatment cognitive characteristics have been shown to be related to eventual weight loss, while "momentary indiscretions" in dieters are often preceded by dysfunc-

153

tional patterns of thought (Saltzer 1981; Sjoberg and Persson 1979; Stuart and Guire 1978; Leon et al. 1977; Mahoney 1975; Mahoney 1974).

Until recently, obesity was viewed primarily as a character disorder manifested as excessive consumption of food. According to this view, the best treatment is restriction of caloric intake coupled with increased levels of exercise, so that fewer calories are taken in than are expended (Bray 1983; Sash 1977). The theory that character is the primary underlying cause for the overweight condition is not, however, sufficient to explain the evidence of extreme variation in weight loss among dieters even when food intake is kept constant (Garrow et al. 1978). Recent research indicates that physiologic and metabolic variables are more relevant to certain individuals' conditions than are personality characteristics and that obesity is a complex disorder of energy metabolism that is affected by biologic, genetic, cultural and cognitive factors (Hirsch 1991; VanItallie and Hirsch 1975).

The process of overcoming these factors and achieving weight loss is inherently a process of developing self-efficacy and control, the cognitive effects of which can be profound. Research has shown that the self-attributed capacity to produce a desired effect increases motivation in goal-oriented situations and that the perception of such control can be predictive of weight loss success (Bandura 1977; Rodin 1974). Yet the importance of control and its cognitive correlates has, to date, been largely ignored by most weight loss theories and programs.

Cognitive therapies, when used in conjunction with behavioral management strategies, have been shown to yield significant success in the treatment of obesity and overweight (Kalodner and DeLucia 1991; Jeffrey et al. 1978). These success rates, when viewed in conjunction with the poor success rates of current weight loss programs, illustrate the need for a more multivariate approach to the treatment of overweight conditions. Although the success rates of primarily cognitive approaches have not been consistent, in general they suggest that such interventions are a viable and necessary part of any weight loss program. Existing data also indicate that differential diagnosis is an important part of successful weight loss programs, despite seemingly higher costs. While individualized treatment programs may appear to be less time- and cost-efficient, food control theory contends that the resultant drop in the long-term costs of recidivism—which often results in repeat treatment and places clients at increased risk of a variety of potentially serious and disabling illnesses—will more than offset the higher "up-front" costs (Brownell and Jeffrey 1987; Bennett 1986). Food control theory demonstrates the clinical use of such a program in food control training.

PSYCHOSOCIAL INFLUENCES ON EATING BEHAVIOR

It is now well-recognized that there are powerful biologic factors underlying weight regulation in humans. Research suggests that each individual has a genetically programmed natural weight range or set point from which the body does not "want" to deviate (Keesey 1986; Corbett 1984; Garner et al 1982). This set point, while marginally influenced by environmental factors such as activity level, food choices, affect and sociocultural programming ultimately controls the body's relative size and shape. There are many genetic studies in man showing a strong heritability of human obesity (Hirsch 1991; Stunkard 1984; Keesey 1986; Corbett 1984; Stunkard 1980; Foch and McClearns 1980). The importance of individual differences in set points and body type to determining long-term weight goals cannot be understated.

Food control theory emphasizes the importance of keeping the genetic and biologic determinants of weight regulation in mind when establishing long-term weight goals. The current "acceptable weight ranges" established by Metropolitan Life Insurance—while generally considered too high for optimal health—may still be too *low* for certain individuals. The author's clinical experience has been that many overweight people become discouraged and return to destructive eating patterns when they cannot reach or maintain an "ideal weight," despite diligent and consistent efforts to control food intake and increase energy expenditure. Age, metabolic changes, prior health problems, and unavoidable lifestyle variables (such as a time-consuming and sedentary job) can all impede efforts to achieve an "ideal weight" goal. In these instances, food control theory advocates establishing a "tolerable weight" goal—one which is sufficiently under the current excessive weight to yield significant health benefits, but which can also be easily maintained within the less flexible parameters of the individual client's life. A weight goal which cannot be realistically maintained can lead to a cycle of yo-yo dieting, which presents health risks that equal (and may even exceed) those of long-term excess weight.

However, it must also be noted that while genetic and physiologic predispositions can set boundaries for upper and lower weight designations and influence food preferences to various degrees, environmental factors play many roles in their actual expression. These factors—ranging from cultural background to individual affect—tend to shape both food preferences and eating behavior in an individual's life.

Sociocultural Influences

Societal attitudes toward food intake, food reward systems and body image have a distinct impact on the development of individual behaviors, cognitions and emotional responses toward food. In people with food control problems, these cognitions are thought to be a primary degenerative force leading to loss of control, prompting impulsive eating-related behavior such as poor menu choices in restaurants and last-minute "grabs" from the shelves in the supermarket.

People may be born with biologic predispositions and food sensitivities, but they are not born with bad eating habits. Infant studies and the documentation of cross-cultural and regional food cravings, demonstrate that instinctual eating habits tend to be more efficient than those demonstrated by adult learned behavior. It has long been recognized that children tend to eat what they need and that eating habits get worse as a person matures (Davis 1930). The overproduction and extensive availability of foods (particularly "nosh" or "finger foods") in our day-to-day lives has created an environment that promotes chronic overeating and many problems of nutrient imbalance. While the roots of many food preferences (including the taste for sweets) are biologically based, the frequency with which individuals act on these preferences is the result of a complex sociocultural value system concerning food. In essence, superimposed societal cognitive schemas and cultural values have weakened our ability to self-regulate eating behaviors.

In America's cultural value system, food still equals success. The majority of today's adults are children of poor and/or Depression era parents, many of whom were themselves immigrants or the children of immigrants. The majority of these people left their countries of origin to escape extreme hardship and poverty—often marked by severe food deprivation. Such deprivation, when coupled with the place food has traditionally held in so many human celebrations, gave food an unprecedented place of importance as a symbol of survival, achievement and freedom from want. The celebration of food and its abundance was based on a very justified survival instinct.

Today, however, the privation of America's agrarian ancestors no longer exists. The problem of food deprivation has been replaced by a new threat of food overabundance, compounded by the retention of the food value system of our ancestors. This value system has promoted a psychological reward system centered on food—particularly the highly refined, sugar-based foods that are traditionally viewed as "goodies" or "treats." As children, we are rewarded for doing the chores or achieving good grades with trips to the ice cream parlor. As adults, our language of love is full of food imagery, from the positive ("honey," "sweetie," "cookie") to the negative ("tart," "crumb"). This food-glorifying value system—which often puts food above considerations of health, appearance or quality of life—is what food control theory refers to as "foodie-ism."

Food control theory hypothesizes that "foodie-ism" is largely responsible for the development of the cognitive schemas which eventually guide food choices. In the tradition of the Italian maxim that "more have perished by the throat than by the sword," food control theory holds that destructive eating patterns evolve from inappropriate beliefs and cognitions concerning food and its powers. People overemphasize food and the pleasure it can bring to the point that they ignore the harmful effects of certain foods on weight, weight control and overall health. Operating within the current societal schema concerning food, people sacrifice control and self-image for the supposed "advantage" of a cookie, despite the available nutritional information on the long-term adverse consequences of these behaviors.

There is, however, a marked inconsistency in society's messages concerning food and those concerning body type. On the one hand, high-calorie foods are craved and promoted, while on the other, a very lean body shape is considered more desirable and acceptable than an overweight or even an average-sized body. This mixed message results in a cultural-biologic dissonance in which people try to obtain a body shape and weight that is physically inappropriate for them as individuals (Callaway 1990).

Instead of acknowledging the essential incompatibility of these messages, many individuals believe that they can have it all—that food glorification and lean body type can coexist. This is a basic denial of reality, a return to the undeveloped, magical thinking of childhood that is inappropriate for mature, functional adults. Weight control therefore requires a shift from the psychology of childhood to the psychology of adulthood. Those with weight problems must realize that they do not live in a world of magic but in a world of reality where compromise and adaptation are a part of life. In order to achieve and maintain weight loss, it is necessary to accept the consequences of decisions made with regard to food and to develop new decision-making processes that promote control.

This process is sometimes impeded by social stimuli which have been shown to promote excessive or uncontrolled eating behavior. Research has shown that social factors and exposure can influence the amount of food eaten, the types of food eaten and how that food is eaten. Mere exposure to certain foods seems to increase preference for those foods (Birch and Marlin 1982; Pliner 1982). There are also many studies that demonstrate an effect of the presence of other people on eating behaviors. One study found that eating with one companion can increase a person's meal size by 28 percent and that eating in a group of six or more can raise it 76 percent.

Such situation-specific influences on food preferences apparently start during infancy. A child's preference for a food can be linked to a social acceptance mechanism learned through observation of the parents' facial expression (Steiner 1977). Observational learning of this type could play a role in the early development and later continuation of food preference responses. The presence of another person in the room has also been shown to play a part in the amount of food and the adjustment of eating behavior of an individual (Herman and Polivy 1979).

All these examples of direct social transmission of food preferences indicate the importance of considering the role of observational learning in the development of such preferences. Observational learning does not even need to be direct to have a measurable effect on preference. Indirect exposure to food—either visually or verbally—can influence food choices in humans, presumably because human beings are the only organisms that rely on printed and recorded information. One of the clearest examples of this indirect influence can be seen in attitudes developed from watching television. Several experiments have reported that children exposed to commercials react with increased preference for foods low in nutritional value (Jeffrey et al. 1980). Unfortunately, they do not exhibit similar preference for foods high in nutritional value when exposed to commercials of that type, perhaps because of differences in the quality and visual power of the commercials themselves.

The sociocultural factors reviewed above condition everything from individuals' underlying belief systems and thoughts about foods (including their internal dialogue or "food talk") to their responses to food cues in specific situations. The power of these underlying schemas should not be underestimated. The food-glorifying values of "foodie-ism" foster a sense of deprivation and loss in those who are attempting to lose weight and prompt a return to destructive eating behaviors in those who are trying to maintain weight loss. In order for weight loss to be permanent, this dysfunctional value system must be replaced with one which puts food in its proper perspective in the overall pattern of a healthy lifestyle.

Psychological Influences

Food control theory does not ascribe to the belief that all overweight individuals eat in response to some underlying emotional or psychological dysfunction. It is true that there is a significant subset of obese individuals whose eating patterns may be influenced by a depressive state. It is also true that many individuals—whether obese or of normal weight—use food as a panacea when they are sad, stressed, or even bored. But under conditions of severe stress or clinical depression, a loss of appetite is far more common than excessive eating and reducing overweight to a symptom of psychological disorder is simplistic.

Individuals with a long-term history of weight problems often experience a situational depression. They feel out of control as their bodies expand and may feel helpless in their efforts to control their own image. This pervasive sense of being out of control can prompt a vicious circle of despair/eating/weight gain/despair. Such individuals usually respond extremely well to weight loss and the increased sense of control they gain from controlling their weight generally leads to a lifting of the situational depressive state.

Individual personality style is significantly related to eating behaviors and the types of foods chosen. Individuals with compulsive tendencies (intense, goal-oriented, often highly successful) often carry these tendencies into their relationship with food. They tend to be "finishers"—with a strong and consistent pattern of consuming all of any food placed in front of them. They eat quickly and—from the perspective of weight control—are better off with an all-or-nothing approach. They find it difficult, if not impossible, to eat only a portion of anything. For them a dietetic model that advises consuming "half of what's on your plate" does not work. They can be defined as "equal opportunity eaters" who have problems with "finger control." Some theorists have called this pattern a food addiction on the basis of its marked behavioral similarity to classic addictive behaviors.

Compulsive types tend to like foods that cater to their personality, ones they can eat quickly and on the run, or small-portioned ones that they can easily finish. Fast foods and snack foods are popular among this group. People with food control problems and compulsive tendencies tend to value only the "finished product." This can have two negative effects on weight control. First, these individuals tend to finish all food placed in front of them; second, they find it hard to appreciate the interim stages of a diet or the importance of developing life management skills in order to achieve long-term weight control.

For these individuals, therefore, it is important to develop an appreciation for the overall process of attaining control over food in the context of permanent weight loss. Cognitive change is generally critical for this group, so that they can control their compulsive tendencies toward food. For those who cannot exercise moderation, abstinence from foods that cause control problems is suggested.

The psychological and emotional underpinnings of food-related behaviors can vary a great deal from person to person, but tend to remain consistent within each individual. Identifying these factors and determining the appropriate measures for changing the destructive cognitions related to food consumption, is one of the most important aspects of food control training.

FOOD CONTROL TRAINING

Need for a Multivariate Approach

The modern dietetic model for weight control was designed to promote weight loss. Its inability to maintain weight loss should not necessarily be interpreted as a complete failure of the model. Many diet programs do succeed at helping overweight individuals lose weight—not because of the diet per se, but because of the control that the diet imposes on eating behavior that was formerly uncontrolled. This control degrades once the "dieting" phase is complete, however, the cognitions and beliefs that are at the root of destructive eating behaviors reassert themselves.

Food control theory maintains that weight control is determined by the interaction of the physiologic, psychosocial and environmental factors that influence food intake. Different factors may assume different roles in various weight control problems. Consideration must therefore be given to all the variables in a client's situation before food control can be achieved. In recognition of this fact, food control theory proposes a new model for weight loss programs that combines the knowledge base of the existing dietetic model with knowledge of the individual's differential response pattern to foods, history of control problems with food and overall cognitive schemas with relation to food. This model is called food control training.

The primary goal of food control training is to protect the quality and length of the client's life. When healthy instinctual control over eating behavior is lost, it is necessary to introduce behavioral choice management training that will enable the client to practice protective behavioral patterns. This is achieved by making clients aware of the unique patterns of their "eating print" and of how to use this knowledge to develop, institute and reinforce alternative food choices, behaviors and—most importantly—cognitions and beliefs concerning food.

Pattern Theory

The pattern theory of food control maintains that behavior predicts behavior. The very same people put on the very same weight, with the very same foods, in the very same instances, at the very same times of the day or week, no matter how many diet programs they may go through. Just as people all have their unique fingerprints, everyone has a unique "eating print," and unless the patterns of this eating print are recognized and adjusted for, it is unlikely that they will ever maintain their ideal weight. As Santayana said, "He who fails to remember the past is doomed to repeat it."

The eating print defines the unique pattern of what, when, where, how and why a person eats. It is influenced by a wide range of biologic, genetic, socioeconomic, cultural and psychological factors. Addressing these factors and the differential response patterns to food has been shown to aid successful weight maintenance (Brownell and Jeffrey 1987; Polivy and Herman 1985; Herman and Mack 1975).

Central to the identification of the eating print is the self-report of the client's previous food history. This increases self-efficacy (Bandura 1977) and also gives information on the specific trigger foods, trigger behaviors and trigger situations that prompt destructive eating patterns in the client.

Trigger foods are those that have been difficult to control in the past. Something in the particular food or category of foods triggers a behavioral control problem. The most common trigger foods are bakery goods (rolls, bagels, muffins, cookies, salty and/or crunchy foods such as pretzels); sweets (especially candy and ice cream); and finger fruits such as cherries or grapes. For some individuals, any food that can be picked up and eaten with the fingers can present a control problem.

Trigger foods tend to have a snowball effect on eating behaviors. Loss of control over a trigger food spreads to other foods and behavioral controls. Patients often feel that once they have lost control over one powerful craving they should surrender to all others.

Trigger behaviors are habitual behavior patterns that lead to the repeated (often unconscious) abuse of certain categories of food. As mentioned earlier, compulsive personality types are particularly prone to trigger behavioral patterns such as "finishing," picking, skipping meals and eating on the run.

Trigger situations are those that promote the eating response regardless of the presence of physiologic hunger. They are predominantly social situations, such as cocktail parties, although situations characterized by large blocks of unstructured time are also powerful triggers for many people. Watching television, going to the movies, or putting away an evening's leftovers are all potential trigger situations, which set up a Pavlovian response leading to overindulgence and loss of control.

Clinical observation has shown some people to report overeating when they are bored, stressed, cooking for their families, given a large variety of foods at a buffet, or when they are in the presence of other people who are eating. Certain times of the day are also commonly reported as trigger situations: mid-afternoon for at-home mothers; evenings after dinner for people with full-time jobs; the middle of the night for anyone; and unfilled blocks of time on weekends.

Establishing Control and Learning Containment

Once the eating print has been defined, food control training seeks to make clients aware of the specific factors that are contributing to their loss of control over food and assist them in developing alternative coping strategies and more healthy decision making skills.

The specific interventions used in food control training will vary depending on the specific eating print of each client. However, the basic coaching model is also applicable to group settings since there is a marked uniformity and predictability in the cognitions, beliefs and triggers of most individuals with weight control problems. Patients in group or individual treatment are required to maintain a detailed food diary which enables both client and coach to monitor progress, analyze difficulties and anticipate future strategies. Whether on a group or individual level, the mission of the coach is to maximize the client's potential in mastering the learned life management skill of food control. The coach is the catalyst for the emergence of new attitudes, values and schemas, while the client is the "star player" in an ongoing process of developing control and containment skills. In each individual, the coach follows these objectives:

1. To track progress by checking weight each week.

2. To check control with the "new scale" (see below).
3. To check the food diary each week.
4. To review the successes and difficulties of the past week to guide and reinforce food control behaviors. (Note: in accordance with the tenet that food control is a skill, there are no value judgments made during this review. Food control training coaches continually remind clients that no one "bats a thousand" in baseball or food control.)
5. To review upcoming events and take the client through cognitive rehearsals to prepare for impending food situations and stress points (including holidays, parties, trips, house guests, etc.).
6. To encourage clients to "air" stress issues with an emphasis on developing adaptive strategies which do not rely on food.
7. To prepare an individualized audio cassette which contains phrases and axioms that reinforce the concept of control and lend motivational support and encouragement to the patient. (Tapes are made during each session. Patients are encouraged to use these tapes as reinforcers in times of stress or food cravings.)

In emphasizing control, food control training makes it clear that gaining control over food does not mean being deprived of food. Patients are made aware of the prevailing sociocultural attitudes toward food and how this unrealistic "foodie-ism" has influenced their weight control problem. This awareness usually proves to be a powerful motivating force and inspiration to change.

Food control training focuses on the importance of becoming "food smart" in dealing with food, so that clients are mastering food instead of the food mastering them. For those who have never been able to adopt moderation when dealing with a particular food, being food smart sometimes means maintaining abstinence. For these individuals, control means eliminating certain trigger foods or behaviors (such as eating with their fingers) from their lives entirely.

Clinical observation has shown that individuals with a long history of abusing a certain food or foods often profit best from complete abstinence. They have learned that where there can be no moderation there must be elimination. These individuals freely admit that they would rather give up a trigger food than give up the control they have over their eating behaviors and their weight. Most have successfully rewritten their internal dialogue (see below) in a way that eliminates the sense of deprivation which might have prompted a return to that food after other diet attempts. This self-chosen abstinence tends to be a strong psychological motivator in that it not only increases the individual's feeling of self-mastery but eliminates any feelings of deprivation that usually develop in the dietetic approach. No person who "chooses" to abstain from certain foods can feel deprived.

For those who are not able to embrace abstinence, or who have very situation-specific problems with a given trigger food, avoidance is the most common option. These individuals employ a "boxing" technique in which they only consume specific trigger foods during special events like weddings or holidays. These clients plan in advance for certain indiscretions and keep these "contained circumstances" outside of their homes and as infrequent as possible. Their willpower must be continuously exercised to keep them psychologically fit.

No weight program can succeed without teaching its participants how to correct errors. The containment strategies of food control training define mistakes not as personal defeats but as teaching tools and learning experiences. As control develops and individuals internalize new choice management behavior and cognitive switching, breaks in control will occur. Most clients who lose most or part of their weight loss goal, no matter how committed, will eventually consume "forbidden" quantities or types of food.

Food control training's emphasis is on developing a skill that allows and anticipates errors as part of the process of self-mastery. It "contains" errors and prevents them from spreading by making it clear that every error is a singular, isolated event. Clients are provided with the cognitive tools necessary to know that breaks in control happen to all people for many reasons aside from and beyond a lack of willpower. The physiologic response to a low-calorie diet is a strong desire for more food. Willpower is at the mercy of biology. Food control training reminds people of how far they have gotten in their lives and that they are by no means psychologically enslaved by a cookie, but that they are probably subject to an as yet undetermined physiologic condition. Food control further maintains that it isn't necessary to identify the exact nature of this biologic predisposition. Identification of its existence and elimination of its triggers is an effective, efficient means of regaining control over the situation.

Cognitive Ambivalence and the Internal Dialogue

Cognitive change is necessary for increased control over food and also for counteracting the destructive thought patterns of "foodie-ism" that often lead to renewed weight gain. Among these patterns are the "tomorrowisms" that sometimes develop after clients experience the satisfaction of the first stage of weight loss.

At this stage, many clients find themselves rationalizing and negotiating with their trigger foods. They want to remain thin and in control, but will do the work necessary for it "tomorrow." They experience a cognitive ambivalence toward trigger foods, in which old cravings compete with new knowledge. They may attempt to have "just a little" of a particular trigger food and come under the control of what food control theory calls the "F-Q principle" of food control.

The F-Q principle refers to the clinical observation that when frequency of consumption increases, quantity inevitably increases as well. Patients begin with "just a little taste" which they believe will happen "just this once." The apparent success of this technique then leads to additional "little tastes" which tend to grow over time. Within a few months, they have slipped back into their old patterns and weight gain ensues.

From the perspective of food control training, initial loss of control (that first "little taste") does not necessarily mean a return to one's original overweight. Instead, these losses of control are viewed as opportunities to reinforce the lessons of the eating print, since they are confirmations of the correct identification of a trigger. Temporary losses of control are therefore used to reinforce clients' efforts to identify and control triggers, rather than making them feel as if they have failed.

Resolving temporary losses of control and avoiding the slippery slope of the F-Q principle require interventions which will help counter cognitive ambivalence and replace an internal dialogue that was conditioned by "foodie-ism" with one that is rooted in control. Much of the food control trainer's time is spent guiding the client toward cognitive switching to a more appropriate and beneficial value system. Successful weight maintenance is dependent on this cognitive restructuring.

Cognitive switching is based on the fact that all people talk to themselves and that this internal dialogue can either undermine or reinforce desired behaviors and choices. Food control training first seeks to identify the client's particular "foodie script" and then develop alternative dialogue which the client can use to counter the old thought patterns and beliefs that led to loss of control. In the final analysis, therefore, it is the client who writes the script.

The new dialogue is recorded onto an audio tape which is typically listened to once or twice per day. The length of the tape from the initial visit is typically less than 15 minutes and includes the basic diet and food guidelines. Subsequent tapes average about 5 to 6 minutes and are deliberately designed to be brief so that the client can listen to the tape daily. It is designed to be listened to in the car or while exercising or relaxing.

The audio cassette is yet another means to advance, control and promote the cognitive shift necessary to maintain weight control. The cassette gives particular emphasis to modulating formerly automatic responses to the sight and smells of trigger foods. The new cognitive framework deemphasizes momentary pleasure and emphasizes the cost of eating a trigger food through questions such as, "Do you like it enough to wear it?"

In using tapes to reinforce alternative cognitive and behavioral patterns in persons with food control problems, food control theory employs elements of what some have called the "principle of overlearning." The cassettes in food control training link a person's triggers with strong, control-oriented aphorisms. The aphorisms used on the food control training cassettes were constructed from many years' observations of what the "successful" vs. the "nonsuccessful" weight program participants tell themselves. Samples of typical destructive cognitions and their food control training switches can be found in Table 1.

The food control training tapes also advocate "affirmative action" by encouraging mental rehearsal of upcoming events. All tapes speak to the clients' personal strengths and accomplishments. The coach applies the same strengths to food control. There is a continuing emphasis on self-mastery and the positive psychological and physical benefits of being in control vs. being controlled by a piece of food.

Maintenance

Food control training's greatest effects are seen after clients have reached their target weight and enter into a lifelong maintenance phase which food control theory calls being a "selective gourmet." The food control theory holds that the eating print is a constant which must be considered throughout an individual's life. Food control training teaches clients that although they have lost the weight, they have not (in the words of one client) "lost the problem." If desired weight is to be maintained, clients must continue to exercise food control in their day-to-day lives.

In order to assist clients in this process, food control training has introduced the concepts of "calorie units" and the "new scale." Calorie units evaluate a given food not in terms of the calories contained in an individual portion, but in terms of the amount of portions likely to be consumed. This serves as a more reliable predictor of a food's actual energy value and is essential to understanding the reality of control problems. Food control would maintain that a person should eat a food with more calories rather than a food with a history of associated control problems. Eating a higher-calorie food represents a "contained," isolated food choice, while the trigger food tends to reactivate the physiologic and psychological desires for that food.

Food control training recognizes that a lifetime of habituation can be very resistant to change and that newly developed food control skills often require reinforcement. This is achieved by measurement of control on the "new scale." The new scale is actually a self-reported reaffirmation of belief in the principles of food control theory. The questions clients asks themselves on at least a daily basis are:

1. Have I indulged or thought of indulging in any of my trigger foods or situations?
2. Am I abusing, in relation to control, any of the allowable foods in my life?

Table 1. Cognitive Switching

Old Internal Dialogue	Cognitive Switch
"The food looks so tempting."	Do I like it enough to wear it?....I've tasted it all before....It didn't make me happy, it only made me fat.
"I'll just have one."	If I could have just one, why have I been fat for 20 years?....I've been eating for decades and one was never enough. Stop lying to myself....If I don't take the first little taste, if I don't begin, I won't have any problem.
"One pretzel won't hurt."	I've gained more weight with my fingers than with my mouth....Remember, I'm a chain eater with finger foods.
"I've had such a stressful day."	Food is not the answer. Happy or sad, rich or poor, it's still better being thin."
"Those rolls look so good."	Stop looking and glorifying the very food that made me fat....What am I looking at? I know what rolls look like — I'm wearing 10 pounds of them now. It's not free, I have to wear it.
"Those desserts must taste good."	Thin tastes better.
"I'll feel deprived if I don't have a dessert."	The only real deprivation is never being thin....I've already spent 10 years being fat due to eating desserts. I'm living my life backwards. I'm putting a piece of food before my body and my right to be thin and healthy....Was I in paradise when I was eating desserts? No! I was fat and miserable.
"I love pizza."	It's better to wear Italian than to eat it.
"I blew it by eating the french fries, so I stopped trying and trying and ate everything. I was very bad!"	I didn't blow it, I had a break in control. Everyone makes mistakes when learning a new skill. I contain the mistakes and move forward.

Table 1 *(continued).*

Old Internal Dialogue	Cognitive Switch
"Every time I see sweets, I crave them."	A craving is a feeling — not a command. Feelings pass. There'll be no pain, no blood loss. I will not have to call 911 for the rescue squad. Studies show cravings pass in minutes. If I don't negotiate or equivocate, isn't thin worth a few minutes?
"I'm not strong enough to resist."	Did I come this far in my life to take orders from a cookie?
"It's so hard to say no."	It's just a piece of food. I've tasted it all before....Only the thin say, "No thank you."
"I wanted to eat those goodies."	What's so good about them? They've given me obesity, hypertension, and misery....It is not whether they look good, but whether they look good on me.
"I bought it for company, but I ate most of it."	Thin starts in the supermarket. If I don't buy it, I don't have to wear it....I'm the easiest client to help....I've gained all my weight in my own kitchen. If I control what I put in that one room I control my weight.

3. Am I negotiating with food or using "tomorrowisms?"
4. Am I thinking like a fat person and allowing the "foodie-isms" of society to influence my judgment?
5. Am I remembering that thin starts in the supermarket and that finger control is more important than mouth control?

In answering these questions, food control clients are performing the control equivalent of taking their vital signs. The information gained from their answers can then be used to make any behavioral, cognitive, or dietetic changes necessary to maintain food control.

CONCLUSION

Food control theory and training constitute a totally new approach to the problem of weight control which emphasizes the importance of control and cognitive restructuring to weight loss and maintenance. Clinical experience with this program indicates that it is an effective technique both for achieving weight loss and for maintaining goal weight for an extended period of time. More than half of the patients currently enrolled in food control training have achieved their target weights and approximately two-thirds of this group have already maintained their weights for a period of 1 to 3 years. The vast majority of these clients also report that they have experienced no feelings of deprivation in following this type of eating regimen. Although a more detailed study of the experience and characteristics of food control training clients is currently underway, existing clinical evidence indicates that a cognitive-behavioral approach to weight control can have a significantly positive impact on the success of weight loss programs.

REFERENCES

Andersen T, Stockholm KH, Backer OG, Quaade F (1988). Long-term (5-year) results after either horizontal gastroplasty or very-low-calorie diet for morbid obesity. Int J Obesity 12:277-284.

Bandura A (1977). Self-efficacy: toward a unifying theory of behavioral change. Psychol Rev 84:191-215.

Bennett GA (1986). An evaluation of self-instructional training in the treatment of obesity. Addictive Behav 11:125-134.

Birch LL, Marlin DW (1982). I don't like it; I've never tried it: effects of exposure on two-year-old children's food preferences. Appetite 3:353-360.

Bjorval H, Rossner S (1986). Long-term effects of commonly available weight reducing programmes in Sweden. Int J Obesity 11:67-71.

Bray GA (1991). Barriers to the treatment of obesity. Ann Intern Med 115(2):152.

Brownell KD, Marlatt GA, Lichtenstein E, Wilson GT (1986). Understanding and preventing relapse. Am Psychol 41:765-782.

Brownell KD, Jeffery RW (1987). Improving long-term weight loss: pushing the limits of treatment. Behav Ther 18:353-374.

Cairella M (1987). Psychological aspects of the drug treatment of obesity. J Obesity 11:5-11.

Callaway CW (1990). The Callaway diet. New York: Bantam Books.

Davis CM (1928). Self-selection of diet by newly weaned infants. Am J Dis Child 36:651-679.

Diener CI, Dweck CS (1978). An analysis of learned helplessness: continuous changes in performance, strategy and achievement cognitions following failure. J Personality Social Psychol 36:451-462.

DiGuiseppe RA, Miller NJ, Trexler LD (1977). A review of rational-emotive psychotherapy outcome studies. Counseling Psychol 7:64-72.

Dryden W (1984). Training in cognitive psychotherapy. Br J Cognitive Psychother 2(1):34-50.

Dryden W (1989). The use of chaining in rational-emotive therapy. J Rational-Emotive Cognitive Behav Ther 7(2):59-66.

Ellis A (1980). Discomfort anxiety: a new cognitive-behavioral construct. Rational Living 15(1):25-30.

Fatis M, Weiner A, Hawkins J, Van Dorsten B (1989). Following up on a commercial weight loss program: do the pounds stay off even after your picture has been in the newspaper? J Am Dietetic Assoc 89:547-548.

Foch TT, McClearns GE (1980). Genetics, body weight and obesity. In AJ Stunkard, Ed, Obesity. Philadelphia: WB Saunders.

Forster JL, Jeffery RW (1986). Gender differences related to weight history, eating patterns, efficacy expectations, self-esteem and weight loss among participants in a weight reduction program. Addictive Behav 11:141-146.

Garner DM, Garfinkel PE, Bemis KM (1982). A multidimensional psychotherapy for anorexia nervosa. Int J Eating Dis 1:3-64.

Garrow JS, Durant MP, Mann S, Stalley S, Warwick P (1978). Factors determining weight loss in obese clients in a metabolic ward. Int J Obesity 2:441-447.

Harris MB, Waschull S, Walters L (1990). Feeling fat: motivations, knowledge and attitudes of overweight women and men. Psychol Rev 67:1191-1202.

Harris MB (1983). Eating habits, restraint, knowledge and attitudes toward obesity. Int J Obesity 7:271-286.

Herman CP, Mack D (1975). Restrained and unrestrained eating. J Personality 43:647-660.

Herman CP, Polivy J (1980). Restrained and unrestrained eating. J Personality 48:647-672.

Hirsch J (1991). Barriers to treating obesity. Editorial response to GA Bray, Barriers to the treatment of obesity. Ann Intern Med 115(2):152.

Jansen A, Van Den Hout M (1991). On being led into temptation: "counterregulation" of dieters after smelling a "preload." Addictive Behav 16:247-253.

Jeffery DB, Boli D, Leminitzer NB, Hickey JS, Hess MJ, Stroud JM (1980). The impact of television advertising on children's eating behavior: an integrative review. Catalog Select Doc Psychol 10:11 (MS No 2011).

Jeffery RW, Wing RR, Stunkard AJ (1978). Behavioral treatment of obesity. The state of the art in 1976. Behav Ther 15:127-142.

Kalodner CR, DeLucia JL (1991). The individual and combined effects of cognitive therapy and nutrition education as additions to a behavior modification program for weight loss. Addictive Behav 16:255-263.

Keasey RE, Corbett SE (1984). Metabolic defense of the body weight set-point. In AJ Stunkard and E Stellare, Eds, Eating and its disorders. New York: Raven Press.

Klesges RC, Klem ML, Epkins C, Klesges LM (1991). A longitudinal evaluation of dietary restraint and its relationship to changes in body weight. Addictive Behav 16:363-368.

Kramer FM, Jeffery RW, Snell MK, Forster JL (1986). Maintenance of successful weight loss over 1 year: effects of financial contracts for weight maintenance of participation in skills training. Behav Ther 17:295-301.

Kramer FM, Jeffery RW, Forster JL, Snell MK (1989). Long-term follow-up of behavioral treatment for obesity: patterns of weight regain among men and women. Int J Obesity 13:123-126.

Kretchmer N (1978). Human nutrition. San Francisco: WH Freeman.

Leon GR, Roth L, Hewitt MI (1977). Eating patterns, satiety and self-control behavior of obese persons during weight reduction. Obesity Bariatric Med 6:172-181.

Logue AW, Smith ME (1986). Predictors of food preferences in humans. Appetite 6:72-83.

Logue AW (1986). The psychology of eating and drinking. San Francisco: WH Freeman.

Mahoney MJ (1975). The obese eating style: bites, beliefs and behavior modification. Addictive Behav 1:47-53.

Mahoney MJ (1974). Cognition and behavior modification. New York: Ballinger.

Marlatt GA, Gordon JR (1980). Determinants of relapse: implications for the maintenance of behavior change. In PO Davidson and SM Davidson, Eds, Behavioral medicine: changing health styles. New York: Brunner/Mazel.

McReynolds WT, Green L, Fisher EB Jr (1983). Self-control as choice management with reference to the behavioral treatment of obesity. Health Psychol 2:261-276.

Moss ND, Dadds MR (1991). Body weight attributions and eating self-efficacy in adolescence. Addictive Behav 16:71-78.

National Institutes of Health Consensus Development Conference (1985). Health implications of obesity. Bethesda, MD: U.S. Department of Health and Human Services.

National Institutes of Health Technology Assessment Conference (1992). Methods for voluntary weight loss and control. Bethesda, MD: Office of Medical Applications of Research, National Institutes of Health.

Paulsen BK, Lutz RN, McReynolds WT, Kohrs MB (1976). Behavior therapy for weight control: long-term results of two programs with nutritionists as therapists. Am J Clin Nutrition 29:880-888.

Pliner P (1982). The effects of mere exposure on liking for edible substances. Appetite 2:283-290.

Polivy J (1976). Perception of calories and regulation of intake in restrained and unrestrained subjects. Addictive Behav 1:237-243.

Polivy J, Herman CP, Younger JC, Erskine B (1979). Effects of a model on eating behavior: the induction of a restrained eating style. J Personality 47:100-117.

Pudel V (1975). Psychological observations on experimental feeding in the obese. In A Howard, Ed, Recent advances in obesity research. London: Newmann.

Rachlin H (1974). Self-control. Behaviorism 2:94-107.

Rodin J (1974). A sense of control. Psychology Today 18:38-39.

Rodin J, Ellias M, Silberstein LR, Wagner A (1988). Combined behavioral and pharmacological treatment for obesity: predictors of successful weight maintenance. J Consult Clin Psychol 56:390-404.

Rodin J (1981). Current status of the internal-external hypothesis for obesity. What went wrong? Am Psychol 86(4):361-372.

Rolls BJ, Rolls ET, Rowe EA (1982). The influence of variety on human food selection and intake. In LM Barker, Ed, The psychobiology of human food selection. Westport, CT: AVI Publishing.

Ruderman AJ (1986). Dietary restraint: a theoretical and empirical review. Psychol Bull 99(2):247-262.

Saltzer EB (1981). Cognitive moderators of the relationship between behavioral intentions and behavior. J Personality Social Psychol 41:260-271.

Sash SE (1977). Why is the treatment of obesity a failure in modern society? Int J Obesity 1:247-248.

Sjoberg L, Persson L (1979). A study of attempts by obese clients to regulate eating. Addictive Behav 4:349-359.

Stang DJ (1975). When familiarity breeds contempt, absence makes the heart grow fonder: effects of exposure and delay on taste pleasantness ratings. Bull Psychonomics Soc 6:273-275.

Steiner JE (1977). Facial expressions of the neonate infant indicating the hedonics of food-related chemical stimuli. In JM Welffenbach, Ed, Taste and development. Bethesda, MD: US Department of Health, Education and Welfare.

Stuart RB, Guire K (1978). Some correlates of the maintenance of weight loss through behavior modification. Int J Obesity 2:225-275.

Stunkard AJ (1980) Obesity. Philadelphia: WB Saunders.

Stunkard SE (1984). The current status of treatment for obesity in adults. In AJ Stunkard and E Stellar, Eds, Eating and its disorders. New York: Raven Press.

VanItallie TB, Hirsch J (1979). Appraisal of excess calories as a factor in the causation of disease. Am J Clin Nutrition 32:2648-2653.

Wadden TA, Stunkard AJ (1988). Three-year follow-up of the treatment of obesity by very-low-calorie diet, behavior therapy and their combination. J Consult Clin Psychol 56:925-928.

Wadden TA, Stunkard AJ, Brownell KD, Day SC (1985). Advances in the treatment of moderate obesity: combined treatment by behavior modification and very-low-calorie diet. In J Hirsch and TB VanItallie, Eds, Recent advances in obesity research IV. London: John Libbey.

Wadden TA, Sternberg JA, Letizia KA, Stunkard AJ, Forbes GD (1989). Treatment of obesity by very-low-calorie diet, behavior therapy and their combination: a five-year perspective. Int J Obesity 13:39-46.

Wilson GT, Brownell KD (1980). Behavior therapy for obesity: an evaluation of treatment outcome. Advances Behav Res Ther 3.49-86.

Wolfe BL (1992). Long-term maintenance following attainment of goal weight: a preliminary investigation. Addictive Behav 17:469-477.

Woody EZ, Constanzo PR, Liefer H, Conger J (1981). The effects of taste and caloric perceptions on the eating behavior of restrained and unrestrained subjects. Cognitive Ther Res 5:381-390.

Wooley SC, Wooley OW, Dyrenforth SR (1979). Theoretical, practical and social issues in behavioral treatments of obesity. J Appl Behav Analysis 12:3-25.

13

The Stages and Processes of Weight Control: Two Replications

John C. Norcross, PhD, James O. Prochaska, PhD
Carlo C. DiClemente, PhD

Obesity and weight control are serious, prevalent and comparatively refractory health problems that involve the complex interaction of biologic, psychologic and sociologic factors (Brownell 1982). Upwards of 50 million Americans are engaged in attempts to control or alter their eating behaviors because of the immense psychosocial significance and dire health ramifications of being overweight. Outcome results from many controlled studies indicate, however, a rather dismal success rate for long-term sustained weight reduction (Brownell and Jeffrey 1987).

As is now widely known, permanent change of one's eating behavior and dietary pattern is a difficult task indeed. Complicating the clinical and research challenge is the wide range of weight control attitudes, behaviors and goals. Some overweight people are actively dieting and exercising; others are preoccupied with the possibility of weight control but are not dieting; still others refuse to diet or to confront their obesity. Predicting who will engage in weight control programs, designing effective messages to engage individuals and matching efficacious treatments to individual needs all depend on the person's stage of change.

Stage models of personal choice (e.g., Janis and Mann 1977; Velicer et al. 1985), psychotherapy process (e.g., Beitman 1987; Cashdan 1983) and self-change of health behaviors (e.g., Horn 1976; Marlatt and Gordon 1985) have received increased attention of late. One such model, the transtheoretical approach (Prochaska and DiClemente 1984, 1986), posits that individuals progress through four stages of change—precontemplation, contempla-

This work was supported in part by grant CA27821 from the National Cancer Institute.

tion, action and maintenance—and if unsuccessful, they relapse and recycle back through the stages. These distinct but interrelated stages can account for the temporal dimension in both self-initiated and treatment-facilitated change efforts (McConnaughy, Prochaska and Velicer 1983; Prochaska and DiClemente 1992).

According to the transtheoretical model, individuals accomplish behavior change by moving through *stages* of change utilizing specific *processes* of change. Support for this stage-by-process relationship has been consistently found in smoking cessation (Prochaska and DiClemente 1983; DiClemente and Prochaska 1982; DiClemente et al. 1991). Stages have been examined in a variety of other behaviors, including head injury rehabilitation (Lam et al. 1988), alcoholism treatment (DiClemente and Hughes 1990), exercise acquisition (Marcus et al. 1992) and sunscreen use (Rossi 1989). Once the stages of change are established for a particular behavior, the relationship between the stages and processes of change can be examined. Furthermore, the stage of change can help determine the intervention of choice and can reliably predict client outcome (see reviews by Prochaska and DiClemente 1992; Prochaska, DiClemente and Norcross 1992).

The stages of change can be briefly characterized as follows (Prochaska, DiClemente and Norcross 1992). *Precontemplation* is the stage in which there is no intention to change behavior in the foreseeable future. Most individuals in this stage are unaware or underaware of their problems. *Contemplation* is the stage in which people are aware that a problem exists and are seriously thinking about overcoming it, but have not yet made a commitment to take action. Serious consideration of problem resolution is the central element of contemplation. *Action* is the stage in which individuals modify their behavior, experiences and/or environment in order to overcome their problems. Modification of the target behavior to an acceptable criterion and significant overt efforts to change are the hallmarks of action. *Maintenance* is the stage in which people work to prevent relapse and consolidate the gains attained during action. For addictive behaviors this stage extends from 6 months to an indeterminate, if not lifetime, period beyond the initial action.

Two methods are currently used to assess the stages of change. A categorical algorithm can be used to classify the person based on several questions inquiring about intention and activity related to changing a particular behavior. This method creates a discrete, mutually exclusive categorization (Prochaska, Norcross and DiClemente 1994). A stage of change questionnaire, called the URICA, yields continuous scores on each stage. This method generates a profile analysis, often using a cluster-analytic procedure and the stage is determined by the most endorsed stage or peak stage (McConnaughy, Prochaska and Velicer 1983; DiClemente and Hughes 1990).

Prochaska and DiClemente (1983), using the categorical algorithm, found that change processes received differential utilization during particular stages of change among smokers and ex-smokers. Specifically, these self-changers used the fewest change processes during precontemplation; emphasized consciousness-raising and dramatic relief during contemplation; emphasized self-liberation, helping relationship and contingency control during action; and used counterconditioning and stimulus control the most in both action and maintenance. Dynamic typologies assessing stage-by-process interactions in smoking cessation show dramatic differences in process activity as people move through the stages of change (Prochaska, Velicer, DiClemente, Guadagnoli and Rossi 1991). These and similar findings suggest that therapeutic interventions need to be tailored not just to the presenting problem, but also to the stage of change. Before that, however, we also need "comparative studies with other problem behaviors to determine the extent to which change processes vary in emphasis as different problem behaviors are being changed" (Prochaska and DiClemente 1983, p. 395).

The present studies attempted to replicate the previous pattern of results and to extend them to the self-initiated and treatment-facilitated modification of body weight. This research applied the transtheoretical model cross-sectionally to investigate the interaction of the stages and processes of change in two populations of obese adults. The stage-by-process relationship will be examined by utilizing a categorical stage classification in one study and the URICA/peak-stage method in the other.

STUDY 1

Method

Participants. Adults from Rhode Island and Texas volunteered to participate in a self-change study in response to newspaper advertisements and articles. Participants were paid $4.00 and became eligible for lottery prizes in return for completing the questionnaire. A total of 608 participants completed the weight control questionnaire. However, 193 of these (32 percent) reported never having weighed 10 percent or more than their ideal weight and were excluded from the study. The remaining 415 participants were asked a series of mutually exclusive questions to determine their current stage of change (DiClemente et al. 1991). All but two (n = 413) were then assigned to one of the following groups.

Precontemplators (PC). Only 9 participants (7 women, 2 men) represented the precontemplation stage, defined as currently weighing 10 percent or more than their ideal weight and reporting no intention of losing weight in the next year. This group was omitted from statistical analyses due to inadequate sample size.

Contemplators (C). These 69 participants (49 women, 20 men) represented the contemplation stage, since they were currently 10 percent or more over their ideal weight, were not actively trying to lose weight, but reported seriously considering trying to lose weight in the next 6 months. The average current weight was 186.8 pounds (SD = 45.4) and the average ideal weight was 146.3 pounds (SD = 30.5), with a mean of 21 percent over their ideal weight.

Action (A). These 191 participants (149 women, 42 men) represented the action stage, defined as currently weighing 10 percent or more than the ideal weight and actively trying to lose weight. The average current weight was 159.6 pounds (SD = 54.1), the average ideal weight was 137.8 pounds (SD = 41.5), with an average 20 percent over their ideal weight.

Maintainers (M). These 102 participants (66 women, 36 men) represented the maintenance stage, since they had previously weighed 10 percent or more than their ideal weight but currently were within 10 percent of their ideal weight and reported trying to maintain the same weight level. These participants had maintained their weight loss for at least 6 months. The average current weight of this group was 144.6 pounds (SD = 29.2), the average ideal weight was 138.4 pounds (SD = 26.5), with an average of 4 percent over their ideal weight.

Relapsers (R). Forty-two participants (30 women, 12 men) represented a relapse group, defined as having lost weight in the past year but then having regained it. The average current weight for this group was 144.6 pounds (SD = 22.3) and the average ideal weight was 135.0 (SD = 21.1).

Demographic data for the entire sample indicated that the participants were largely middle-age and middle income white adults. The mean age was 42.2 years (SD = 12.2) with a range from 18 to 75. Twenty percent of the total sample had a high school education or less, 41 percent had some college, 20 percent had a college degree and 18 percent had some postgraduate education or a graduate degree. Practically all (97 percent) of the participants were Caucasian.

Instruments

The Weight Control Processes of Change Scale (WCPS) is a 60-item, Likert-type instrument that measures 11 change processes in a statistically well-defined and highly reliable manner (Prochaska and DiClemente 1983, 1985; Prochaska, Velicer, DiClemente and Fava 1988). The change processes have been labeled: consciousness-raising, self-liberation, social liberation, self-reevaluation, environmental reevaluation, counterconditioning, stimulus control, reinforcement management, dramatic relief, helping relationship and substance use. Analyses of response distortions on the processes of change scores have found no evidence for centrality, extremity, or halo effects (Prochaska et al. 1988). In the WCPS, participants rated how frequently they use each item on a five-point scale (1 = never; 2 = seldom; 3 = occasionally; 4 = often; 5 = repeatedly).

The 60×60 item correlation matrix (n = 413) was subjected to a principal component analysis. The multiple average partial (MAP) procedure (Velicer 1976; Zwick and Velicer 1986) indicated that 10 components merited retention and these were then rotated to an orthogonal solution. The 10 components accounted for 66.4 percent of the total variance. Fifty-two items loaded .40 or greater on only one component, five items were complex (i.e., loaded .40 or greater on two or more components) and three items were singular (i.e., loaded less than .40 on any component).

The resultant components closely resembled the original 11 processes. Self-liberation and self-reevaluation items merged into one large component. The reinforcement management items combined with several others to form an expanded dimension labeled contingency control. The remaining eight components represented the other change processes and were so named. Estimates of internal consistency (alpha) ranged between .68 and .97 and averaged .82. Table 1 presents sample items and the alpha coefficients of the 10 processes.

Weight Measures. Participants answered 10 items concerning their weight history and intentions. Items included current weight, ideal weight, heaviest lifetime weight, past and present attempts to lose weight, current goals and plans about weight control.

Self-report measures of physical weight were utilized and considered preferable in this study for several reasons. First, self-report measures were available for all participants. Second, the inclusion criterion was the relative difference between the participants' current (or heaviest lifetime) weight and their self-perceived ideal weight, not pounds based on actuarial tables. Third, inclusion criteria depended on prior weights not subject to current measurement.

Results

A multivariate analysis of variance (MANOVA) was performed on the 10 change processes across the four groups representing the contemplation, action, maintenance and relapse stages. The MANOVA was statistically significant [$F (30, 1148) = 6.25, p < .001$, Wilk's value = .64] and was followed by separate ANOVAs since the change processes have been found to be relatively independent (Prochaska et al. 1988) and since the ANOVAs more clearly communicated the results than a discriminant function analysis.

Table 2 presents the T scores, ANOVA results, and group comparisons on each of the 10 processes of change. Nine of the 10 ANOVAs were statistically significant and were examined further by Newman-Keuls comparisons ($p < .05$). On all the significant ANOVAs except contingency control, the maintainers reported using significantly less of the change

Table 1. Sample Items and Alpha Coefficients for the Processes of Change

Process	Alpha Coefficients		Sample Item
	Study 1	Study 2	
Self-Liberation and Reevaluation	.94	.79	I make commitments to lose weight.
Dramatic Relief	.91	.86	Warnings about health hazards of being overweight move me emotionally.
Stimulus Control	.87	.78	I keep things around my place of work that remind me not to eat.
Substance Use	.97	.77	I take diet aids to help me lose weight.
Counterconditioning	.80	.77	I do something other than eating when I need to relax or deal with tension.
Contingency Control	.71	.73	I am rewarded by others if I don't overeat.
Helping Relationship	.78	.90	I have someone whom I can count on when I have problems with overeating.
Environmental Reevaluation	.76	.84	I stop and think that I am eating more than my share of the world's food.
Consciousness Raising	.78	.81	I read about people who successfully lose weight.
Social Liberation	.68	.57	I find society more supportive of thin people.
Self-Blame	-	.88	I blame myself for overeating.
Minimize Threat	-	.76	I make light of my weight situation; I refuse to get too serious about it.
Wishful Thinking	-	.72	I wish that I could change what happens with my weight.

Table 2. T Scores, ANOVA Results, and Group Comparisons of the Processes of Change (Study 1)

| Process | Group Mean | | | | $F(3,400)$ | Significant Group Differences |
	C (n=69)	A (n=191)	M (n=102)	R (n=42)		
Self-Liberation and Reevaluation	50.5	54.5	42.0	50.6	46.9 ***	A > RL, C > M
Dramatic Relief	52.5	51.9	45.9	48.5	10.6 ***	C, A > RL > M
Stimulus Control	49.9	51.8	47.7	49.2	3.9 **	A > M
Substance Use	48.6	52.2	47.2	49.9	6.1 ***	A > C, M
Counterconditioning	49.9	52.8	45.6	50.0	12.6 ***	A, RL, C > M
Contingency Control	48.1	51.6	45.1	54.8	17.4 ***	M > A > RL, C
Helping Relationship	48.9	52.1	47.0	50.2	6.6 ***	A > M
Environmental Reevaluation	49.9	49.9	50.1	50.8	1.1 *	
Consciousness Raising	50.3	52.9	45.1	49.7	15.0 ***	A, C, RL > M
Social Liberation	52.5	52.2	45.0	49.6	14.7 ***	C, A, RL > M

C = contemplation, A = action, M = maintenance, R = relapse

* p < .05 ** p < .01 *** p < .001

process. Participants in the action and contemplation stages generally reported employing the various change processes most frequently. This pattern closely parallels the earlier findings on smoking cessation. In no case did the recent relapsers employ the process most frequently.

The relationships between the processes of change and the stages of change are clearer if the relapser group is temporarily dismissed. The relapsers were included as an exploratory group without a priori predictions. Equally importantly, the results indicate that relapsers behave rather uniquely.

Despite stage disparities in utilization of the change processes, there was a consistent pattern of employment. Social liberation (M = 3.6), helping relationship (M = 3.4) and self-liberation (M = 3.1) were the processes used most frequently across groups for weight control, as indicated by mean scores between 3 (occasionally) and 4 (frequently) on the five-point response scale. By contrast, substance use (1.3), environmental reevaluation (1.5), stimulus control (1.7) and contingency control (1.9) were used the least frequently in weight control, all with mean scores below 2 (rarely).

STUDY 2

Method

Participants. The initial sample was composed of 104 hospital staff members in Rhode Island who enrolled in a work-site behavioral program for weight control and who completed all pretreatment research measures. The clients were recruited through announcements enclosed in the payroll, rosters displayed throughout the hospital and articles published in the hospital newsletters. All data reported in this study were collected prior to active treatment (see Prochaska, Norcross, Fowler, Follick and Abrams 1992 for a summary of the treatment study). All participants were at least 10 percent overweight as calculated by the revised Metropolitan Life Insurance Norms (1983). The average percent overweight for the sample was 35 percent (SD = 21) and ranged between 10 and 114 percent.

The 104 clients completed the stages of change (or URICA) questionnaire, which provides scores for each of the stages. Only subjects who had a clear peak scale were classified. Using this method, six could not be reliably classified in terms of their stage and five were in the precontemplation stage; both these groups were omitted from the statistical analyses. The remaining 93 clients were categorized on the basis of their highest scale scores as being in the contemplation stage (n = 59), action stage (n = 21) and maintenance stage (n = 13). There were no significant differences among the three groups on average current weight or on average normative weight.

Demographically, 91 percent of the sample was female; 63 percent were married and 19 percent were never married. The mean age was 40 years and the average years of formal education was 14.7. Most (95 percent) of the clients were Caucasian.

Instruments

The same weight control processes of change scale was administered as in Study 1 with the addition of three subscales. Self-blame, wishful thinking and minimize threat—three "emotion-focused" coping methods derived from the Ways of Coping Checklist (Folkman and Lazarus 1980, 1986)— were included since they tap relatively defensive and affective coping strategies not assessed by the processes of change scale. Items were tailored to weight control and participants responded on the same five-point Likert scale in terms of frequency of use during the past month (1 = never; 5 = repeatedly). In this sample, the internal consistency (alpha) coefficients of the scales ranged from .57 to .90 and averaged .78 (see Table 1).

The Stages of Change (or URICA) Questionnaire, a 32-item instrument, assesses four robust and statistically well-defined stages: precontemplation, contemplation, action and maintenance (McConnaughy, Prochaska and Velicer 1983; McConnaughy, DiClemente, Prochaska and Velicer 1989). The instrument was developed and validated with a sample of 150 clients presenting for outpatient psychotherapy and cross-validated with another sample of 350 adults. Clients responded to a weight control version of this scale using a five-point Likert format in which 1 = strongly disagree and 5 = strongly agree.

Results

A MANOVA was performed on the change processes across the three groups of participants representing the contemplation, action and maintenance stages of change. The significant MANOVA (p < .05, Wilk's value = .58) was followed by univariate ANOVAs, four of which were statistically significant (p < .05). The mean scores and significant group differences (Newman-Keuls p < .05), as shown in Table 3, reveal that efforts to minimize threat are the most pronounced during contemplation. Helping relationships are used significantly more during both contemplation and action than during maintenance. Counterconditioning and stimulus control are favored by participants in the action stage.

DISCUSSION

These results provide further evidence of the differential utilization of change processes across the stages of change and additional support for developmental-temporal models of weight control. Despite differences between the two studies in method of weight assessment (self-report vs.

Table 3. Mean Scores and Group Comparisons of Significantly Different Processes of Change (Study 2)

Process	Group Mean C (n=59)	A (n=21)	M (n=13)	F (2,900)	Significant Group Differences
Stimulus Control	1.8	2.4	2.1	3.6*	A > M > C
Counterconditioning	2.5	3.0	2.6	3.6*	A > M, C
Helping Relationship	3.4	3.8	2.8	3.8*	A, C > M
Minimize Threat	2.4	2.1	2.0	5.8*	C > A, M

C = contemplation, A = action, M = maintenance
* p < .05, ** p < .01

Table 4.   Stages of Change in which Processes of Change are Most
Emphasized

Contemplation	Action	Maintenance

Minimize Threat
      Dramatic Relief
      Helping Relationship
      Consciousness Raising
      Social Liberation

                              Self-Liberation
                              & Reevaluation
                              Stimulus Control
                              Substance Use
                              Counterconditioning
                                          Contingency Control

physical measurement), in time perspective (retrospective vs. current), in measure of stage of change (discrete categorical measure vs. continuous measure) and in method of behavior change (self-mediated vs. treatment-facilitated), the stages and processes interaction for obese adults in both investigations was quite similar. Compared to previous findings with smokers, the current patterns of process utilization in weight reduction provide essential replications with a few twists.

Table 4 presents a schematic interaction of the processes of change and the stages of change in weight control. Specifically, this table shows the stages in which particular processes of change are emphasized the most. The contemplation stage is characterized by threat minimization. Dramatic relief, helping relationships, consciousness-raising and social liberation appear to bridge contemplation and action insofar as they are emphasized equally in both stages. When individuals commit to action, self-liberation, stimulus control, substance use and counterconditioning are differentially emphasized. Contingency control then bridges the action and maintenance stages. No change process in either study was used most often by obese adults in the maintenance stage. The absence of any change process distinctive to maintenance portends future difficulties in maintaining weight control and poses serious challenges to relapse prevention plans.

The results of these two studies support using a transtheoretical model in weight control. The first study replicated for obese adults what has been found repeatedly for smokers and the cross-behavior consistency provides strong support for a stage by process interaction. The second study demonstrated stage differences among a treatment-seeking sample using a different method of stage assessment and adds further support for using a change process analysis to study weight control. This focus on the mechanism of behavior change may enlarge our understanding of achieving and maintaining weight loss and may also enhance prescriptive matching of interventions to the individual patient's stage of change (see, for example, DiClemente 1992; Norcross 1991; Prochaska 1991).

REFERENCES

Beitman BD (1987). The structure of individual psychotherapy. New York: Guilford Press.

Brownell KD (1982). Obesity: understanding and treating a serious, prevalent and refractory disorder. J Consulting Clin Psychol 50:820-840.

Brownell KD, Jeffrey RW (1987). Improving long-term weight loss: pushing the limits of treatment. Behav Ther 18:353-374.

Cashdan S (1983). Interactional psychotherapy: stages and strategies in behavioral change. New York: Grune & Stratton.

DiClemente CC (1992). Motivational interviewing and the stages of change. In WR Miller and S Rollnick, Eds, Motivational interviewing: preparing people for change. New York: Guilford Press.

DiClemente CC, Hughes SL (1990). Stages of change profiles in alcoholism treatment. J Substance Abuse 2:217-235.

DiClemente CC, Prochaska JO (1982). Self-change and therapy change of smoking behavior: a comparison of processes of change in cessation and maintenance. Addictive Behav 7:133-142.

DiClemente CC, Prochaska JO, Fairhurst SK, Velicer WF, Velasques MM, Rossi JS (1991). The process of smoking cessation: an analysis of precontemplation, contemplation and preparation stages of change. J Consulting Clin Psychol 59:295-304.

Folkman S, Lazarus R (1980). An analysis of coping in a middle-aged community sample. J Health Social Behav 21:219-239.

Folkman S, Lazarus RS (1986). Stress processes and depressive symptomatology. J Abnormal Psychol 95:107-113.

Horn D (1976). A model for the study of personal choice behavior. Int J Addictions 19:89-98.

Janis IL, Mann L (1977). Decision making: a psychological analysis of conflict, choice and commitment. New York: Free Press.

Lam CS, McMahon BT, Priddy DA, Gehred-Schultz A (1988). Deficit awareness and treatment performance among traumatic head injury adults. Brain Injury 2:235-242.

Marcus BH, Rossi JS, Selby VC, Niaura RS, Abrams DB (1992). The stages and processes of exercise adoption and maintenance. Health Psychol 11:386-395.

Marlatt GA, Gordon JR (1985). Relapse prevention: a self-control strategy for the maintenance of behavior change. New York: Guilford Press.

McConnaughy EA, DiClemente CC, Prochaska JO, Velicer WF (1989). Stages of change in psychotherapy: a follow-up report. Psychotherapy 26:494-503.

McConnaughy EA, Prochaska JO, Velicer WF (1983). Stages of change in psychotherapy: measurement and sample profiles. Psychotherapy 20:368-375.

Metropolitan Life Insurance Company (1983). Revised standards for overweight. New York: Metropolitan Life Insurance Company.

Norcross JC (1991). Prescriptive matching in psychotherapy: psychoanalysis for simple phobias? Psychotherapy 28:439-443.

Prochaska JO (1991). Prescribing to the stage and level of phobic patients. Psychotherapy 28:463-468.

Prochaska JO, DiClemente CC (1983). Stages and processes of self-change of smoking: toward an integrative model of change. J Consulting Clin Psychol 5:390-395.

Prochaska JO, DiClemente CC (1984). The transtheoretical approach: crossing traditional boundaries of therapy. Chicago: Dow Jones/Irwin.

Prochaska JO, DiClemente CC (1985). Common processes of self-change in smoking, weight control and psychological distress. In S Shiffman and T Wells, Eds, Coping and substance abuse. New York: Academic Press.

Prochaska JO, DiClemente CC (1986). Toward a comprehensive model of change. In W Miller and N Heather, Eds, Treating addictive behaviors: processes of change. New York: Plenum.

Prochaska JO, DiClemente CC (1992). The transtheoretical approach. In JC Norcross and MR Goldfried, Eds, Handbook of psychotherapy integration. New York: Basic Books.

Prochaska JO, DiClemente CC (1992). Stages of change in the modification of problem behaviors. In M Hersen, RM Eisler and PM Mokker, Eds, Progress in behavior modification. Sycamore, IL: Sycamore.

Prochaska JO, DiClemente CC, (1994). Changing for good. New York: William Morrow.

Prochaska JO, DiClemente CC, Norcross JC (1992). In search of how people change: applications to addictive behaviors. Am Psychologist 47:1102-1114.

Prochaska JO, DiClemente CC, Velicer WF, Ginpil S, Norcross JC (1985). Predicting change in smoking status for self-changers. Addictive Behav 10:395-406.

Prochaska JO, Norcross JC, Fowler JL, Follick MJ, Abrams DB (1992). Attendance and outcome in work site weight control program: processes and stages of change as process and predictor variables. Addictive Behav 17:35-45.

Prochaska JO, Velicer WF, DiClemente CC, Fava J (1988). Measuring the processes of change: applications to the cessation of smoking. J Consulting Clin Psychol 56:520-528.

Prochaska JO, Velicer WF, DiClemente CC, Guadagnoli E, Rossi JS (1991). Patterns of change: dynamic typology applied to smoking cessation. Multivariate Behav Res 26:83-107.

Rossi JS (1989). The hazards of sunlight: a report of the Consensus Development Conference. Health Psychologist 11:3-7.

Velicer WF (1976). Determining the number of components from the matrix of partial correlations. Psychometrika 41:321-327.

Velicer WF, DiClemente CC, Prochaska JO, Brandenburg N (1985). A decisional balance measure for assessing and predicting smoking status. J Personality Social Psychol 48:1279-1289.

Zwick WR, Velicer WF (1986). Comparison of five rules for determining the number of components to retain. Psychol Bull 99:432-444.

14

Compulsive Eating: Applying a Medical Addiction Model

Ellen S. Parham, PhD, RD

...this sandwich triggered off something in me. I don't know why it is, but this has happened to me before; that's why when I go on a diet it's best for me to just drink liquids; then this *craving* for all sorts of yummy foods doesn't get to me. Well, I gave in just a little.... I couldn't stop, I was so hungry... (Roth 1982, p. 89).

The woman quoted above is a compulsive eater,* describing her experience of losing control over eating. If she is like many other compulsive eaters, she will also describe herself as addicted to a particular food or to food in general. Does the behavior she describes fit a medical model of substance dependence? This chapter will examine the evidence supporting and refuting such an application of the addiction model.

DEFINITION OF TWO KEY CONCEPTS

Wardle describes compulsive eating (CE) as "a disturbed eating pattern with an excessive food intake and abnormalities of hunger and satiety" (1987, p.47) and considers CE as almost synonymous with binge eating which, in turn, is described in the DSM III-R definition of bulimia (1987, p.64) as "rapid consumption of a large amount of food in a discrete period of time." The DSM IV adds the specificity that binge eating is recurrent, involves amounts of food definitely larger than what is eaten by most people in a finite (2-hour) period and is accompanied by a sense of lack of control. Bulimics practice binge/purge behavior, but not all compulsive

---

* Although the designation binge eating disorder (BED) has come into wide use, this chapter uses the term compulsive eating (CE) as a means of emphasizing the possible addiction connection.

eaters purge or otherwise compensate for their binge and therefore, do not meet the criteria for bulimia (Wardle 1987; White 1991). It is anticipated that the DSM IV will include a new category, binge eating disorder, that will distinguish noncompensating binge eaters from bulimics (Fairburn and Wilson 1993). In spite of the support that has led to the potential recognition of binge eating disorder, there is still widespread consideration of binge or compulsive eating as a form of addiction (Wilson 1993).

According to White (1991), CE may take the form not only of binge eating, but also of overeating at meals or of graze eating. The meal-time compulsive eater starts the meal with hunger, but eats far beyond satisfaction at several meals per day. Grazers pick at food constantly or during a few hours daily, never allowing themselves to experience hunger. Although these two types of behavior meet some of the criteria for the disorder proposed for the DSM IV, it is not clear that they would satisfy the criterion related to the amount of food consumed at one time.

Obviously, if practiced frequently and if not accompanied by compensatory behavior, CE will lead to obesity, but only 20 to 30 percent of obese persons who present for treatment are compulsive eaters (Spitzer et al. 1992; Marcus 1993). Females are over-represented among compulsive eaters (Kagan and Squires 1984; Spitzer et al. 1992). This chapter will focus on this group of obese, mostly female, compulsive eaters.

Although various addiction models are currently in use (Lewis, Dana and Blevins 1988), the medical or addiction-as-disease (AAD) model, with its emphasis upon a biologic vulnerability to the substance in question, is the most applicable for this examination because it is a guiding principle of Overeaters Anonymous (OA) (Yeary 1987), the most prominent example of treatment of CE in the United States at this time (Wilson 1991). The AAD model assumes that addiction is the product of a defect, usually thought to be genetic, that alters the individual's response to the substance under question. Having this vulnerability is thought to condemn the individual to inevitable loss of control whenever the substance is used. Therefore, total abstinence is necessary. Since total abstinence from food is impossible, compulsive eaters may be urged to discover which particular food items they are addicted to. White sugar and white flour are often suggested as good candidates for the offending foods (McDowell 1980). The AAD model further assumes that the addiction is irreversible and follows a progression with distinct phases (Lewis, Dana and Blevins 1988).

According to the DSM III-R (1987), diagnosis of substance dependence requires that the individual display at least three of a list of nine characteristics. Six of these reflect various aspects of a pathologic pattern of usage, whereas the remainder reflect tolerance and withdrawal experiences. Symptoms must have persisted for at least a month or have occurred repeatedly over a longer time. These criteria are not model-specific. Therefore, this chapter will consider first whether food can be considered psychoactive and then will examine evidence not only for the occurrence of these criteria among compulsive eaters, but also for a biologic vulnerability that predisposes to the development of the dependence.

FOOD AS A PSYCHOACTIVE SUBSTANCE

The DSM III-R (1987) does not use the term addiction, but instead refers to dependence on psychoactive substances. In the revision of DSM III there was apparently an effort to exclude food from consideration as an addictive substance through the substitution of the term "psychoactive substance" for the earlier used and more generic term substance (Rounsaville, Spitzer and Williams 1986).

Should food be considered psychoactive? There is no question that eating can affect mood, that severe deficiencies of certain vitamins are characterized by dementia and that starvation, whether in a famine victim or an anorexic adolescent, produces a characteristic loss of rationality (Mahan and Arlin 1992). In searching for an intoxicating effect of CE, we obviously can eliminate those effects associated with undereating. Further, although foods selected by compulsive eaters most frequently are items with low nutrient density, the sheer quantity is such that nutrient deficiencies are unlikely.

Hypoglycemic Responses as Intoxication

The popular notion of food as a psychoactive substance involves a sensitive individual eating particular foods, usually white sugar and/or white flour and experiencing a sudden elevation of blood glucose (McDowell 1980). This effect feels at least mildly good, but is fleeting (lasting about an hour), being followed by low glucose levels produced by overcompensation in insulin release. The resulting hypoglycemia is accompanied by feelings of being tired, jittery, anxious, confused, dizzy or worse. The individual then eats again to relieve the symptoms and to return to the better feeling associated with the high glucose levels. Anticipation of the cycle may soon lead to avoiding it by continuous eating or by eating huge quantities.

Controlled observations show that in response to the ordinary sporadic eating patterns of meal-eating humans, blood levels of glucose rise sharply after eating and fall slowly to the fasting level (Mahan and Arlin 1992). Monitoring of these fluctuations is one of the several mechanisms the body uses to trigger hunger and satiety. Normally, the rise and fall in glucose levels are closely regulated by the reciprocal actions of insulin and glucagon even when eating is irregular or when the quantity or nature of the food eaten varies widely.

Although the mental and emotional effects of hypoglycemia are well-documented (Taylor and Rachman 1988), only a few individuals who experience the symptoms are confirmed as hypoglycemic when given a 5-hour glucose tolerance test, the explanation probably being that the symptoms overlap those of a general response to stress (Mahan and Arlin 1992). Reactive hypoglycemia can be readily diagnosed and treated with a diet similar to that used with diabetes mellitus. Should a hypoglycemic state occur, it can be corrected with a modest amount of food, such as a glass of juice. Studies of the effect of individual foods on glucose levels indicate that white sugar and flour are no more likely to produce an intoxicating hypoglycemic state than their less-processed analogs or than any other carbohydrate-rich food (Jenkins, Wolever and Jenkins 1988).

Dietary Influences on Neurotransmitters as Intoxication

Wurtman's group (Lieberman, Wurtman and Chew 1986) has identified two distinct groups of obese individuals who practice compulsive eating of the grazing form—carbohydrate cravers and noncravers. The two groups differ in their mood response to high-carbohydrate foods. The cravers feel less depressed after eating, whereas the noncravers report feeling both more depressed and more fatigued and sleepy. In contrast to those who support a hypoglycemic mechanism, Wurtman's group suggests that changes in serotoninergic neurotransmission in the cravers may be responsible for their snacking behavior. The increased carbohydrate intake may represent an attempt to enhance serotonin transmission centrally. Eating carbohydrate lowers the levels of substances competing with tryptophan, the precursor of serotonin, for transport across the blood/brain barrier and thereby promotes serotonin synthesis in the brain. Normally, the raised serotonin levels are associated with satiety, especially for carbohydrates (Wurtman 1987).

Although they do not suggest it as evidence of intoxicating properties, Drewnowski and co-workers (1992) found that the opioid antagonist naloxone had a significantly greater effect on the taste preferences and food consumption of binge eaters than of control subjects. Consistent with the general understanding that endogenous opioids stimulate food intake, naloxone reduced taste pleasantness and reduced voluntary consumption of offered snacks. The consumption effect was most pronounced for sweet, high-fat foods, foods often selected for binges.

Mitchell (1990) reviewed the evidence of abnormalities in control of serotonin and several other neurotransmitters as part of the psychobiology of bulimia nervosa and concluded that understanding is still at the theory-building stage. He notes that several investigators have found responders and nonresponders, suggesting a heterogeneity among the bulimics studied. Heterogeneity often obscures reality and makes interpretation difficult. Presumably, his observations apply generally to compulsive eating.

EVIDENCE OF FOOD DEPENDENCE
AMONG COMPULSIVE EATERS

Inability to Cut Down or Stop

The description of pathologic use patterns as part of dependence includes the inability to cut down or stop usage. Personal accounts of compulsive eaters speak of feeling driven and helpless to change their eating behavior (Roth 1982). Herman and Polivy (1984) state that binge eating stops not when eating becomes unpleasant, but when it becomes impossible. However, Wilson (1991) reviews several studies that have observed that under some circumstances almost all compulsive eaters do control their eating.

Temporary Abstinence or Restriction

Numerous independent observations strongly establish that CE meets the temporary abstinence or restriction characteristic of substance dependence. Yanovski (1993) has pointed out that there is a high level of dieting among binge eaters, apparently as a compensatory response. Alternation of binge eating with periods of inappropriate compensatory behavior such as purging, rigid dieting, or fasting is part of the diagnostic criteria for bulimia, but not of binge eating disorder (Fairburn and Wilson 1993).

Herman and his colleagues (Herman and Polivy 1984; Wardle 1987; Heatherton, Polivy and Herman 1991) have developed the concept of dietary restraint to describe individuals who use cognitive processes to attempt to restrict their food intake in order to achieve or maintain a lower weight. Restrained eaters have been observed to vacillate between periods of intense caloric restriction and bouts of disinhibited eating. Binge eaters score higher on the disinhibition and hunger sections than on the restraint section of the Three-Factor Eating Inventory (Yanovski 1993).

Continued Use Despite Serious Physical Disorders

Compulsive eaters who do not purge are at risk of weight gain and its effects on mental and physical well-being (Brownell and Wadden 1992). Although purging and other compensatory behaviors may help to avoid fatness, they do so at the cost of other health impairments (Mitchell 1990). It is clear that the experience of serious health impairments does not end CE.

Daily Need in Order to Function

The common understanding of CE is that it serves as a means of buffering emotional pain, reducing anxiety, coping with stress, or expressing hostility. Orbach (1978) explained that CE is an almost exclusively female disorder because the social conditioning of women to play subordinate roles con-tributes to feelings of anger and hostility, but deprives females of acceptable means of expressing these feelings. Stuffing food is seen as a means of stuffing down emotions.

Kagan and Squires (1984) demonstrated this relationship through a survey of college students, finding a positive correlation between several measures of hostility and CE practices, especially among females. They concluded that CE was like an addiction, a narcotic that the users depended upon to cope.

On the other hand, Katzman (1989) compared hourly reports of eating and feelings of stress experienced by bulimic and control college women during the midterm examination period. Stress levels reported by bulimics were higher chronically, as well as before and after eating. There was no evidence that stress was highest before eating or that it was reduced by eating. Just anticipating eating may have reduced anxiety. Moreover, given the extreme level of anxiety about weight that almost always accompanies CE, it is not surprising that stress was higher after eating. Undoubtedly, the immediate gratification of eating is a stronger motivator than the guilt that follows.

Heatherton and Baumeister (1991), in a major critical review of the literature, concluded that binge eating is motivated by a desire to escape from self-awareness. Binge eaters are characterized by the perception of a major and insurmountable discrepancy between what they are and what they should be. Weight or fatness becomes a symbol of this gulf. Falling far short of their own standards, they develop an acute but extremely negative self-awareness. Their binge is accompanied by focus on immediate stimuli, low-level or deconstructed thinking and rejection of meaningful thought. The authors noted that some treatment programs that focus on reducing CE without dealing with the cognitive processes and causes that set the escapist pattern in motion are associated with increases in alcohol and drug abuse among their patients.

Use Patterns That Interfere With Social/Occupational Functioning

Stunkard (1955) described night eaters who eat little or nothing throughout the day, but consume huge quantities late at night, sometimes staying up alone until 2 or 3 a.m. to eat. Some wake up in the night and get up to eat. Stunkard described night eating among 80 percent of his obese patients in a psychiatric service, but in a more diverse cross-section of obese persons night eating is much more rare, this author having seen only one case among more than 200 individuals participating in a community weight management program. Much more common are the practices of maintain-ing hidden hordes of food and eating in secrecy.

Cathy is a slim young bulimic: "Visions of cookies and chocolate eclairs appear in front of me as I'm trying to do my work....We went on this wonderful honeymoon and even while we were making love all I could think of was when would we stop so that I could eat" (Meadow and Weiss 1992).

In our weight-conscious and puritanic culture eating huge amounts of food is highly unacceptable. Compulsive eaters feel horror at their behavior and go great lengths to hide it (Roth 1982). This results in social contortions to provide the opportunity for CE.

Tolerance

One characteristic of addiction is the requirement of increasingly higher levels to get the effect. Some compulsive eaters start quite suddenly to binge, while others increase their eating more gradually. Nevertheless, there is a tendency to increase the amount or the frequency of uncontrolled eating. There are well-documented physiologic responses to a continued energy intake beyond expenditure (Brownell and Wadden 1992). These include an increase in metabolic rate (but not so great as to prevent fat accumulation in most cases) and increases in the size and number of fat cells. These changes accompany any prolonged overeating and are not specific to CE.

More specific to CE is the observation by Geliebter and co-workers (1992) that binge eaters had an enlarged stomach capacity. Since one component of satiety is triggered by stomach distention, this enlargement could not only make it possible to eat more, but also could lessen satiety. The investigators were unable to determine whether the stomach enlargement was a cause or effect of the binge eating.

Withdrawal

In the case of CE, withdrawal must be modified to mean avoidance of certain foods or certain behaviors (binges) or restriction of intake to a certain level or diet pattern. Although these constraints can be highly disturbing psychologically, there is little or no evidence of physiologic withdrawal symptoms specific to CE.

Reducing one's energy intake to below energy expenditure will result in loss of fat stores. As fat cells shrink and the body otherwise responds to the negative energy balance, the body's homeostatic systems are activated, reducing the metabolic rate and increasing food-seeking behavior (Brownell and Wadden 1992). These processes occur not only in emaciated people, but also in the obese and are sometimes interpreted as evidence of a setpoint for fatness. However, once again we must note that these processes are not exclusive to withdrawal from CE, but are responsive to any undereating.

Cephalic insulin secretion, the release of insulin in response to thinking about eating, has been proposed as a mechanism of withdrawal that may affect compulsive eaters more than the general population (Wilson 1991). The resulting hypoglycemia could be experienced as hunger or craving. However, many investigators have been unable to demonstrate the existence of cephalic insulin secretion and there certainly is no evidence that it is a characteristic unique or universal to compulsive eaters. Furthermore, as pointed out in the above discussion of hypoglycemia, eating modest amounts of ordinary foods should provide relief.

SUMMARY OF THE GOODNESS OF
FIT OF THE ADDICTION MODEL

We have seen that there are many commonalities between CE and dependence on psychoactive substances. These commonalities are compelling in regard to some of the characteristics of pathologic use, namely eating at inappropriate times and in inappropriate ways, feeling that the behavior is beyond control, temporary abstinence or restriction and continuing use despite serious physical disorders. The reliance on the behavior to cope with demands of daily living also may be interpreted as a good fit to the addiction model.

On the other hand, there are major flaws in the analogy in regard to consideration of food as intoxicating. In addition, the evidence for tolerance and for withdrawal is extremely weak. Furthermore, the addiction model does not easily accommodate the extreme dissatisfaction with their body size and shape that plagues most compulsive eaters (Meadows and Weiss 1992).

In addition to the characteristics explored above, a medical model of addiction presumes the existence of a biologic factor that predisposes the individual to dependence on the substance (Lewis, Dana and Blevins 1988). Although most of the behaviors we have seen can be better explained by cultural, social and psychological influences, there have been a few candidates for the disease factor: abnormalities in insulin secretion, differences in neurotransmitter function and enlarged stomach size. There has been limited search for a biologic factor for CE not associated with bulimia. The much greater volume of literature available on bulimia suggests that the disorder has a multiple etiology including both physiologic and psychological factors (Heatherton and Baumeister 1991). Heatherton and Baumeister (1991) point out that while a biopsychosocial theory integrates numerous findings, no strictly physiologic explanation is compelling.

There is a large volume of literature documenting both that compulsive eaters and addicts share many characteristics and that co-morbidity is high (Wilson 1991, 1993). These observations need not be interpreted as evidence that CE is an addictive disorder, but rather they may indicate that another factor affects both the compulsive eaters and the individuals dependent on psychoactive substances. Heatherton and Baumeister (1991) believe that this factor is the drive to escape self-awareness. That compulsive eaters attempt to satisfy this drive through the paradoxical, self-defeating behavior of excessive eating may be the result of the juxtaposition of several social, cultural and psychological factors, not least of which may be being female.

CLINICAL SIGNIFICANCE OF USE OF THE ADDICTION MODEL

It has been advanced that regardless of the theoretical fit of CE to a medical addiction model, there may be advantages to treatments based on that model (Wardle 1987; Yeary 1987). White (1991), while recognizing that therapy based on the addiction model may be the only effective approach for a minority, has found that an approach that de-emphasizes abstinence is a more appropriate first measure for most compulsive eaters. Her thinking reflects that of Wilson (1991) as well as Heatherton and Baumeister (1991): promoting abstinence exacerbates restraint and feelings of deprivation, triggering a vicious circle of restraint and disinhibition. Furthermore, for many individuals, defining abstinence may be highly artificial, obscuring the significant behaviors. Fundamental to the addiction-as-disease model is the concept of no cure. We do not know that this is true in regard to CE. Certainly, relapse is common and must be planned for, but this does not mean that the individual is never free of CE.

It must be concluded that there are major problems of fit of compulsive eating to a medical addiction model. Further, there is a real potential that application of that model in therapy may worsen the condition. Other addiction models may be a better fit, but as food cannot truly be considered psychoactive, attempts to define CE as addiction may be inhibiting an understanding of the problem.

REFERENCES

American Psychiatric Association Task Force on Nomenclature and Statistics (1987). Diagnostic and statistical manual of mental disorders (3/e, rev). Washington, DC: American Psychiatric Association.
American Psychiatric Association (1994). Diagnostic ans statistic manual of mental disorders, 4/e. Washington, DC: American Psychiatric Association.
Brownell KD, Wadden TA (1992). Etiology and treatment of obesity: understanding a serious, prevalent and refractory disorder. J Consult Clin Psychol 60:505-517.
Drewnowski A, Krahn DD, Demitrack MA, Nairn K, Gosnell BA (1992). Taste responses and preferences for sweet high-fat foods: evidence for opioid involvement. Physiol Behav 51:371-379.
Fairburn CG, Wilson GT (1993). Binge eating: definition and classification. In CG Fairburn and GT Wilson, Eds, Binge eating: nature, assessment and treatment. New York: Guilford Press.
Geliebter A, Melton PM, McCray RS, Gallagher DR, Gage D, Hashim SA (1992). Gastric capacity, gastric emptying and test-meal intake in normal and bulimic women. Am J Clin Nutrition 56:656-561.

194   *Obesity*

Heatherton TF, Baumeister RF (1991). Binge eating as escape from self-awareness. Psychol Bull 110:86-108.

Heatherton TF, Polivy J, Herman CP (1991). Restraint, weight loss and variability of body weight. J Abnormal Psychol 100:78-83.

Herman CP, Polivy J (1984). A boundary model for the regulation of eating. In AJ Stunkard and E Elliott, Eds, Eating and its disorders. New York: Raven Press.

Jenkins DJA, Wolever TMS, Jenkins AL (1988). Starchy foods and glycemic index. Diabetes Care 11:149-153.

Kagan DM, Squires RL (1984). Compulsive eating, dieting, stress and hostility among college students. J College Student Personnel 25:213-220.

Katzman MA (1989). Is it true eating makes you feel better? A naturalistic assessment of food consumption and its effect on stress. J College Student Psychol 3:75-87.

Lewis JA, Dana RQ, Blevins GA (1988). Substance abuse counseling: an individualized approach. Pacific Grove, CA: Brooks/Cole.

Lieberman HR, Wurtman JJ, Chew B (1986). Changes in mood after carbohydrate consumption among obese individuals. Am J Clin Nutrition 44:772-778.

Mahan LK, Arlin MT (1992). Krause's food, nutrition and diet therapy. Philadelphia: WB Saunders.

Marcus MD (1993). Binge eating in obesity. In CG Fairburn and GT Wilson, Eds, Binge eating: nature, assessment and treatment. New York: Guilford Press.

McDowell M (1980). Appetite control: an addiction-like component in overeating and its cure. Obesity Bariatric Med 9:138-142.

Meadow RW, Weiss L (1992). Women's conflicts about eating and sexuality. Binghamton, NY: Harrington Park Press.

Mitchell JE (1990). Bulimia nervosa. Minneapolis: University of Minnesota Press.

Orbach S (1978). Fat is a feminist issue. New York: Paddington Press.

Roth G (1982). Feeding the hungry heart: the experience of compulsive eating. New York: New American Library.

Rounsaville BJ, Spitzer RL, Williams JBW (1986). Proposed changes in DSM-III substance use disorders: description and rationale. Am J Psychiatry 143:463-468.

Spitzer RL, Devlin M, Walsh BT, Hasin D, Wing R, Marcus M, Stunkard A, Wadden T, Yanovski S, Agras S, Mitchell J, Nonas C (1992). Binge eating disorder: a multisite trial of the diagnostic criteria. Int J Eating Disorders 11:191-203.

Stunkard AJ, Grace WJ, Wolff HG (1955). The night-eating syndrome. A pattern of food intake among certain obese persons. Am J Med 19:78-86.

Taylor LA, Rachman SJ (1988). The effects of blood sugar level changes on cognitive function, affective state and somatic symptoms. J Behav Med 11:279-291.

Wardle J (1987). Compulsive eating and dietary restraint. Br J Clin Psychol 26:47-55.

White F (1991). Compulsive eating: new treatment approaches. Houston: Nutrition Health Services.

Wilson GT (1991). The addiction model of eating disorders: a critical analysis. Advance Behav Res Ther 13:27-72.

Wilson GT (1993). Binge eating and addictive disorders. In CG Fairburn and GT Wilson, Eds, Binge eating: nature, assessment and treatment. New York: Guilford Press.

Wurtman RJ (1987). Circulating nutrients and neurotransmitter synthesis. J Appl Nutrition 39:7-28.

Yanovski SZ (1993). Binge eating disorder: current knowledge and future directions. Obesity Res 1:306-324.

Yeary J (1987). The use of Overeaters Anonymous in the treatment of eating disorders. J Psychoactive Drugs 19:303-309.

15

The Benefits of an Interdisciplinary Approach in a Nutrition Medicine Clinic

George L. Blackburn, MD, PhD, Sharon L. Gallagher, RD, CDE
Amy E. Peterson, MS, RD, Mary L. Rowan, MS, RD
Martha G. Pontes, RN, MAA-HCA, MBA

According to the National Health and Nutrition Examination Survey (NHANES II, 1976-80), 26 percent of U.S. adults are overweight (VanItallie 1985). Overweight is defined as a body mass index of 27.8 kg/m^2 or greater for men and 27.3 kg/m^2 or greater for women. As many as 40 percent of women and 24 percent of men are trying to lose weight at any given time (NIH Technology Assessment Conference Panel 1992). Unfortunately, the success rates of weight reduction programs have been poor (Goodrick and Foreyt 1991).

Health care professionals are advised to extend the duration of their weight control programs and to address reasons for attrition. According to the NIH Technology Assessment Conference panel, the duration of most programs is from several weeks to a few months and the drop-out rates can be as high as 80 percent, varying considerably (NIH Technology Assessment Conference Panel 1992). It has been noted that duration of treatment has been associated with a positive outcome (Brownell and Wadden 1992); therefore, major challenges to health care providers are to provide longer programs and to investigate reasons for attrition, then design weight reduction programs accordingly.

Research indicates that participants who drop out have higher initial expectations of weight loss and a higher level of anxiety about losing weight than those who remain in the program (Bennett and Jones 1986; Atkinson, Russ, Ciavarella, Owsley and Bibbs 1984; Kolotkin and Moore 1983). Pratt (1990) suggests that to improve program retention rates, professionals should promote motivation and learning skills of the participants, offer lessons that promote commitment to the program, clarify the program's weight loss goals and discuss with participants their expected outcomes for the program. Clarification of patients' goals is especially relevant because many patients seek treatment with unrealistic expectations of weight loss.

The Michigan Health Council's Task Force to Establish Weight Loss Guidelines suggests that weight reduction programs use a multidisciplinary approach with an emphasis on screening patients for appropriateness of weight loss (Michigan Health Council 1990). Physicians have the responsibility of explaining the rationale for weight loss and its health implications to participants (Council on Scientific Affairs 1988). The dietitian can play a key role in helping patients set realistic weight loss goals and develop treatments to meet their needs (Pace, Bolton and Reeves 1991). It could be hypothesized that the dietitian/physician partnership can produce a greater impact in reinforcing program goals and evaluating patients' progress than either discipline alone. For this reason we decided to examine the retention rate of a nutrition clinic offering this model of treatment. We compared this clinic to a traditional hospital outpatient system to see if the dietitian/physician collaboration is indeed associated with a higher retention rate.

METHODS

We examined the medical records of all patients who sought nutrition counseling for weight loss between September 1992 and February 1993 at the Deaconess Hospital in Boston. A total of 116 patients with medically significant obesity were studied; 65 patients from the Nutrition Counseling Service (NCS) program and 51 from the Nutrition Medicine Clinic (NMC). (The Nutrition Counseling Service is a traditional hospital outpatient program where physicians refer patients to dietitians. The Nutrition Medicine Clinic provides coordinated physician/dietitian services with an interdisciplinary approach.) Patients were self-selected for each group and therefore could not be randomly assigned. Patients were considered "active" if they had two or more visits in the specified time period and if they had been seen in the last 6 weeks of the study period. Those patients who did not meet these requirements were considered "inactive." Patients were excluded from the study if their initial visit was after January 28, 1993. This was done in order to avoid including those patients who had not yet had the opportunity to return for a follow-up visit and thus might be considered "inactive." The retention rate for each clinic was determined by dividing the number of active patients by the total number of patients who sought treatment during this period.

Because the patient characteristics vary between the two groups, we compared age, sex, body mass index (BMI) and number of comorbidities in patients from each clinic and their effect on retention. These variables were predicted to be potentially confounding variables. All subjects were mailed confidential surveys in which they were asked to identify the strengths and weaknesses of their particular program. The questions were identical for both groups and were designed with a rating scale ranging from 1 (strongly agree) to 5 (strongly disagree). The intent was to quantitate patient perceptions and look for a correlation with retention rates in each clinic.

RESULTS

A total of 116 medical records were reviewed. The NMC tends to have a better retention rate as compared to the NCS (Table 1).

In the NMC there were a total of 37 females (22 active) and 14 males (5 active). In the NCS there were a total of 43 females (20 active) and 22 males (6 active). Women tend to have a better retention rate than men in both clinics (Table 2).

We looked at four variables that may have affected retention rate: sex, age, body mass index (BMI) and the number of comorbidities other than obesity (Tables 3, 4 and 5 and Figures 1, 2, 3 and 4).

Sex, Age, BMI and Comorbidity

There were more females than males in both clinics: 73 percent in the NMC and 66 percent in the NCS. However, there was no real difference between

Table 1. Overall Retention Rate

Active Patients	Percent Retention
NMC (n=51)	53
NCS (n=65)	42

Table 2. Retention Rate by Gender and Clinic

	Females	Males
NMC	59%	36%
NCS	47%	27%
Both clinics combined	53%	32%

the number of females in either clinic. The NMC active females tended to be slightly younger than the NCS active females and both were younger than active NMC and NCS males. The mean BMI tended to be slightly higher in the NMC patients than the NCS patients. This was particularly true in males. There was no real difference in the mean number of comorbidities between the two clinics. However, NMC males had slightly more comorbidities than NMC females.

Survey Results

The survey return rate was 26 percent, thus making it difficult to generalize interpretation of results. The rate of return was 25 percent in each clinic, with active patients returning a higher proportion of the surveys. When comparing the modes for each survey question between the two clinics, there was no difference in the most common responses. Qualitative results reflected the answer to the question, "Which features did you like best/least about the program?" Patients noted "helpful and supportive atmosphere" and "personal approach" most often. The number of times these features were mentioned was similar for both clinics. Survey results, although enlightening, did not support patient preference for one clinic over the other.

DISCUSSION

Sex was the only variable that was associated with retention in both nutrition clinics. According to four federal surveys of health practices, 33 to 40 percent of adult women in the United States are currently trying to lose weight, compared to 20 to 24 percent of men (NIH Technology Assessment Conference Panel 1992). Women in the United States are also at a greater risk of major weight gain during adulthood than men. Factors related to this weight gain may include childbearing, cessation of smoking, diet, physical activity and patterns of morbidity and mortality (NIH Technology Assessment Conference Panel 1992; Williamson, Kahn, Remington and Anda 1990).

Cultural and societal pressure to be thin, especially among women, may also explain the higher percentage of women in the two nutrition clinics. Today's society equates beauty, success and happiness with being thin. Rolla (1992:7) states, "It is ironic that the same society that facilitates obesity demands thinness for social acceptance." This emphasis on being thin combined with the fear of becoming obese has been termed "The Thinderella Syndrome." In addition, these pressures on women often increase the risk of developing eating disorders. Bruce (1993) found that 12 percent of women surveyed were binge eaters (those who reported uncontrolled eating) and that episodes of binge eating were often triggered by

Table 3. Patient Characteristics by Clinic

	NMC (n=51)	NCS (n=65)
Mean age	45	49
Female/male ratio	2.6	2
Mean BMI	42	36
Mean no. comorbidities	1.9	1.5

Table 4. Patient Characteristics by Clinic and Program Status

	Active		Inactive	
	NMC	NCS	NMC	NCS
Mean age	44.0	50.0	46.0	48.0
Female/male ratio	4.4	3.3	1.7	1.4
Mean BMI	42.6	38.0	41.3	35.9
Mean no. comorbidites	1.9	1.5	1.8	1.4

Table 5. Patient Characteristics by Clinic, Program Status and Gender

	Active				Inactive			
	NMC		NCS		NMC		NCS	
	F	M	F	M	F	M	F	M
Mean age	43.0	51.2	51.0	47.2	42.3	51.7	47.4	49.2
Mean BMI	41.0	51.2	39.0	35.0	39.5	44.5	36.0	36.0
Mean no. comorbidties	1.9	2.2	1.6	1.5	1.2	2.8	1.3	1.6

depression, loneliness and cravings. Many female patients in the NMC exhibit these same characteristics.

The other three variables (age, BMI and number of comorbidities) were not associated with retention in either nutrition clinic. We suggest that the higher retention rate in the NMC may involve other factors (Table 6). We suspect that the retention rate in the NMC may have been lowered due to a large number of patients seeking medication as the primary mode of obesity therapy. These patients may have higher attrition rates than other NMC patients because they were dissatisfied with our non-drug-oriented empha-

Table 6. Potential Variables Influencing Retention Rate

Characteristics	NMC	NCS
Interdisciplinary approach	+	inconsistent
Physician reinforcement	+	inconsistent
Concomitant presentation of expectations by health professional	+	nonexistent
Special medical services	+	inconsistent
Telephone correspondence with patients	frequent	inconsistent

sis. Unfortunately, we were unable to support this hypothesis with survey results, since only three inactive NMC patients returned their surveys.

The NMC uses an interdisciplinary approach to help patients treat and deal with various nutrition-related diseases and disorders. We chose patients with medically significant obesity for our study because the majority of patients referred to the NMC have this disease. The NMC interdisciplinary "team" consists of a physician, a dietitian, a nurse and a behavior therapist (psychologist) who are trained and knowledgeable in weight management. The functions of the NMC team members are similar to those outlined in the Michigan Health Council's guidelines for adult weight loss (Michigan Health Council 1990). Other adjunct health professionals may be involved, such as an exercise physiologist, physical therapist, or psychiatrist. Several studies have shown that an interdisciplinary approach to weight control is beneficial in providing effective treatment to the obese patient (Fitzwater, Weinsier, Wooldridge, Birch, Liu and Bartolucci 1991; Atkinson, Russ, Ciavarella, Owsley and Bibbs 1984; Wadden, Foster, Letizia and Stunkard 1992; Hudiburgh 1984).

The physician is the medical director of the NMC and is responsible for completing a medical history and physical evaluation; prescribing the individualized nutrition and activity program; prescribing any medication; ordering and interpreting laboratory and medical tests (such as body composition analysis and indirect calorimetry); and supervising the other team members. The physician may also "outsource" patients to other physicians or programs as part of treatment.

The dietitian completes a nutritional assessment and weight history; obtains a diet recall and food frequency; determines food preferences, food preparation practices and dining-out practices; outlines the goals of treatment; and executes the nutrition prescription as determined by the physi-

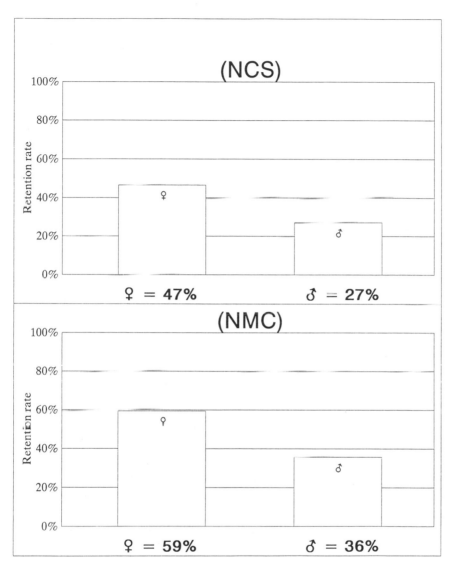

Figure 1. Gender vs. retention rate.

cian. Throughout the patient's course of treatment, the dietitian provides nutrition education and counseling, assesses compliance to the program and addresses any barriers to treatment. The physician may be asked to intervene at any time if the dietitian perceives a problem (i.e., poor compliance or frequent cancellations), if an eating disorder or emotional issues are revealed, or if any medical complications develop.

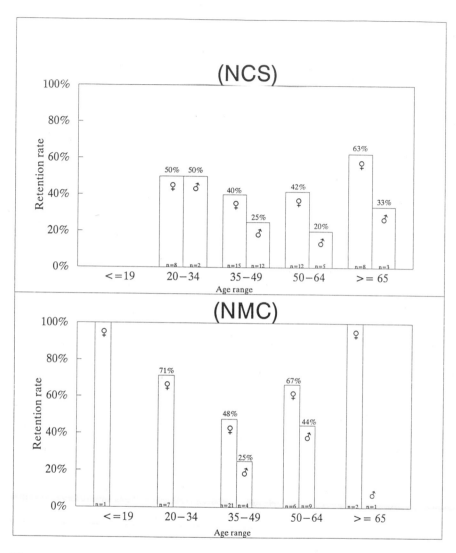

Figure 2. Age vs. retention rate.

The nurse in the NMC determines if the patients are "diet-ready" to begin the program, using a specially designed questionnaire. This is based on the premise as determined by Ferguson, Brink, Wood and Koop (1992) that "cognitive and behavioral readiness for weight control are important factors in successful weight loss and maintenance." She also obtains a more detailed medical history; identifies any additional medical factors that may impede treatment; monitors patients for potential adverse health effects;

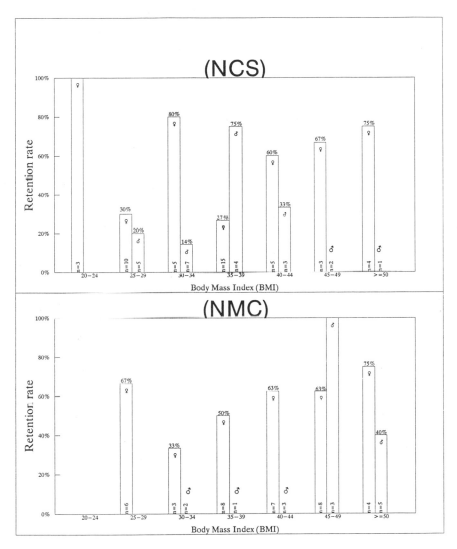

Figure 3. Body mass index (BMI) vs. retention rate.

orders further laboratory and medical tests, if necessary; and determines if additional medical intervention is needed.

Although the dietitian and nurse utilize behavior modification techniques and teach coping skills for eating control, it is often necessary for a therapist to intervene for issues such as depression, stress reduction, body

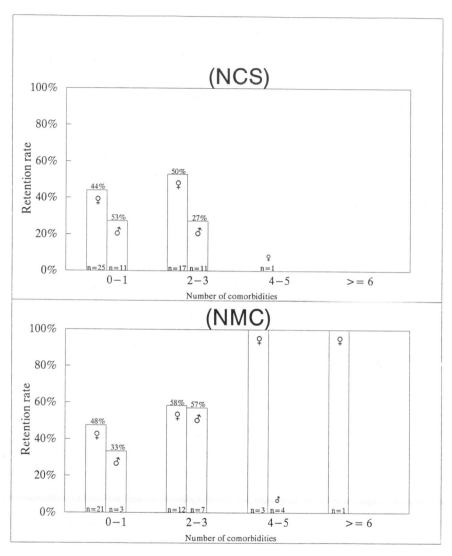

Figure 4.   Comorbidities vs. retention rate.

image disturbance, eating disorders and other psychological factors that may be interfering with weight loss. The therapist may also refer patients to a psychiatrist or stress management program.

The expectations of the program are outlined for the patient during the first visit to the NMC. Patients are informed that treatment will consist of approximately 14 to 29 visits, spread out over the course of a year; visits are scheduled with the dietitian and/or nurse every 1 to 3 weeks on average. Patients who are unable to come as often, due to schedule conflicts or long distances, are monitored by telephone. Daily food records and regular monitoring for optimal success are strongly reinforced by all disciplines. All team members in the NMC are consistent in their recommendations of diet, exercise and behavioral changes and stress that a lifelong commitment to these changes is necessary.

There are no "canned" diets used in the NMC. Rather, the NMC strives to develop a realistic, yet effective, individualized program for every patient. Depending on the patient's degree of obesity, health status and lifestyle, several options are available:

1. Low-fat, high-fiber plan
2. Balanced-deficit diet
3. Protein-sparing modified fast
4. Meal replacements
5. Very-low-calorie liquid diets (e.g., Optifast)
6. Gastric-bypass surgery

In some situations the physician may also prescribe an appetite suppressant as an adjunct to one of the above diets. Treatment, then, is highly structured to meet the individual's needs and includes education, guidance and continued support to enhance adherence.

The NCS may offer some of the same features as the NMC, such as physician reinforcement, special medical services and telephone correspondence, but these are inconsistent. In addition, because the physician is not present concomitantly with the dietitian during the initial visit, patients may not fully realize their own role and responsibilities as partners in the program.

The higher retention rate in the NMC suggests that this type of nutrition clinic possesses certain characteristics not always evident in a traditional nutrition clinic. We feel that patients with medically significant obesity seeking sound nutritional and medical treatment can benefit from a nutrition clinic using an interdisciplinary approach, as exemplified by the NMC.

REFERENCES

Atkinson RL, Russ CS, Ciavarella PA, Owsley ES, Bibbs ML (1984). A comprehensive approach to outpatient obesity management. J Am Dietetic Assoc 84(4):439-444.

Bennett GA, Jones SE (1986). Dropping out of treatment for obesity. J Psychosom Res 30(5):567-573.

Brownell KD, Wadden TA (1992). Etiology and treatment of obesity: understanding a serious, prevalent and refractory disorder. J Consulting Clin Psychol 60(4):505-517.

Bruce B (1993). Beyond the clinic: binge eating in the community. Weight Control Digest, January/February, 3(1):230-232.

Council on Scientific Affairs (1988). Treatment of obesity in adults. JAMA 260(17):2547-2551.

Ferguson KJ, Brink PJ, Wood M, Koop PM (1992). Characteristics of successful dieters as measured by guided interview responses and restraint scale scores. J Am Dietetic Assoc 92(9):1119-1121.

Fitzwater SL, Weinsier RL, Wooldridge NH, Birch R, Liu C, Bartolucci AA (1991). Evaluation of long-term weight changes after a multidisciplinary weight control program. J Am Dietetic Assoc 91(4):421-429.

Fowler JL, Follick MJ, Abrams DB, Richard-Figueroa K (1985). Participant characteristics as predictors of attrition in a worksite weight loss program. Addictive Behav 10(4):445-448.

Goodrick GK, Foreyt JP (1991). Why treatments for obesity don't last. J Am Dietetic Assoc 91(10):1243-1247.

Hudiburgh NK (1984). A multidisciplinary approach to weight control. J Am Dietetic Assoc 84(4):447-450.

Kolotkin RL, Moore JM (1983). Attrition in a behavioral weight control program: a comparison of dropouts and completers. Int J Eating Disorders 2(3):93-100.

Michigan Health Council (1990). Toward safe weight loss: recommended interim guidelines for adult weight loss programs in Michigan, final report. East Lansing: Michigan Health Council.

NIH Technology Assessment Conference Panel (1992). Methods for voluntary weight loss and control. Ann Intern Med 116(11):942-949.

Pace PW, Bolton MP, Reeves RS (1991). Ethics of obesity treatment. J Am Dietetic Assoc 91(10):1258-1260.

Pratt CA (1990). Factors related to the completion of a weight reduction program. J Am Dietetic Assoc 90(9):1268-1270.

Rolla AR (1992). Obesity: an eating disorder. Paper presented at Treatment of Obesity and Eating Disorders: An Interdisciplinary Approach, Technology Assessment of Medical/Surgical Treatment, Boston, November 12-14.

VanItallie TB (1985). Health implications of overweight and obesity in the United States. Ann Intern Med 150:665-672.

Wadden TA, Foster GD, Letizia KA, Stunkard AJ (1992). A multicenter evaluation of a proprietary weight reduction program for the treatment of marked obesity. Arch Intern Med 152:961-966.

Williamson DF, Kahn HS, Remington PL, Anda RF (1990). The 10-year incidence of overweight and major weight gain in U.S. adults. Arch Intern Med 150:665-672.

Wooley SC, Garner DM (1991). Obesity treatment: the high cost of false hope. J Am Dietetic Assoc 91(10):1243-1247.

16

Weight Management Activities Among Black Women

Janet D. Allan, PhD, RNC, FAAN

Currently in the United States, over 24 percent of women are overweight (Stephenson, Levy, Sass and McGarvey 1987). Moreover, obesity is most prevalent among black and working-class women (Dawson 1988). In a 1985 national study, Dawson found that 35 percent of black women were obese, in contrast to 20 percent of white women and 26 percent of Hispanic women. Despite some contradictory evidence (Walker and Segal 1980; Ernsberger and Haskew 1986), ecologic data demonstrate greater obesity-related health risks in black women compared to white women (Kumanyika 1987; VanItallie 1992). Obesity in women also increases the risk of psychological difficulties resulting from stereotyping of the overweight and the greater cultural pressure on women to maintain "ideal weight" (Attie and Brooks-Gunn 1987; Lakoff and Scherr 1984; Streigel-Moore, Silberstein and Rodin 1986).

Despite extensive research, obesity continues to elude effective understanding and treatment. One reason for this lack of knowledge can be attributed to the narrowly focused research on obesity which has neglected to examine the relationship between sociocultural-environmental variables and weight management patterns among vulnerable groups such as black women. Most weight control research has involved individuals, primarily white women, in treatment programs and has focused on a few physiologic or psychological variables within these skewed populations (Colvin and Olson 1983; Schachter 1982; Wooley and Wooley 1984). Therefore, little is known about the weight management activities of black

Preparation of this chapter was supported by a five-year First Award from the National Institute for Nursing Research.

women or about the environmental milieus within which weight management activities occur.

The focus of this chapter is on the methods black women use to manage weight and factors that influence the selection, use and success of these methods. The results reported here are one aspect of a study of the patterns and processes of weight management among 31 working- and middle-class black women. The specific research questions were:

1. Under what conditions (e.g., marriage, pregnancy) do black women gain weight?
2. What are the weight management methods used by black women?
3. What are black women's explanatory models of weight?
4. What are black women's values about body size?
5. What factors (e.g., socioeconomic status, reasons for losing weight) influence the selection, use and success of weight management methods?

This study builds upon a previous study of weight management among working- and middle-class white women (Allan 1986; Allan 1988; Allan 1989; Allan 1991).

LITERATURE

The cultural-ecological approach to weight and weight management for this study is adapted from the work of Ritenbaugh (1982a) on the macroenvironmental influences on weight and Pelto's (1981) concept of lifestyle, the distillation of macro-environmental influences at the level of the household. In addition, the concept of explanatory model (Kleinman 1980) and the concept of individual coping (Bennett 1976; Lazarus and Folkman 1984) guided the exploration of weight management. Weight, from an ecological perspective, is a function of adaptation to the environment through both physiologic and cultural means (Stini 1981). A variety of macro-environmental factors are considered salient influences on weight management in the United States; technologically produced sedentariness (Ritenbaugh 1982a), changes in the American diet (Jerome 1981) and the cultural meanings and values attached to biologic phenomena like weight (Cassidy 1991; Dawson 1988; Ritenbaugh 1982b). American society constitutes a stressful environment in which to manage weight.

Dominant cultural values about body size and beauty in women influence perceptions of weight and weight management activities. MacKenzie (1985) suggests that obese individuals, particularly women, contradict many American values related to beauty and self-control and thus become "culturally diagnosed as out of control, lazy and incompetent." Fat women internalize these norms and develop very critical views of themselves (Davis 1986). There is also evidence of differential standards of weight based upon gender. Several researchers (Streigel-Moore, Silberstein and Rodin 1986; Ritenbaugh 1982b) found a steady decline over 40 years in what has been considered "ideal weight" for women to the point that currently the average women is considered to be overweight. Ritenbaugh (1982b) views these standards of weight as originating from culturally shaped biomedical categories such as ideal weight, which values youth and thinness in women and promotes unrealistic images of beauty. There is some evidence that women do not adopt these thin ideals. In my study of white women (Allan 1988), I found that women developed personalized weight norms or explanatory models of what to weigh that were not based upon biomedical standards. These norms, as models of physical identity, represented a creative way to deal with the perceived pressure to be thin and rigid biomedical weight standards. There also is growing evidence that ethnic differences exist in relation to weight perception (Massara 1979; Stern, Pugh, Gaskill, et al. 1982; Kumanyika, Wilson and Guilford-Davenport 1993). Dawson (1988) reported that black women were less likely than white women to perceive themselves as overweight. Allan, Mayo and Michel (1993), in a study comparing body size values of 36 white and 31 black women, reported that black women of lower socioeconomic status had to become a great deal heavier than black women of higher socioeconomic status and white women, regardless of status, before they defined themselves as overweight.

Bennett (1976) suggests that coping is a process through which an individual manages the demands of an environment that is appraised as stressful. American women are faced with initiating weight management in an environment that places tremendous stresses on their ability to maintain weight stability through physiologic mechanisms alone (Bradley 1982). In response, they must adopt behavioral and cognitive methods of coping with environmental stresses. Although minimal, there are some data suggesting that black women make fewer attempts at weight loss than white women (Dawson 1988; Stephenson, Levy, Sass, et al. 1987).

Factors triggering weight loss activities include the desire for physical attractiveness (White 1984; Laffrey 1986; Ferguson, Brink, Wood and Koop 1992) and social situations such as a new job or expectations of friends (Colvin and Olson 1983; Saltzer 1980; Gillet 1980). Several researchers (Allan 1989; Davis 1986; Laffrey 1986) reported that health concerns were not strong motivators for weight loss because overweight individuals did not define themselves as unhealthy.

METHODS

A naturalistic study design (Lincoln and Guba 1985) using ethnographic interviewing techniques (Spradley 1979) and anthropometric measures was employed. A combination of snowball and theoretical nonprobability sampling techniques (Field and Morse 1985; Lincoln and Guba 1985) was used to make contact with 31 working- and middle-class black women living in central Texas. A variety of contacts such as occupational health nurses, personnel directors and women's church groups was used to advertise the study, reach potential informants and obtain a broad community sample. The sampling criteria included being black; being between the ages of 18 and 55; being normal weight to moderately obese; living in the study area; being without major health problems; and not being pregnant.

STUDY GROUP

The study group exhibited modal patterns of being young, well-educated, Protestant, married and native-born Texans. The mean age was 35 with a range of 18 to 55 years. All women were employed, mostly in sedentary occupations such as clerical, sales and education. However, the study group did represent a wide range of occupations from domestic to assembly line worker to policewoman to university professor. Individual income ranged from $10,000 to $70,000. Eighteen women were categorized as middle-class and 13 as working-class (as determined by the Hollingshead Four-Factor Index of Social Status 1975). The majority of the study group were overweight or obese (18) and more working-class women than middle-class women were obese (9 vs. 4).

Data Collection and Analysis

Data were collected through use of a semi-structured interview and anthropometric measures of height and weight. Participants were asked to respond the question, "Tell me about the history of your weight starting at whatever age you want and describe your experiences." Probes were used to elicit further elaboration of informants' experiences such as sources of information about weight, ideas about what to weigh and types and content of weight management methods. All informants participated in multiple interviews (mean number, 2.3; mean, 3 hours in length) which were audiotaped and transcribed verbatim to maintain the integrity of the data and to reduce analytic bias (LeCompte and Goetz 1980). Content analysis and theme techniques (Field and Morse 1985; Lincoln and Guba 1985) were used to identify categories and themes related to types of weight management activities and factors influencing the selection, use and success of weight management methods.

RESULTS

All of the women used a complex variety of weight management methods to cope with weight. In this study, I defined weight management as all of an individual's efforts (behavioral, cognitive and emotional) to deal with actual or potential weight gain. This is based upon the assumption that in this society with the high value placed upon appearance and thinness, all women, regardless of weight, are aware of their weight and are dealing with their weight in some way.

Efforts to Lose Weight

All of the women, regardless of weight, had tried to lose weight at some time in their life and many had been trying for years. A total of 11 specific methods for weight loss were elicited from analysis of the informants' past and current experiences. These methods were coded into two categories: dieting and changing one's whole life. Dieting represented a variety of short-term tactics that ranged from simple to complex, from fasting to going to Mexico for diet drugs to joining Weight Watchers. Although most informants, both heavy and thin, at some point in their lives had tried most of the 11 methods, they only used three repeatedly and successfully for long-term weight loss and maintenance: skipping meals, reducing the intake of high-calorie foods and exercise.

Dieting

Simple tactics like fasting and skipping meals involved common sense and only minor alterations in established eating patterns. Informants could implement such methods without recourse to professional resources. As one informant stated,

> I dieted, nothing professional, just common sense. It's like I'm going to go on a diet this week, so that means I'm not going to eat some days or eat one meal and drink lots of coffee and smoke to reduce my appetite.

More complex tactics, such as reducing the intake of high-calorie foods, fad diets, over-the-counter diet drugs or products and exercising on one's own involved the use of some specialized knowledge from the mass media, diet or nutrition books, family or peers. Although these methods are more complex, they are used for very short periods of time, a day to a month.

Reducing the intake of high-calorie foods was the most commonly used tactic. This method of weight loss involved not only cutting out desserts, chips and other goodies, but also exercising micro-environmental control such as not eating in restaurants, not snacking from the machine at work, or not keeping the usual high-calorie foods in the home. Essentially, informants temporarily rearranged their usual lifestyle patterns to avoid tempting eating opportunities. For example, a 32-year-old, married (obese) assembly line worker discussed this tactic and her comment illustrates its properties very well.

> Well I do this little diet, not a real diet, all the time. You go for a week or so and that's it. I'll say I'm going to lose weight so I stop eating potato chips, desserts, buying cookies from the machine on my breaks and all that good stuff.

Despite their tremendous coverage in the mass media, fad diets and diet drugs were used by surprisingly few women. If they were used, it was never for longer than a week at the most. The comments of this 40-year-old married (currently normal-weight) policewoman captures the problems with fad diets:

> I have a drawer full of all the diets that I've tried. I've been on the Mayo diet, that's a bad diet. Who wants to eat 15 eggs a day. The whole family went on the Dolly Parton diet, because my son's football coach gave it to him. After one day of fruit, like I gave my husband 10 bowls of fruit in one day, we were all sneaking around, let me get a piece of cheese but don't tell.

The study group was not as sedentary as these data imply. A total of 10 informants were involved in exercising on their own, either walking, biking, aerobic dancing, or weight lifting, and one woman attended a fitness program. However, only six used exercise to lose weight. They all walked. The others exercised for health problems, socializing and appearance. Exercise as a tactic was always short-term. If exercise became a routine activity for weight management, I classified it as a strategy, either used alone or as one aspect of a new lifestyle.

Sources of Information

The women in this study obtained most of their information about how to lose weight from the mass media and peers. Although most of us would perceive this information to be pervasive in the mass media, several women stated that the black media, specifically women's magazines, only started to focus on weight and health in the last 5 years. Prior to that time, the focus in these magazines was on getting screened and treated for hypertension. These informants used this to explain why in their view black women as a group were so heavy; they did not have an awareness of the importance of losing weight or the knowledge of how to do it. In fact, most women in the study viewed overweight as unattractive rather than unhealthy. Direct contact with the health care system was not perceived as a major source of information about weight loss. In fact, heavier women, the only ones who ever had weight mentioned during a health visit, seemed to perceive health professionals as judgmental, giving commands ("you've got to get that weight off") rather than assistance.

The most complex tactics used by informants involved seeking professional services for weight loss. Weight reduction programs, specifically Weight Watchers, were the most frequently used professional service. The infrequent use of professional services for weight loss is similar to the findings in my previous study and support a growing body of literature (Schachter 1982; Colvin and Olson 1983; Jeffery, Folsom, Luepker, et al. 1984) that most individuals try to lose weight on their own.

Changing One's Whole Life

In contrast, to dieting, changing one's whole life represented a series of complex, long-term strategies for weight loss that involved making permanent changes in a variety of lifestyle behaviors. There were three major strategies used by informants to lose and then maintain their weight: new eating patterns, habitual exercise and new lifestyle. New eating patterns involved a major alteration in established eating patterns that consisted of smaller portions, more lower-calorie foods, altered preparation style and a consistent meal pattern. New eating patterns evolved over time as women experimented with minor changes in their eating routines, incorporated information on "healthy foods" from the mass media and lost weight. A 26-year-old, married (normal-weight) data processor illustrates the strategy of new eating patterns:

> I used to eat a really fatty diet. In general, black families eat more fatty and fried foods. My family ate that way, too. I call it soul food grease. Well, since I left home, I have discovered that you can eat chicken and greens and cornbread without all the grease. I eat all that stuff but plain.

Interestingly, informants clearly differentiated between the tactic of reducing high-calorie foods and new eating patterns. For many, they were descriptively the same. However, when informants talked about the tactic they always called what they were doing dieting, whereas when they talked about new eating patterns, they stated that they were watching their weight, not dieting. Dieting to the women in this study and in the study of white women, meant deprivation, denial, restricting and not having the things you liked. It seemed to connote the imposition from outside of a rigid eating pattern, such as "my doctor put me on this diet." By contrast, "watching my weight" seemed to connote a moderate limitation or restriction of usual eating patterns decided upon by the informant. Watching my weight was also discussed in a positive way. In my view, this is an example of a tactic being transformed and relabeled as part of the informants' routine activities.

New lifestyle involved a cluster of routines for living, such as habitual exercise, new eating patterns and reduced or no alcohol intake, that enabled women to lose and maintain their weight loss for longer than a year. New lifestyle, as developed by six of the women, also incorporated the tactics of skipping meals and reducing the intake of high-calorie foods. These tactics were used for weight maintenance. The development of a new lifestyle started with one change, most frequently exercise and then led to other changes. The concept of new lifestyle is exemplified by the statements of a 35-year-old, married, formerly obese disability examiner:

> I figured that if I wanted to stay at this weight, I couldn't have the same lifestyle I had before. I had eaten a certain way growing up and I thought that's how you're supposed to eat. I went to Weight Watchers and learned a different way of eating and since then I have completely changed my eating habits and my exercise habits. I don't consider that I'm on a diet anymore. I consider it a way of living.

The relationship between new lifestyle and Weight Watchers was interesting. Three of the six women who developed a new lifestyle initially attended Weight Watchers, learned new eating patterns, adapted them over time to their own personal tastes and then maintained a life membership as a form of what they called "external control." This involved attending one meeting a month as a way to help support their new lifestyle.

Before discussing the success of these methods for weight loss and some of the factors influencing success, let us consider another type of tactic used by informants to manage their weight.

De-Emphasizing Weight

In addition to attempting to managing weight gain through the behavioral methods already presented, informants, particularly heavier women, also used several tactics to de-emphasize their weight. These tactics were coded into two categories: avoidance and isolating. Avoidance tactics included not weighing, wearing larger and larger clothing and avoiding health appointments. Isolating tactics involved not participating in certain activities such as social events and sports activities. One woman's comments illustrate avoidance tactics:

> I got bigger and bigger and bigger. But I didn't think about it. I'd just go out and buy more clothes. I stopped wearing pants and got into flared dresses and mu-mus.

Another informant talked about not going to the neighborhood pool in the summer because she was embarrassed about her size and felt her kids would be embarrassed as well.

De-emphasizing tactics functioned to minimize women's awareness of their weight or body size and in my view deal with the negative self-feelings expressed by every overweight women in the study. Essentially, these tactics enabled women to temporarily ignore their weight by not invoking the process of appraisal; in other words, being cognizant of one's weight as measured by a scale, clothing size, general appearance, or comments from a health professional.

The Success of These Methods and the Contributing Factors

Three less complex tactics—skipping meals, reducing the intake of high-calorie foods and exercising—were successful for short-term, modest weight loss (e.g., 5 to 15 pounds) in all women regardless of weight or age. However, heavier women of all ages were never able to lose large amounts of weight with such simple tactics. They needed to use more complex methods such as weight reduction programs, new eating patterns, or new lifestyles. Thus weight was a major factor influencing the success of methods for weight loss.

Essentially, the three tactics enabled small amounts of weight loss because they involved only minor alterations in established routines of eating and activity. They were easy to initiate, seemed like common sense, were palatable, inexpensive, caused no harm and worked. Fad diets, fasting and diet pills were not successful or used frequently because of the unpalatable content, the total lack of similarity with women's usual eating patterns and, in the case of the diet drugs, the unpleasant side effects.

Normal-weight women who wished to maintain weight or overweight women who wished to lose weight could successfully use these tactics. Thinner women could manage their weight fairly easily by alternating between their usual high-calorie routines of eating and sedentary lifestyle and their dieting. However, the findings suggest that heavier women must adopt permanent alterations in their routines of eating and activity in order to lose major amounts of weight and sustain that weight loss. They simply have more weight to lose than thinner women. In fact, four of the six women who developed a new lifestyle had been obese. Most heavier women in this study had, as the saying goes, lost the same 10 or 20 pounds many times over. This is the revolving door of dieting. There are several reasons why few women in the study were able to develop new lifestyles. The most relevant reasons related to time and energy. Routines such as eating and physical activity are patterns that are familiar, recurring and do not require much attention. Many women in this study perceived that they did not have the time or energy required to alter their eating and activity routines. As one 30-year-old married woman with three school-age children stated,

> When I get off work in the evening and the past 6 months we've had to work 10-hour shifts, I come home, fix dinner, get the kids ready for bed and collapse. I don't have time to exercise or make a different meal for me.

Sennott-Miller and Miller (1987), in several studies of weight reduction programs, found that the greater the perceived difficulty of adopting a particular activity, the lower the likelihood of adoption. The gap between heavier women's routines of eating and exercise and those required for major weight loss was so great that attempting to do so was perceived as too difficult. The concept of "hierarchies of resort" is also applicable here (Schwartz 1969). This concept suggests that when individuals are confronted with a problem, routine, well-known solutions are attempted, such as the simple dieting tactics described and as these attempts fail to resolve the problem, newer solutions are undertaken. Moreover, individuals do not move from old routines to new ones, but instead old routines are transformed into new ones. The other aspect of the concept is the bigger the problem, the greater the cost to address it. For heavier women, developing new eating and exercise patterns involves a tremendous alteration in routines, such as preparation style, shopping patterns, meal patterns and socializing. To lose major amounts of weight and then to sustain this weight loss, heavier women must make major alterations in their micro-environment.

In addition to weight, several other factors were interactive in influencing weight management activities. In this study, factors such as environmental and financial resources, climate and peer and family support were not major influences on weight management. However, class or socioeconomic status and weight perception did influence weight management.

There were class differences in the use of particular methods for weight loss. More middle-class women than working-class women used exercise and more middle-class women used the strategies of new eating patterns and new lifestyle. It is not clear exactly how class influences the use of different methods. Since financial resources were not defined by women as a problem, it would seem that the other indicators of class, education and occupation may be more influential. Education and occupation are interrelated and may expose individuals to different information as well as different values. Women in blue-collar jobs seemed to feel no peer or management pressure to be a certain weight, whereas women in white-collar occupations did feel the need to conform to what they called white body sizes. The well-educated professional black women in this study used methods very similar to their white counterparts.

Perception of weight was the other major influence on weight management. Before informants could initiate weight management activities, they had to define themselves as overweight. Many women in this study, although overweight for years by biomedical standards, did not view themselves as overweight. They described themselves as always big, the smallest in the family, like all their aunts, or strong rather than fat. Defining oneself as overweight or becoming aware of one's weight occurred through a variety of social or health encounters, role and physiologic transitions. For heavier women, the awareness of being overweight seemed to be triggered by a situation occurring outside their natal family. It is possible that these women did not perceive themselves as overweight because they evaluated their weight or body size not in relation to the white ideal portrayed in the media but in comparison to other black women who on average are heavier than white women. The existence of a wider normative weight range for many women of lower socioeconomic status created a social environment which did not encourage weight loss activities (Allan, Mayo and Michel 1993).

CONCLUSIONS

Clinical interventions related to weight control rely on two assumptions: that being overweight is detrimental to health and that normal weight or the healthiest weight is that which is defined by the biomedical standard of ideal weight. Contrary to the first assumption, most black women did not define being overweight as unhealthy. What bothered them the most about being overweight was appearance, either not being able to wear nice clothes or just not looking good. That health concerns are not a motivator for weight loss is supported in other studies of white populations (Allan 1988; Laffrey 1986). Health providers and health educators need to reconsider their traditional use of the threat of ill health as a motivator for weight loss.

Many black women, although obese by biomedical standards, did not define themselves as overweight. They essentially had a definition of normal weight that was at odds with biomedical norms. Therefore, using ideal weight to guide weight loss interventions will be ineffective for many women and in addition will alienate them from the care system. Feminists would suggest that basing clinical interventions on ideal weight standards, standards which have been severely criticized as being nonrepresentative and lacking a clear relationship to health (Allan 1988), is a form of oppression of women and promotes unrealistic images of what is a normal and desirable body size. Clinicians need to elicit client perspectives about weight and weight norms.

The findings of this study also suggest the relevance of examining weight management within the context of lifestyle. Using this broader focus is one way to identify the environmental opportunities and barriers confronting women as they attempt to lose weight and the common-sense, effective methods women develop as they experiment with their usual routines of eating and exercise to lose weight.

REFERENCES

Allan J, Mayo K, Michel Y (1993). Body size values of white and black women. Res Nursing Health 16:323-333.
Allan J (1988). Knowing what to weigh: women's self-care activities related to weight. Adv Nursing Sci 11(1):47-60.

218   *Obesity*

Allan J (1986). Patterns and processes of weight management among urban dwelling women. Unpublished doctoral dissertation, University of California at Berkeley.

Allan J (1991). To lose, to maintain, to ignore: weight management among women. Health Care Women Int 12(2):223-235.

Allan J (1989). Women who successfully manage their weight: a naturalistic study. Western J Nursing Res 11(6):657-675.

Attie I, Brooks-Gunn J (1987). Weight concerns as chronic stressors in women. In L Biener and G Baruch, Eds, Gender and stress. New York: The Free Press.

Bennett J (1976). Ecological transition: cultural anthropology and human adaptation. New York: Pergamon Press.

Bradley PJ (1982). Is obesity an advantageous adaptation? Int J Obesity 6:43-52.

Cassidy C (1991). The good body: when big is better. Med Anthropol 13:181-214.

Colvin R, Olson S (1983). A descriptive analysis of men and women who have lost significant weight and are highly successful at maintaining the loss. Addictive Behav 8:287-295.

Davis D (1986). Changing body aesthetics: exercise fads in a Newfoundland outpost community. Paper presented at the American Anthropological Association Meetings, Philadelphia.

Dawson D (1988). Ethnic differences in female overweight: data from the 1985 National Health Interview Survey. Am J Public Health 78(10):1326-1329.

Ernsberger P, Haskew P (1986). News about obesity. N Engl J Med 315:130-131.

Ferguson K, Brink P, Wood M, Koop P (1992). Characteristics of successful dieters as measured by guided interview responses and restraint scale scores. J Am Dietetic Assoc 92(9):1119-1121.

Field PA, Morse JM (1985). Nursing research: the application of qualitative approaches. Rockville, MD: Aspen.

Gillet P (1988). Self-reported factors influencing exercise adherence in overweight women. Nursing Res 37(1):25-29.

Hollingshead A (1975). Four-factor index of social status. Unpublished paper, Department of Sociology, Yale University.

Jerome N (1981). The U.S. dietary pattern from an anthropological perspective. Food Technol 14:37-42.

Kleinman A (1980). Patients and healers in the context of culture. Berkeley: University of California Press.

Kumanyika S (1987). Obesity in black women. Epidemiol Rev 9:31-50.

Kumanyika S, Wilson J, Guilford-Davenport M (1993). Weight-related attitudes and behaviors of black women. J Am Dietetic Assoc 93(4):416-422.

Laffrey S (1986). Normal and overweight adults: perceived weight and health behavior characteristics. Nutrition Res 35(3):173-177.

Lakoff R, Scherr R (1984). Face value: the politics of beauty. Boston: Routledge and Kegan Paul.

Lazarus R, Folkman S (1984). Stress, appraisal and coping. New York: Springer.

LeCompte M, Goetz J (1982). Problems of reliability and validity in ethnographic research. Rev Ed Res 52:31-60.

Lincoln YS, Guba EG (1985). Naturalistic inquiry. Beverly Hills, CA: Sage.

MacKenzie M (1985). The pursuit of slenderness and addiction to self-control: an anthropological interpretation of eating disorders. Nutrition Update 5:174-194.

Mallick MJ (1981). The adverse effects of weight control in teenage girls. Adv Nursing Sci 3(2):121-123.

Massara E (1979). Que gordita! A study of weight among a Puerto Rican community. Unpublished doctoral dissertation, Bryn Mawr College.

Pelto G (1981). Anthropological contributions to nutrition education and research. J Nutrition Ed 13:1-8.

Ritenbaugh C (1982a). New approaches to old problems: interactions of culture and nutrition. In N Chrisman and T Maretzki, Eds, Clinically applied anthropology. Dordrecht, Holland: Reidel.

Ritenbaugh C (1982b). Obesity as a culture-bound syndrome. Culture Med Psychiatry 6:347-381.

Saltzer EB (1980). Social determinants of successful weight loss: an analysis of behavioral intentions and actual behavior. Basic Appl Soc Psychol 1(4):329-341.

Schachter S (1982). Recidivism and self-cure of smoking and obesity. Am Psychol 37(4):436-444.

Schwartz L (1969). The hierarchy of resort in curative practices: the Admiralty Islands, Melanesia. J Health Soc Behav 10:302-309.

Sennott-Miller L, Miller J (1987). Difficulty: a neglected factor in health promotion. Nursing Res 36(5):268-272.

Spradley J (1979). The ethnographic interview. New York: Holt, Rinehart and Winston.

Stephenson M, Levy A, Sass N, MacGarvey W (1987). 1985 NHIS findings: nutrition knowledge and baseline data for the weight-loss objectives. Public Health Rep 102(1):61-67.

Stern M, Pugh J, Gaskill S, Hazuda H (1982). Knowledge, attitudes and behavior related to obesity and dieting in Mexican Americans and Anglos: the San Antonio heart study. Am J Epidemiol 115(6):917-928.

Stini W (1981). Body composition and nutrient reserves in evolutionary perspective. In D Walcher and N Kretchmer, Eds, Food, nutrition and evolution. New York: Mason.

Streigel-Moore RH, Silberstein LR, Rodin J (1986). Toward an understanding of the risk factors for bulimia. Am Psychol 41(3):246-263.

VanItallie T (1992). Body weight, morbidity and longevity. In P Bjorntorp and B Brodoff, Eds, Obesity. Philadelphia: JB Lippincott.

Walker A, Segal I (1980). The puzzle of obesity in the African black female. Lancet 1:263-265.

White JH (1984). The process of embarking on a weight control program. Health Care Women Int 5:77-91.

Wooley S, Wooley O (1984). Should obesity be treated at all? In A Stunkard and E Stellar, Eds, Eating and its disorders. New York: Raven Press.

17

Phenylpropanolamine in the Management of Moderate Obesity

David E. Schteingart, MD

Management approaches to the treatment of obesity include nutritional intervention, exercise and behavioral therapy. While weight reduction occurs with any of these techniques given singly or in combination, recidivism is high. When the success rate of people undertaking weight reduction with diet alone, behavior therapy alone, or combinations of the two is measured at the end of therapy after 1 year and after 5 years, it becomes clear that the weight loss is quickly reversed so that by the end of 5 years less than 10 percent of patients have continued to maintain a lower weight level. The addition of pharmacologic agents has the potential for more effective initial weight loss and long-term maintenance of weight reduction. Ultimately, the treatment of obesity should be based on principles similar to those used in the treatment of hypertension and non-insulin-dependent diabetes. Nonpharmacologic approaches including diet, exercise and behavioral therapy can reduce blood pressure or blood glucose in these two conditions. However, effective antihypertensive drugs and hypoglycemic agents have taken the predominant role in their management.

Several categories of drugs are currently available for treatment of obesity. These include (1) drugs that decrease food intake; (2) thermogenic stimulants; and (3) drugs that decrease intestinal absorption through inhibition of specific enzymes involved in carbohydrate or lipid digestion. Among the drugs that decrease food intake phenylpropanolamine (PPA), a sympathomimetic drug without central nervous system stimulating effect, has been studied the most over the past 30 years. In preclinical studies, phenylpropanolamine has been shown to decrease food intake and cause weight loss in a dose-dependent fashion. Twenty-eight clinical studies have tested the effectiveness of PPA in humans. Twenty-one were placebo-controlled (16 with a parallel design and five with a cross-over design); four were prescription drug-controlled (one study compared the effectiveness of PPA with or without caffeine and three studies were uncontrolled, long-term studies). The 16 placebo-controlled parallel studies ranged in duration from 2 to 16 weeks. These studies comprised 924 patients of which 484 were on PPA and 440 were on placebo. The PPA-treated group had greater weight loss than the placebo-treated group and the difference in weight loss was statistically significant (p < .05) in 11 of the 16 studies.[1-6] More recently, the Food and Drug Administration (FDA) in its April 1, 1991 Federal Register on PPA indicated that an FDA panel had reviewed a number of studies which had concluded that PPA-HCl was effective as an over-the-counter weight control drug product. The agency considered these studies as supportive but insufficient to establish this claim. However, more recently the agency reviewed two adequate and well-controlled studies that support the effectiveness of PPA-HCl. One of these studies was conducted by us at the University of Michigan;[7] the other study was conducted by Greenway and co-workers.[3]

The objective of our study was to determine the effectiveness of PPA as an adjunct in the dietary management of obesity. We wished to compare the effectiveness and safety of PPA to that of placebo in inducing weight loss when administered in addition to a hypocaloric diet to moderately obese men and women once a day for at least 42 consecutive days.

METHODS

Subjects

A total of 101 ambulatory subjects were selected for study; 85 were female and 16 were male. They ranged in age from 21 to 61 years and they were 15 to 45 percent overweight. Overweight criteria were established on the basis of desirable weight calculated from the Metropolitan Life Insurance Company Weight Tables[8] and were determined by the following formula: actual weight minus desirable weight/desirable weight x 100. Patients were excluded from the study if they were taking medications other than analgesics on an occasional basis, or drugs containing sympathomimetic amines. Also excluded were subjects with known endocrine, renal, hepatic, or thyroid disease; diabetes; cardiac disease; hypertension (blood pressure above 150/90 mm Hg) or glaucoma. Likewise excluded were known alcoholics, pregnant or lactating women, and patients who had participated in another weight reduction program which included drugs that promoted weight loss within 1 month prior to the start of this study. Informed consent was obtained and eligibility requirements were assessed prior to randomization.

STUDY DESIGN

A double-blind, placebo-controlled design was used. Following an initial detailed clinical evaluation which consisted of a structured interview and a complete physical examination, patients were randomly assigned to one of two treatment groups: (1) 75 mg PPA (sustained release); or (2) an identically appearing, pharmacologically inert placebo. Subjects took one capsule daily at 10:00 a.m. with 30 ml of water. Following the random assignment to one of the two treatment groups, patients participated in a 2-week placebo lead-in. They then took the drug or the placebo for at least 6 weeks without interruption. Patients were re-evaluated at weeks 2, 4, 6 and 8. Body weight was measured on each individual patient without outer clothing, and sitting blood pressure and pulse rate were determined each time on the same arm with a sphygmomanometer. Assessment of compliance was made by counting the number of capsules left in each bottle at the time of each visit. Patients who did not comply were excluded from the study. Patients were also given instruction on a 1200-calorie diet containing 54 percent of the calories as carbohydrate, 26 percent as protein and 20 percent as fat. The diet was also high in dietary fiber. Patients were given a specific daily diet pattern for three main meals and a snack. They were also given general guidelines concerning food exchanges, preparation of meals, types of vegetables and fruits to be consumed and the type of low-calorie beverages that were allowed. Patients started their diet at the beginning of the 2-week placebo lead-in period. They were not specifically monitored for compliance with the prescribed diet in an attempt to reproduce the situation which prevails with the use of an over-the-counter drug. Patients were also required to complete an appetite suppression questionnaire daily every 2 hours between 8:00 a.m. and midnight using a four-point scale (1 = no suppression; 2 = mild; 3 = moderate; 4 = complete).

DATA ANALYSIS

Treatment was evaluated for both efficacy and safety. Efficacy was determined by comparing weight loss over time for each treatment group. The amount of weight lost in the medication group was used as a measure of effectiveness. Both expected and unexpected untoward experiences while taking the drug were recorded based on the signs and symptoms detected at the time of the clinical interview and the physical examination. Particular attention was given to changes in blood pressure and heart rate as well as to symptoms of adrenergic stimulation.

Similarities between the two treatment groups and effectiveness of randomization were evaluated by comparing the background characteristics of the patients using a one-way analysis of variance, a Fisher's exact test, and a chi-square test. Differences in overall weight changes and differences between the active drug and placebo groups with respect to the trend in weight reduction were analyzed by univariate analysis of variance with repeated observations. An analysis of covariance test was also used to determine the level of significance of differences in weight loss between the two treatment groups observed at each visit. Patients who did not complete the study were considered dropouts and were reported accordingly. The data were reported for the entire patient sample, using an end-point analysis, which included each participant up to the point of leaving the study as well as completers.

RESULTS

The groups were found to be comparable with respect to age, race, marital status, body frame, height, initial body weight, ideal body weight, and percentage overweight (Table 1), indicating adequate randomization. Table 2 depicts cumulative mean weight loss during the first 6 weeks of treatment. These data were recorded following the 2-week placebo lead-in control period. It is clear that at each point of observation, patients on PPA had experienced a greater weight loss than those on placebo. For a second stage, patients were kept on the same groups in an extended double-blind study for up to 20 weeks; 24 patients from the PPA group and 12 from the placebo group chose to participate. The background characteristics for the two groups in terms of age, height, weight and percentage overweight were not significantly different. The cumulative weight loss for the PPA-treated patients continued to increase, reaching a mean loss of 5.1 1.48 kg by week 20 (Figure 1). In contrast, no significant weight loss was observed in the placebo group (0.39 0.9 kg) (p .05). A significant dropout occurred throughout the study. During the initial 8 week double-blind study, more patients dropped out from the placebo group (44 percent) than from the PPA-treated group (29.4 percent). This difference was not statistically significant but indicated a trend toward greater dropout among those on placebo. In the 8-week study more patients on placebo were lost to follow-up than those on PPA. Two patients in the placebo group indicated dissatisfaction with results, while none in the PPA group had this reason for dropping out. No significant difference in systolic or diastolic blood pressure, pulse rate, or subjective complaints (e.g., palpitations, dry nose, irritability, tiredness, nausea, constipation) was noted between the two groups. The mean weight loss during each of the two study phases was generally greater in male than female subjects when examined at weeks 8, 12, 16 and 20. This was particularly true in the placebo-treated group. There were no significant differences between the two treatment groups in their response to either the daily appetite suppression questionnaire or the questions regarding appetite asked at the time of their clinic visits. In spite of a greater weight loss on PPA, patients did not report a greater anorexic effect.

Table 1. Background Characteristics of All Selected Patients
(mean values)

	PPA Group	Placebo Group [*]
Number of patients	51.0	50.0
Sex		
Male	7.0	9.0
Female	44.0	41.0
Age	37.7	37.9
Weight (kg)	78.8	84.8
Height (cm)	163.0	165.5
Overweight (percent)	31.1	35.2

[*] Differences between PPA and placebo groups were not significant.

Table 2. Cumulative Weight Loss Achieved During the Initial 6-week
Treatment with PPA or Placebo Following a 2-Week Placebo
Lead-in Period*

	Weight Lost (kg) (Mean ± SEM)		
Week	PPA	Placebo	P
4	1.25 ± 0.18 (n=36)	0.24 ± 0.10 (n=28)	< .001
6	2.23 ± 0.23	1.0 ± 0.24	< .001
8	2.59 ± 0.35	1.07 ± 0.4	< .01

*Weight loss was calculated taking as baseline the weight observed in each
group at the end of week 2.

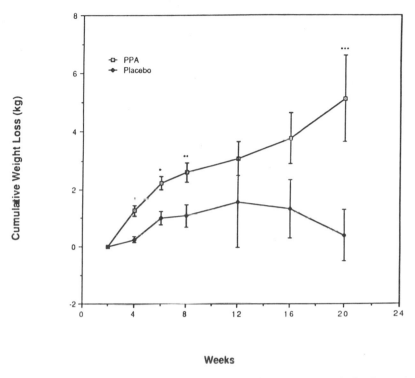

Figure 1. Difference in cumulative weight loss between PPA- and placebo-treated groups during the extended double-blind period (* $p < .001$; ** $p < .01$; *** $p < .05$).

COMMENT

These studies demonstrate that when PPA was added to a hypocaloric diet, weight loss was greater than with placebo. These results are consistent with several published and unpublished reports which indicate that PPA is an effective adjunct in weight reduction programs.[1-6] While the design of previous studies had been variable and the results not always comparable because of problems with ancillary therapy, inclusion criteria, treatment group comparability, duration of treatment, and dropouts, the present study had controlled these factors and shows significantly greater weight loss with PPA than with placebo for up to 20 weeks of treatment. Although the rate of additional weight loss experienced by patients on PPA when compared to placebo was relatively small, a comparison of PPA with prescription anorexics revealed comparable effectiveness in inducing weight loss.[9,10] In addition, in some cases, a decrease in weight of as little as 10 percent may have significant clinical consequence in terms of improvement in glucose tolerance and hypertension. Of interest is that no significant differences were reported by patients in terms of suppression of appetite between the two treatment groups. It is possible that enhancement of weight loss by PPA may be mediated by both mild appetite suppression and a mild sympathomimetic effect causing increased thermogenesis. In a study reported by Alger, patients who had been placed on a hypocaloric diet and PPA experienced a lesser decrease in 24-hour energy expenditure than those who were given the same hypocaloric diet and placebo.[11] This potential dual effect of PPA on appetite suppression and thermogenesis needs to be further defined.

NOTES

1. Weintraub M (1985). Phenylpropanolamine as an anorexiant agent in weight control: a review of published and unpublished studies. In JP Morgan, DV Kagan and JS Brody, Eds, Phenylpropanolamine: risks, benefits and controversies. Clinical pharmacology and therapeutic series, Vol 5. New York: Praeger Scientific.

2. Altschuler S, Frazer DL (1986). Double-blind clinical evaluation of the anorectic activity of phenylpropanolamine hydrochloride drops and placebo drops in the treatment of exogenous obesity. Curr Ther Res 40:211-217.

3. Greenway F (1989). A double-blind clinical evaluation of the anorectic activity of phenylpropanolamine versus placebo. Clin Ther 11:584-589.

4. Griboff S, Berman R, Silverman HI (1975). A double-blind clinical evaluation of a phenylpropanolamine-caffeine-vitamin combination and a placebo in the treatment of exogenous obesity. Curr Ther Res 17:535-543.

5. Sebok M (1985). A double-blinded, placebo-controlled, clinical study of the efficacy of a phenylpropanolamine-caffeine combination product as an aid to weight loss in adults. Curr Ther Res 37:701-708.

6. Weintraub M, et al. (1986). Phenylpropanolamine OROS (Acutrim) vs. placebo in combination with caloric restriction and physician-managed behavior modification. Clin Pharmacol Ther 39(5):501-509.

7. Schteingart DE (1992). Effectiveness of phenylpropanolamine in the management of moderate obesity. Int J Obesity 16:487-493.

8. Metropolitan height and weight tables (1984). Stat Bull Metro Life Ins Co 64:2-9.

9. Scoville BA (1991). Review of amphetamine-like drugs by the Food and Drug Administration. In GA Bray, Ed, Obesity in perspective. Fogarty International Center for Advanced Studies in the Health Sciences series on preventive medicine, Vol II. Washington DC: U.S. Government Printing Office.

10. Bray G (1985). Current status of drug therapy in obesity. In JP Morgan, DV Kagan and JS Brody, Eds, Phenylpropanolamine: risks, benefits and controversies. Clinical pharmacology and therapeutic series, Vol 5. New York: Praeger Scientific.

11. Alger S, Larson K, Boyce VL, Seagle H, Fontvielle A, Ferraro R, Rising R, Ravussin E (1991). Effect of phenylpropanolamine (PPA) on energy expenditure and weight loss in overweight Caucasian women. Presented at the Satellite Symposium to the 6th International Congress on Obesity: Pharmacological treatment of obesity, Yokohama, Japan, October 18-20.

18

Dexfenfluramine for the Long-Term Management of Obesity

Stanley Heshka, PhD

The research evidence on the success of weight reduction programs presents a fairly consistent picture. In the short term, substantial weight reduction can be achieved through a variety of treatment modalities, including very-low-calorie diets, medications and nutrition and exercise counseling. In the longer term, however, noncompliance, dropping out, side effects and difficulty in adhering to the treatment regimen lead to weight regain, so that after 4 to 5 years a large percentage of participants are back near their pretreatment starting weight. The initial steep decline in weight is followed by a gradual but almost inexorable trend upward (Brownell and Jeffery 1987).

The confluence of several factors, including the lack of long-term success in the maintenance of reduced weight, has obliged researchers to consider new approaches to the management of obesity. Some of these factors are: (1) a model of obesity as a chronic condition requiring continuing, long-term care rather than a brief intervention; (2) the need for effective weight reduction and maintenance with high success rates and low dropout rates for the efficacious treatment of such weight-related conditions as hypertension and non-insulin-dependent diabetes mellitus (NIDDM); (3) the identification of risk factors in obese individuals, such as a very high body mass index (BMI), large waist-to-hip ratio, substantial visceral fat deposits, or a family history of health problems exacerbated by obesity, which are strongly associated with eventual development of obesity-related pathologies; (4) the development of new anti-obesity drugs with novel modes of action and low abuse potential; and (5) evidence that improvements in health indices can occur after modest amounts of weight reduction (e.g., 10 to 15 percent) and, therefore, that attainment of "ideal" weight is an unnecessary and, for many, an unrealistic goal (Goldstein 1991).

Many promising new medications with interesting modes of action are at various stages of investigation and development. Among these are fat absorption blockers, lipid oxidation stimulators, carbohydrate digestion blockers, gastric emptying retardants, thermogenic agents and appetite suppressants.

One of the most promising of the new anti-obesity drugs is dex-fenfluramine (dFF). Its pharmacologic properties were the subject of a recent review (McTavish and Heel 1992). It is the dextrorotatory isomer of difenfluramine, which has been available for short-term treatment of obe-sity in the United States for several decades. Both dexfenfluramine and the racemic dl- fenfluramine stimulate serotonin (5-hydroxytryptamine, 5-HT) release and inhibit reuptake. Serotonin is stored in vesicles at synaptic sites and when released it acts on postsynaptic receptors. It is then transported out of the synaptic cleft back into the nerve terminal via specific membrane uptake carriers. Fenfluramine as well as other well-known compounds (e.g., fluoxetine, fluvoxemine, imipramine, clomipramine) inhibit the up-take carrier thereby increasing 5-HT concentrations in the synaptic cleft. Although the dexfenfluramine molecule is similar to amphetamine, there is no abuse potential or central nervous system stimulation; rather, a slight drowsiness may be induced.

The involvement of the serotonergic system in appetite and food regu-lation is well known. Complicating matters somewhat is the fact that there appear to be different classes of serotonin receptors (types 1, 2 and 3), that one of these classes has at least four distinct subtypes (1A-1D) and that the serotonergic system is also involved in numerous other functions such as depression, anxiety, pain and sleep (Whitaker-Azmitia and Peroutka 1990). The precise causal chain leading from increased serotonergic activity to suppression of food intake is unknown.

In the United States, fenfluramine (available under the trade name Pondimin) has received renewed interest as a result of a series of studies conducted recently by Weintraub and colleagues at the University of Roch-ester (Weintraub 1992). In these studies, fenfluramine was used in combi-nation with phentermine, a sympathomimetic agent, in a complex, multimodal weight loss program. The aspect which caught most public attention was the fact that medication was used in a long-term program and that some patients successfully reduced and maintained their lower weight for a period of 4 years. Previously, there were only a few reports in the research literature on the use of fenfluramine alone or in alternation with other medications for extended periods of 36 to 48 weeks, showing successful weight loss and maintenance (Douglas et al. 1983; Steel et al. 1973).

The Weintraub study was complex and involved many combinations and changes in medication regimen; however, two observations are of interest here. In the first phase, after a 6-week run-in, 121 patients were

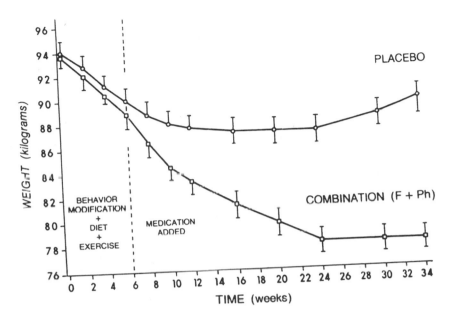

Figure 1. Participant body weight (kg) by study week. Open circles represent placebo group SEM ± (n = 54). Open squares represent fenfluramine plus phentermine group mean ± SEM (n = 58). (Reprinted with permission from M Weintraub, Long-term weight control. Clin Pharmacol Therapeutics 51:581 1992.)

randomly assigned into either combination treatment using 60 mg fenfluramine plus 15 mg phentermine, or placebo, along with caloric restriction, for 28 weeks. By week 34 the active group lost a mean of 14.2 kg, while the placebo group lost 4.6 kg. Only 9 patients dropped out and their decision did not appear to be related to adverse effects. Note that the plateau or leveling-off of the curve is not evidence for the development of tolerance to the medication (Figure 1). Rather, it should be interpreted as a new equilibrium in energy balance resulting from reduced food intake and reduced expenditure as a consequence of lower body weight. However, if we skip ahead to a point later in the protocol, between weeks 159 and 190, we note unmistakable upward trends in both the placebo and active medication groups (Figure 2). Assuming continued compliance with the medication regimen, such a trend suggests an eventual decline in efficacy resulting from development of tolerance or some other process.

Compared with fenfluramine, dexfenfluramine is effective at about half the dose level. At its effective dose level it has fewer adverse effects than

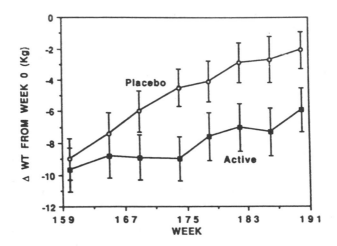

Figure 2.   Clearly observable upward trends in placebo and active medication groups between weeks 159 and 190. (Reprinted with permission from M Weintraub, Long-term weight control. Clin Pharmacol Therapeutics 51:581, 1992).

fenfluramine and its therapeutic index (ratio of active dose to toxic dose) is much more favorable. Dexfenfluramine has been approved for use in obesity treatment by regulatory agencies in many European countries including France, Belgium, Switzerland and the United Kingdom.

A number of recent studies have investigated various effects of dFF with some very interesting results. First, some acute effects which would likely be beneficial to the typical obese patient have been demonstrated. There is increased insulin sensitivity in NIDDM patients (Scheen et al. 1991), lower fasting blood glucose and lower serum insulin in obese, nondiabetic patients (Andersen et al. 1993). There is an immediate lowering of blood pressure (Andersson et al. 1991), increased free fatty-acid oxidation (Mingrone et al. 1991) and a lowering of the respiratory quotient (Even, Coulaud and Nicolaides 1988). There may also be increased dietary induced thermogenesis (Schutz et al. 1992). There is a substantial reduction in meal size and frequency of snacking and the reduction may be in the carbohydrate component for those subjects who describe themselves as "carbohydrate cravers" (Blundell and Hill 1992). Dexfenfluramine has been shown to delay stomach emptying of a solid meal (Horowitz et al. 1990).

Short-term studies (1 to 3 months) of dexfenfluramine have almost unanimously shown efficacy and safety. In one such study, conducted at the New York Obesity Research Center, 86 obese patients were randomized (double-blind) into active (n = 57) and placebo (n = 29) conditions, were instructed to follow a moderately restricted diet and were followed as outpatients for 3 months. The dropout rate was relatively high, almost one-third and was related to lack of efficacy in the placebo group. With respect to safety and adverse experiences, only one patient left the study for reasons related to medication (gastrointestinal discomfort and diarrhea). Few of the adverse events reported were judged to be severe and all of the subjects reporting such events nevertheless chose to continue in the study. No significant adverse changes in biochemistry or electrocardiograms (including corrected QT interval) were detected. A small decline in blood pressure (5 to 6 mm Hg) and a heart rate decrease (3 to 4 beats per minute) were observed during the first month.

With regard to efficacy, at 1 month the placebo group's weight had decreased by 1 kg, while that of the active group had decreased by about 2.5 kg. At 3 months, the placebo group had lost 2.4 kg, while the dexfenfluramine group had lost 3.8 kg. During the study, dietitians rated how well patients appeared to be adhering to the restricted-calorie diet. Upon the completion of the study the medicated patients were found to have shown better adherence. An improved total cholesterol to HDL cholesterol ratio was observed in the dFF group compared to the placebo group (4.5 vs. 4.2) after 3 months of medication. Also, body composition as measured by pooled total body electrical conductivity (TOBEC) and bio-impedance analysis (BIA) showed no change in percent body fat in the placebo group but a decline in percent body fat in the dexfenfluramine group. This latter result suggests greater conservation of fat free mass during weight loss in the medicated group. Such an effect would be consistent with a finding reported by Van Gaal and co-workers (1991) that resting metabolic rate decreased less after weight loss in the dFF group than placebo and also with the effect noted earlier of increased free fatty-acid oxidation under dFF (Mingrone et al. 1991).

Another recent 3-month study was conducted by Lafreniere and colleagues (1993). Thirty men and women participated in a double-blind, placebo-controlled trial. The dFF group lost 4.6 kg, while the placebo group maintained their initial weight. A most interesting aspect of this study was that participants were not explicitly instructed to restrict their calorie intake, yet the magnitude of the weight loss in the medicated group was comparable to that seen in studies where explicit dietary restriction was included. It would appear then that either instruction to restrict caloric intake is not usually followed, or that such an effort is unnecessary to achieve weight losses. In view of the frequent reports by patients of a sense of hunger, deprivation and effort that accompany restricted-calorie diets, the effortlessness of weight loss in the medicated group may be a very important aspect of such programs.

Only one large, long-term (1 year), multi-center study of dFF has been reported (Guy-Grand et al. 1989). A group of 822 obese patients in nine European countries were randomized to dFF or placebo and restricted diet, for 1 year. Initial weights of the participants were in the range of 96 to 98 kg. After 1 year there were more dropouts from the placebo group than from the dFF group (45 percent vs. 37 percent) and more of these dropouts in the placebo group expressed dissatisfaction with their rate of weight loss. Weight loss of completers (n = 483) amounted to 9.8 kg in the dFF group and 7.1 kg in the placebo group. The latter group showed a significant regain between the 6-month and 12-month measures. The active medication group was also beginning an upward trend, although it was not statistically significant by the end of the study period.

The most frequent side effects associated with dFF are abdominal discomfort (including diarrhea, nausea and constipation), dry mouth and tiredness or drowsiness. The effects are most prominent at the start of medication and appear to diminish over time. Of course, with long-term medication in large populations, there is the ever-present danger of infrequent but serious adverse effects. With dFF these concerns have focused on several cases of pulmonary hypertension (*Lancet* 1992) and on the possible depletion of brain serotonin (*Science* 1989a, 1989b).

In summary, dFF is a promising medication for use in a program of long-term weight loss and maintenance. The immediate side effects are mild and the weight loss seems to be achieved without great effort on the part of the subject. Additional data are needed to establish whether, after periods of 3 or 4 years, medications show loss of efficacy as suggested by the gradual upturn in the weight curves. If so, long-term medication programs may require intermittent medication or alternating among different medications with different modes of action to maintain a lower weight.

The risks involved in medicating for very long periods are also not well known. Obviously, these risks are most justifiably assumed with persons who, if untreated or unsuccessfully treated, are at high risk of developing pathologies, such as persons with a very high BMI, a large waist-to-hip ratio, substantial visceral fat deposits, or a family history of health problems related to, or exacerbated by, obesity.

REFERENCES

Andersen PH, Richelsen B, Bak J, Schmitz O, Sorensen NS, Laveille R, Pedersen O (1993). Influence of short-term dexfenfluramine therapy on glucose and lipid metabolism in obese non-diabetic patients. Acta Endocrinol 128(3):251-258.

Andersson B, Zimmermann ME, Hedner T, Bjorntorp P (1991). Haemodynamic, metabolic and endocrine effects of short-term dexfenfluramine treatment in young, obese women. Europ J Clin Pharmacol 40(3):249-254.

Blundell JE, Hill AJ (1992). Dexfenfluramine and appetite in humans. Int J Obesity 16(Suppl3):S51-S59.

Brownell KD, Jeffery RW (1987). Improving long-term weight loss: pushing the limits of treatment. Behav Ther 18:353-374.

Douglas JG, Gough J, Preston PG, et al. (1983). Long-term efficacy of fenfluramine in treatment of obesity. Lancet 1:384-386.

Even P, Coulaud H, Nicolaides S (1988). Lipostatic and ischymetric mechanisms originate dexfenfluramine-induced anorexia. Pharmacol Biochem Behav 30:89-99.

Goldstein DJ (1992). Beneficial effects of modest weight loss. Int J Obesity 16:397-415.

Guy-Grand B, Apfelbaum M, Crepaldi G, Gries A, Lefebvre PJ, Turner P (1989). International trial of long-term dexfenfluramine in obesity. Lancet 2:1142-1144.

Horowitz M, Maddox A, Wishart J, Vernon-Roberts J, Chatterton B, Shearman D (1990). Effect of dexfenfluramine on gastric emptying of a mixed solid-liquid meal in obese subjects. Br J Nutrition 63(3):447-455.

Lafreniere F, Lambert J, Rasio E, Serri O (1993). Effects of dexfenfluramine treatment on body weight and postprandial thermogenesis in obese subjects: a double-blind placebo-controlled study. Int J Obesity 17:25-30.

Lancet (1992). Pulmonary hypertension and dexfenfluramine (letters). Feb 15:436-437

McTavish D, Heel RC (1992). Dexfenfluramine: a review of its pharmacological properties and therapeutic potential in obesity. Drugs 43(5):713-733.

Mingrone G, Greco AV, Tataranni A, Raguso C, Finotti E, Tacchino RM, Marino F, De Gaetano A, Castagneto M, Ghirlanda G (1991). Effect of acute and chronic administration of d-fenfluramine on free fatty acid mobilization and oxidation. Paper presented at 3rd European Congress on Obesity, Nice, May 30-June 1.

Schutz Y, Munger R, Deriaz O, Jequier E (1992). Effect of dexfenfluramine on energy expenditure in man. Int J Obesity 16(Suppl3):S61-S66.

Science (1989a). Neurotoxicity creates regulatory dilemma. Jan 6:29-39.

Science (1989b). Fenfluramine studies (letters). Feb 24:991.

Sheen AJ, Paolisso G, Salvatore T, Lefebvre PJ (1991). Improvement of insulin-induced glucose disposal in obese patients with NIDDM after 1-week treatment with d-fenfluramine. Diabetes Care 14(4):325-332.

Steel JM, Munro JF, Duncan LJP (1973). A comparative trial of different regimens of fenfluramine and phentermine in obesity. Practitioner 211:232-236.

Van Gaal L, Vansant G, Van de Voorde K, De Leeuw I (1991). Positive effects of dexfenfluramine on energy expenditure during long-term weight reduction in obese women. Paper presented at 3rd European Congress on Obesity, Nice, May 30-June 1.

Weintraub M (1992). Long-term weight control: the National Heart, Lung and Blood Institute funded multimodal intervention study. Clin Pharmacol Therapeutics 51:581-646.

Whitaker-Azmitia PM, Peroutka SJ, Eds (1990). The Neuropharmacology of Serotonin. New York: New York Academy of Sciences.

19

Individualizing Pharmacologic Therapy for Weight Reduction: The Lovan Example

David J. Goldstein, MD, PhD, Paul J. Roback, MS
Susan L. Holman, MS, Michael G. Wilson, MS
Gary D. Tollefson, MD, PhD, Rocco L. Brunelle, MS
Alvin H. Rampey, Jr., PhD

Obesity is a common health problem in the United States. Although attempts at weight reduction are frequent, reduced weight is rarely maintained even when the attempt is associated with a complete program which incorporates nutritional and behavioral counseling and exercise. Individuals have difficulty losing and maintaining weight despite the health benefits and social incentives that accompany reduction in overweight.

Because weight loss and maintenance are typically unsuccessful, pharmacologic therapy has been utilized in an effort to improve outcomes. Scoville (1976) reviewed the results from 105 New Drug Applications of agents for weight reduction. The trials compared the effects of pharmacologic agents to placebo over 6 to 20 weeks. Scoville noted that the pharmacologic agents available at that time were similar in their weight loss effects. In summary, he stated that "the administration of an anorectic drug will result in a weight loss of approximately 0.5 pounds (0.23 kg) more each week than if he or she were taking placebo." In 1987, Ferguson and Feighner reported on an 8-week, double-blind trial of fluoxetine, benzphetamine and placebo in obesity over 8 weeks of double-blind therapy (Figure 1). Both agents induced superior weight loss over placebo by about 0.18 kg per

The authors gratefully acknowledge the many contributions of Mary E. Sayler, MS, Gregory G. Enas, PhD, and Janet Potvin, PhD in the preparation of this chapter.

week. Thus, fluoxetine is probably similar in its weight-reducing effects to the adrenergic agents assessed by Scoville.

In his analyses, Scoville failed to recognize two important variables which influence outcome: dose and length of therapy. Evidence suggests that pharmacologic agents have a dose-related effect on weight loss. In a dose-response study (Levine 1989) investigating 0, 10, 20, 40 and 60 mg of fluoxetine, the correlation coefficients for linear regression of change in weight versus dose were 0.995 and 0.940 at weeks 4 and 8, respectively (Figure 2), demonstrating a significant linear component in the dose-response relationship for fluoxetine.

Length of therapy provides additional insights into the effectiveness of pharmacologic agents. Long-term therapy produces a characteristic profile of weight loss. Mean maximal weight loss is achieved after about 6 months of therapy; thereafter, weight stabilizes or gradually is regained. In addition to demonstrating this characteristic therapeutic profile, long-term trials also demonstrate variability of results between trials, effects of adjunctive therapy and individualized response. The following trials illustrate these effects.

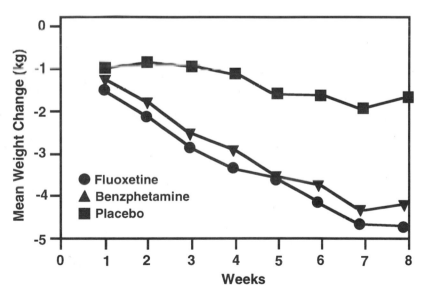

Figure 1. Comparison of the effects of floxetine, benphetamine and placebo on weight over 8 weeks. (Adapted from JM Ferguson and JP Feighner, Fluoxetine-induced weight loss in overweight non-depressed humans. Int J Obesity 11S:163-170, 1987.)

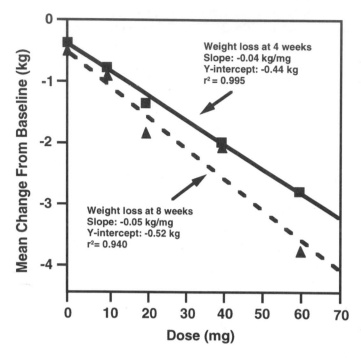

Figure 2. Dose-response analysis of fluoxetine over 8 weeks in a double-blind, placebo-controlled trial.

The long-term effectiveness of active therapy and 24-week weight loss plateau were observed in a 36-week trial of phentermine, intermittent phentermine and placebo (Munro 1968). At the end of the study, the active therapy-treated patients had lost about 9 kg more than the placebo-treated patients.

Long-term effectiveness, the 24-week weight loss plateau and slow regain were observed by Guy-Grand (1989) in a 52-week double-blind, placebo-controlled trial with dexfenfluramine. Among the completers, weight loss plateaued at 6 months with slight regain after 32 weeks. About 40 percent of patients prematurely discontinued treatment. At 52 weeks, dexfenfluramine was associated with about 4 percent greater weight loss from baseline than placebo.

The 24-week weight loss plateau, weight regain and the variability among trials are apparent from another trial using dexfenfluramine. Mathus-Vliegen (1992) reported on a double-blind, placebo-controlled 52-week study of dexfenfluramine and a very-low-calorie diet. Mean maximal weight loss occurred at 24 weeks; thereafter, weight began to be regained.

At the end of the trial the mean weight loss was about 6 kg for both groups. There was no separation between treatment groups at any time during the study. The differences in results of these dexfenfluramine trials show the variability in results that can occur, possibly due to differences in design and patient populations.

The weight loss plateau, effect of adjunctive therapy and individualized response are demonstrated by a 5-year trial by Weintraub (1991). This long-term trial had multiple phases. Patients were rigorously screened prior to selection for the trial. A 6-week, no-drug, lead-in period showed a mean 5 kg weight loss attributable to the comprehensive adjunctive dietary, behavioral and exercise therapy program. In the 28-week, double-blind, placebo-controlled phase, the combination of phentermine and fenfluramine was compared with placebo. Mean weight loss plateaued after 18 weeks of double-blind therapy. After 28 weeks of therapy, the active therapy-treated patients had lost about 12 kg more than the placebo-treated patients. During the next phase, a 26-week open-label extension, the initial placebo-treated cohort received combined therapy which induced a mean weight loss of about 10 kg; no additional weight loss was achieved in subsequent phases. Of the initial combined therapy cohort, patients not losing weight on the combination (nonresponders) were treated with a higher dose for an additional 26 weeks without achieving additional weight loss. The lack of response in these nonresponders suggests that some individuals are resistant to certain therapies despite dose escalation. Responders from the initial combined therapy cohort, who continued active therapy over the 5 years of the study, generally regained some of the weight lost.

Clinical trials with fluoxetine have shown similar outcomes to the above trials. Marcus (1990) reported on a 52-week, double-blind, placebo-controlled trial with fluoxetine as an adjunct to behavioral counseling. Mean weight loss plateaued at 36 weeks and at 52 weeks the fluoxetine-treated patients lost about 15 kg more than the placebo-treated patients. Darga (1991) reported on a study using the same design with nutritional counseling instead of behavioral counseling. The weight loss peaked at 28 weeks after which weight was gradually regained. At 52 weeks the fluoxetine-treated patients lost about 3.5 kg more than the placebo-treated patients. These and other studies suggest that results may vary with different adjunctive therapies.

Pharmacologic therapy appears to be characterized by a weight loss plateau after 6 months of therapy and a tendency for weight regain thereafter. However, variability across studies and probable subgroup differences limit the generalization of these conclusions to individuals.

To better compare the effectiveness of various therapies, we defined a clinically meaningful pattern of weight loss consistent with successful pharmacologic therapy. Figure 3 shows the characteristics of a successful pattern of weight loss. Although an early possibility of weight gain due to

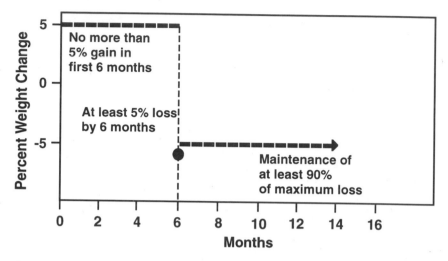

Figure 3.   Characteristics of a successful pattern of weight loss induced by a pharmacologic weight loss agent.

normal variation is permitted, the weight loss after 6 months of therapy must be at least 5 percent of baseline weight. This amount of weight loss has been shown to be clinically relevant (Goldstein 1992). Subsequently, the patient must maintain at least 90 percent of the maximum weight loss achieved. We evaluated the weight loss patterns from all long-term patients (n = 1026) in four double-blind, placebo controlled clinical trials lasting at least 36 weeks. A greater proportion of fluoxetine-treated patients (8.6 percent) than placebo-treated patients (5.4 percent) achieved a successful weight loss pattern (Holman 1994).

Since we have seen that not everyone accrues benefit from each specific agent, it would be helpful if we could predict which patients had a greater likelihood of success from a given therapy. We investigated the relationship between long-term outcome and baseline variables collected in our weight loss studies, including demographics; smoking and drinking habits; historic, chronic and comorbid conditions; concomitant medications; and laboratory values (Roback 1994). The baseline predictors associated with a long-term treatment effect on weight loss are age, smoking status and plasma uric acid concentrations. Patients who were older, did not smoke and had higher uric acid concentrations lost the most weight over comparable placebo-treated patients. These predictors are associated with a higher plasma level of fluoxetine and its active major metabolite norfluoxetine.

Use of the predictors can enrich the treatment population so that a greater proportion of treated patients will be successful.

The relationship of early treatment response to long-term outcome can also be used to reduce ineffective patient exposure. Only 17 percent of the patients who had not lost any weight after 4 weeks of fluoxetine therapy had lost weight after 52 weeks of therapy (Rampey, unpublished data 1993). Thus, since the likelihood of later benefit is low, patients who do not benefit by 4 weeks should be discontinued from therapy.

Once a patient has been selected to receive pharmacologic therapy, how should that patient's progress be monitored? Figure 4 shows a graph based on the data from the fluoxetine-treated patients who had successful weight loss patterns over 52 weeks as described above. A realistic percent weight loss goal should be set for each patient prior to initiation of therapy and marked on the graph. The patient's percent weight loss should be plotted at each visit and compared to the data from the successful patterns. One should evaluate the progress at each visit against the long-term goal. If the patient does not seem to be approaching the long-term goal, the therapy should be reevaluated. The reevaluation should include the following considerations: reassessment of the goal, more frequent visits, more intensive counseling, more intensive exercise, alternative therapy, higher dose, or addition of another agent.

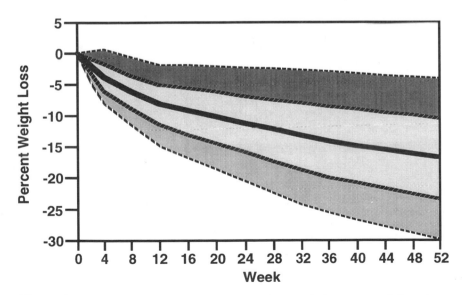

Figure 4. Data from patients with a successful weight loss pattern (plotted as a mean ± 1 and 2 SD).

240 *Obesity*

Existing pharmacologic therapy for weight reduction and weight maintenance offers promise for many individuals who are unable to succeed with nonpharmacologic programs. Strategies such as selection of patients most likely to benefit from treatment, use of adjunctive therapies and monitoring of therapy against guidelines need to be developed for maximizing the benefit of these therapies. It is hoped that agents with novel mechanisms of action will demonstrate greater efficacy than existing agents. Until that time, strategies will need to be developed to maximize the benefits of existing therapies.

REFERENCES

Darga LL, Carroll-Michals L, Botsford SJ, Lucas CP (1991). Fluoxetine's effect on weight loss in obese subjects. Am J Clin Nutrition 54:321-325.

Ferguson JM, Feighner JP (1987). Fluoxetine-induced weight loss in overweight nondepressed humans. Int J Obesity 11S:163-170.

Goldstein DJ (1992). Beneficial health effects of modest weight loss. Int J Obesity 16:397-415.

Guy-Grand B, Apfelbaum M, Crepaldi G, Gries A, Lefebvre P, Turner P (1989). International trial of long-term D-fenfluramine in obesity. Lancet ii:1142-1144.

Holman SJ, Goldstein DJ, Enas GG (1994). Pattern analysis method for assessing successful weight reduction. Int J Obes 18:281-285.

Levine LR, Enas GG, Thompson WL, et al. (1989). Use of fluoxetine, a selective serotonin-uptake inhibitor, in the treatment of obesity: a dose response study (with a commentary by Michael Weintraub). Int J Obesity 13:635-645.

Marcus MD, Wing RR, Ewing L, Kern E, McDermott M, Gooding W (1990). A double-blind placebo-controlled trial of fluoxetine plus behavior modification in the treatment of obese binge eaters and non-binge-eaters. Am J Psychol 147:876-881.

Mathus-Vliegen EMH, Van De Voore K, Kok AME, Res AMA (1992). Dexfenfluramine in the treatment of severe obesity: a placebo-controlled investigation of the effects on weight loss, cardiovascular risk factors, food intake and eating behavior. J Intern Med 232:119-127.

Munro JF, MacCuish AC, Wilson EM, Duncan LJP (1968). Comparison of continuous and intermittent anorectic therapy in obesity. Br Med J 1:352-354.

Roback, PJ, Goldstein DJ, Rampey AH, Wilson MG (1994). Baseline predictors of success when comparing two treatments. Obes Res 2:337-347.

Scoville BA (1976). Review of amphetamine-like drugs by the Food and Drug Administration: clinical data and value judgments. In GA Bray, Ed, Obesity in perspective. Proceedings of the Fogarty Conference. Washington, DC: U.S. Government Printing Office.

Weintraub M, Sundaresan PR, Ginsberg G, Madan M, Balder A, Stein EC, Byrne L (1991). Long-term weight control study II (weeks 34 to 104): an open-label study of continuous fenfluramine plus phentermine versus targeted intermittent medication as adjuncts to behavior modification, caloric restriction and exercise. Clin Pharm Ther 51:595-601.

Weintraub M, Sundaresan PR, Madan M, Schuster B, Balder A, Lasagna L, Cox C (1991). Long-term weight control study I (weeks 0 to 34): the enhancement of behavior modification, caloric restriction and exercise by fenfluramine plus phentermine versus placebo. Clin Pharm Ther 51:586-594.

20

Evolutionary Aspects of Diet: Fatty Acids, Insulin Resistance and Obesity

Artemis P. Simopoulos, MD

The health of the individual and the population[1] as a whole is the result of interactions between genetic and environmental factors and the milieu in which development occurs[1,2] (Figure 1). Advances in genetics and molecular biology have contributed to our understanding of many of the chronic diseases, including obesity. Obesity is the most common disorder of the developed world[3] and is becoming prevalent in the developing world as well.[4] Obesity is not a new disorder—Hippocrates was concerned about obesity and noted that "sudden death is more common in those who are naturally fat than in the lean."[5] Hippocrates did not define obesity in terms of what is desirable body weight, but the artists of the period emphasized a small waist and muscle development for males and a small waist with a more rounded figure for females.

In defining the concept of positive health, Hippocrates stated:

> Positive health requires a knowledge of man's primary constitution and of the powers of various foods, both those natural to them and those resulting from human skill. But eating alone is not enough for health. There must also be exercise, of which the effects must likewise be known. The combination of these two things makes regimen, when proper attention is given to the season of the year, the changes of the winds, the age of the individual and the situation of his home. If there is any deficiency in food or exercise the body will fall sick.

Food as a source of energy intake was recognized by Hippocrates. The statement that if there is any dificiency in food or exercise the body will fall sick is as true today as it was 2500 years ago. Restating this concept in today's scientific terms obesity is the result of an imbalance between energy intake and energy expenditure involving metabolic defects, genetic suscep-

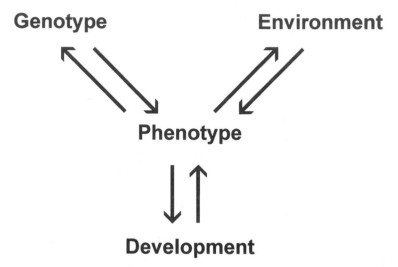

Figure 1.   Relationships among genes, environment, and development are dynamic. Adapted from B Childs, Genetic variation and nutrition. Am J Clin Nutrition 48:1500-1504, 1988.

tibility, and environmental factors. Nutrition is an environmental factor of major importance as is physical activity. The prevalence of obesity in a population depends on the definition of obesity or the standard of desirable body weight selected for use.

This chapter discusses the evolutionary aspects of diet and the major changes that have occurred in the food supply in terms of protein, carbohydrate, and fat intake, with an emphasis on the type and amount of fatty acids: isomeric trans fatty acids, essential fatty acids (EFAs), and their contribution to, or interplay with, hyperinsulinemia or insulin resistance (decreased sensitivity to insulin) and obesity.

EVOLUTIONARY ASPECTS OF DIET AND
THE OMEGA-6/OMEGA-3 BALANCE

Information on the diet of early man is obtained from archaeological studies and from observations of present-day hunter-gatherer societies. Based on estimates from studies in paleolithic nutrition and contemporary hunter-gatherer populations, man evolved on a diet that was much higher in protein, lower in carbohydrate, but higher in fruits and vegetables, and much lower in saturated fat than today's conventional diet (Tables 1 and 2).[6-10]

Sugar and particularly free fructose have increased in the diet of Ameri-

Table 1. Characteristics of Hunter-Gatherer and Western Diet
and Lifestyles

Characteristic	Hunter-Gatherer Lifestyle	Western Lifestyle
Physical Activity Level	high	low
Diet		
Energy density	low	high
Energy intake	moderate	high
Protein	high	low-moderate
animal	high	low-moderate
vegetable	very low	low-moderate
Carbohydrate	low-moderate (slowly absorbed)	moderate (rapidly absorbed)
Fiber	high	low
Fat	low	high
vegetable	very low	moderate to high
animal	low polyunsaturated	high saturated
ω6/ω3 ratio	low (2.4)	high (12)
linolenic and linoleic acids*	low (3.3)	high (12.3)
long-chain ω6 and ω3 PUFA*	high (2.3)	low (0.2)

* Expressed in grams of fatty acid per person per day.
From AP Simopoulos, Dietary risk factors for hypertension. Comp Ther
18(10):26-30, 1992.

cans over the past 25 years because of the wide introduction of high-fructose corn sweetener in 1967. Fructose is a component of many fruits,
vegetables and sweeteners. Intake of fructose from sweeteners such as
sucrose, high-fructose corn syrup and honey accounts for about 8 percent

Table 2. Comparison of the Late Paleolithic Diet and the Current American Diet

Characteristic	Late Paleolithic Diet[1]	Current American Diet
Total dietary energy (%)		
Protein	34.0	12.0
Carbohydrate	45.0	46.0
Fat	21.0	42
P:S ratio[2]	1.41	0.44
Cholesterol (mg)	591	600
Fiber (g)	45.7	19.7
Sodium (mg)	690	2300-6900
Calcium (mg)	1580	740[3]
Ascorbic acid (mg)	392.3	87.7[3]

[1] Assuming the diet contained 35 percent meat and 65 percent vegetables.
[2] P:S denotes the ratio of polyunsaturated to saturated fats.
[3] U.S. Department of Agriculture Food Consumption Survey, 1977-1978.

of the total calories consumed.[11] Consumption of fructose favors synthesis of fat over gluconeogenesis. This is the result of increased hepatic synthesis of glycerol and fatty acids compared to glucose, as has been demonstrated in rats.[12] In humans, fructose increases plasma triglycerides and under some conditions dietary fructose may increase plasma cholesterol concentration.[13] Postmenopausal women are more likely to become hypertriglyceridemic after fructose consumption.[12]

It is important to understand the evolutionary forces in dietary development and the consequences of deviating sharply from the diet that humans were genetically programmed for during their long evolutionary period. New information clearly shows that high-carbohydrate diets raise serum triglyceride levels and lower high-density lipoprotein (HDL) concentration.[12,14-16] High triglycerides are associated with obesity. Considering that the average American woman today is 20 percent above desirable body weight,[3] which translates into a body mass index (BMI) of 27, it is obvious why the majority of women in this country have elevated triglycerides. A high-carbohydrate diet rich in fructose further raises their triglyceride levels. The combination of low HDL and high triglyceride concentrations constitutes a risk factor for cardiovascular disease, particularly in postmenopausal women.[17]

The paleolithic diet contained roughly equal amounts of omega-6 and omega-3 polyunsaturated fatty acids [6,8,10,18,19] (Figure 2). Modern agriculture with its emphasis on production has decreased the omega-3 fatty acid

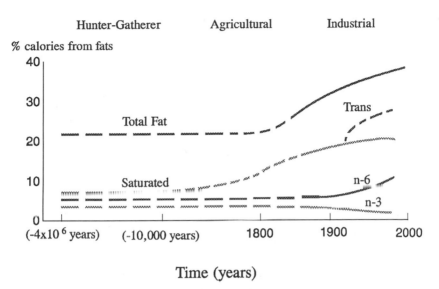

Figure 2. Relative percentages of fat and different fatty acid families in human nutrition as extrapolated from cross-sectional analyses of contemporary hunter-gatherer populations and from longitudinal observations and their putative changes during the preceding 100 years. Adapted from A Leaf and PC Weber, A new era for science in nutrition. Am J Clin Nutrition 45(suppl):1048-1053, 1987.

Table 3. Polyunsaturated Fatty Acid Content* in Typical Western and Hunter-Gatherer Diets

Diet	Linoleic and Linolenic Acids	Long-chain ω6 and ω3 PUFA	ω6/ω3 Ratio
Western diet	12.3	0.2	12
Hunter-gatherer diet	3.3	2.3	2.4

* Expressed in grams of fatty acid type per person per day.
Modified from AJ Sinclair and K O'Dea, Fats in human diets through history. In JD Wood and AV Fisher, Eds, Reducing fat in meat animals. London: Elsevier, 1990.

content in many foods: green leafy vegetables, animal meats, eggs and even fish.[20-22] Wild animals and birds who feed on wild plants are very lean with a carcass fat content of only 3.9 percent[23]; their bodies contain about five times more polyunsaturated fat per gram than is found in domestic livestock. Edible wild plants contain a good balance of omega-6 and omega-3 fatty acids and are rich in vitamin C and carotenoids.[10,18] Wild purslane, for example, contains 10 times as much omega-3 fatty acids as cultivated green vegetables and is richer in vitamins C and E and glutathione than spinach.[18]

An absolute and relative change of omega-6/omega-3 fatty acids in the food supply of western societies has occurred over the last 100 years[8] (Figure 2). A balance existed between omega-6 and omega-3 for most of human history, and the genetic changes that occurred did so partly in response to changing dietary influences.[6]

The ratio of omega-6 to omega-3 fatty acids that was about 1:1 from vegetable and animal sources during the hunter-gatherer of human evolution is now estimated by Hunter[24] to be between 10 and 11:1 from vegetable sources. From evidence that the per capita consumption of major foods in 1987 was 135 lb (61.4 kg) red meat, 63 lb (28.6 kg) chicken and 15 lb (6.8 kg) fish plus the increases in omega-6 fatty acids from vegetable oils, the ratio of omega-6 to omega-3 fatty acids is closer to 20 to 25:1 from vegetable and animal sources. From per capita quantities of foods available for consumption in the U.S. national food supply in 1985, the level of eicosapentaenoic acid (EPA) is reported to be approximately 50 mg per person per day and the level of docosahexaenoic acid (DHA) is 80 mg per person per day. The two main

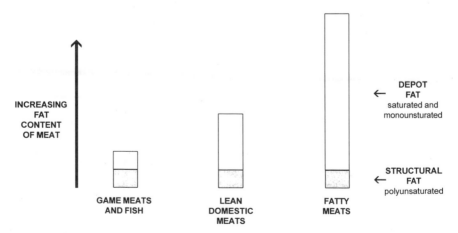

Figure 3.   The relationship between total fat content in meat and the relative proportion of structural lipid. The higher the total fat content, the lower the proportion of structural lipid.

sources are fish and poultry,[25] whereas the intake of arachidonic acid (AA) from meat, eggs and dairy products is between 500 and 1000 mg.[16,26]

However, rapid dietary changes over short periods of time, as have occurred over the past 100 to 150 years, is a significant new phenomenon in human evolution (see Tables 1 and 2; Figure 2). In addition to the changes in the ratio of omega-6 to omega-3, there has been a decrease in the ratio of EPA and DHA to linolenic acid and of AA to linoleic acid[10] (Table 3).

The indiscriminate recommendation to replace saturated fats with poly-unsaturated fatty acids (PUFAs) from vegetable oils and margarines has led to increased amounts of omega-6 fatty acids, mainly 18:236 from oils and trans fatty acids from margarine in standard diets over the past 50 to 60 years. Therefore, humans have been exposed to pharmacologic doses of omega-6 fatty acids for the first time in their evolution. Our paleolithic ancestors consumed more structural and less depot fat[10] (Figure 3). Further-more, the trans fatty acids that today account for about 5 to 7 percent of energy from fat[27,28] occur rarely in nature and are the result of the hydro-genation process developed on a large scale after the World War I.

Elongation and Desaturation of Omega-3 and Omega-6 Fatty Acids

Omega-3 and omega-6 fatty acids are also known as essential fatty acids (EFAs) because humans, like all mammals, cannot make them and must obtain both from their diet. Omega-6 fatty acids are represented by linoleic acid (LA) and omega-3 fatty acids by alpha-linolenic acid (LNA).

LA is plentiful in nature and is found in the seeds of most plants except for coconut, cocoa and palm. LNA, on the other hand, is found in the chloroplasts of green leafy vegetables and in the seeds of flax and rape. Both EFAs are metabolized to longer-chain fatty acids of 20- and 22-carbon atoms. LA is metabolized to AA and LNA metabolized to EPA and DHA, increasing the chain length and degree of unsaturation by adding extra double bonds to the carboxyl group (Figure 4).

Humans and animals, except for obligate carnivores such as lions, can convert LA to AA and LNA to EPA and DHA.[29] This conversion was shown by using deuterated LNA.[30] There is competition between omega-3 and omega-6 fatty acids for the desaturation enzymes. However, both delta-4 and delta-6 desaturases prefer omega-3 to omega-6 fatty acids.[29,31,32] There is some evidence that delta-6 desaturase decreases with age.[29] DHA, like EPA, can be derived only from direct ingestion or by synthesis from dietary EPA or LNA. Similarly, AA can be derived only from direct ingestion or by synthesis from dietary LA. Premature infants,[33] hypertensive individuals[34] and some diabetics[35] are limited in their ability to make EPA and DHA from LNA. These findings are important and need to be considered when making dietary recommendations. EPA and DHA are found in the oils of

Linoleate series		Linolenate series	
C18:2w6	Linoleic acid	C18:3w3	Alpha-linolenic acid
$\triangle^6$ desaturase		$\triangle^6$ desaturase	
↓		↓	
C18:3w6	Gamma-linolenic acid	C18:4w3	
↓		↓	
C20:3w6	Dihomo-gamma-Linolenic Acid	C20:4w3	
$\triangle^5$ desaturase		$\triangle^5$ desaturase	
↓		↓	
C20:4w6	Arachidonic acid	C20:5w3	Eicosapentaenoic acid
↓		↓	
C22:4w6		C22:5w3	Docosapentaenoic acid
$\triangle^4$ desaturase		$\triangle^4$ desaturase	
↓		↓	
C22:5w6	Docosapentaenoic acid	C22:6w3	Docosahexaenoic acid

Figure 4. Essential fatty acid metabolism, desaturation, and elongation of omega-6 and omega-3 fatty acids.

fish, particularly fatty fish.[36] AA is found predominantly in the phospholipids of grain-fed animals.

LA, LNA and their long-chain derivatives are important components of animal and plant cell membranes. In mammals and birds the omega-3 fatty acids are distributed selectively among lipid classes. LNA is found in triglycerides, in cholesteryl esters and in very small amounts in phospholipids. LA is found in phospholipids in larger amounts than LNA. EPA and AA are found mostly in phospholipids. In mammals, including humans, the cerebral cortex,[37] retina,[38] and testis and sperm[39] are particularly rich in DHA. It is one of the most abundant components of the plasma membranes of brain neurons.

Eicosanoid Metabolism

Arachidonic acid and eicosapentaenoic acid are precursors of metabolic products that consist of 20-carbon atoms and are known collectively as eicosanoids (prostaglandins, thromboxanes and leukotrienes)[40,41] (Figure 5). The discovery of prostaglandins and subsequently the recognition that AA is the precursor of the 2-series of prostanoids (prostaglandins and thromboxanes) and of leukotrienes of the 4-series expanded the horizons of research on omega-6 and omega-3 fatty acids because LA, the precursor of AA, is the predominant PUFA in the Western diet. EPA and DHA are precursors of the prostanoids of the 3-series and leukotrienes of the 5-series. The discovery by Needleman and co-workers[42] in 1979 that prostaglandins

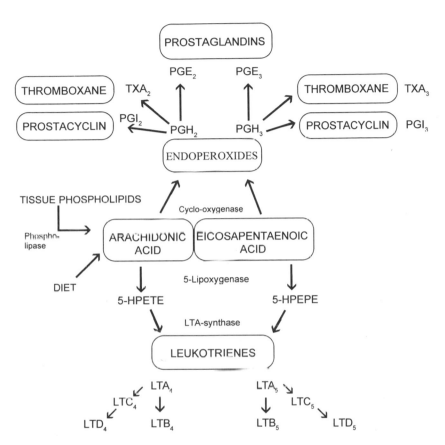

Figure 5. Oxidative metabolism of arachidonic acid and eicosapentaenoic acid by the cyclooxygenase and 5-lipoxygenase pathways. 5-HPETE denotes 5-hydroperoxyeicosatetraenoic acid and 5-HPEPE denotes 5-hydroxyeicosapentaenoic acid.

derived from EPA have different biologic properties than do those derived from AA stimulated further research on fish oils and on the nutritional aspects of prostaglandins.

Competition between the two different classes of PUFAs occurs in prostaglandin formation: EPA competes with AA for prostaglandin and leukotriene synthesis at the cyclooxygenase and lipoxygenase level. When humans ingest fish or fish oil, the EPA and DHA from the diet partially replace the omega-6 fatty acids, especially AA, in the membranes of probably all cells (especially in the membranes of platelets, erythrocytes, neu-

250 Obesity

trophils, monocytes and liver cells.) In animals, diet influences the PUFA phospholipids of muscle cells.[43] As a result, ingestion of EPA and DHA from fish or fish oil leads to:

- a decreased production of prostaglandin E_2 (PgE$_2$) metabolites
- a decrease in thromboxane A_2, a potent platelet aggregator and vasoconstrictor
- a decrease in leukotriene B_4 formation, an inducer of inflammation and a powerful inducer of leukocyte chemotaxis and adherence
- an increase in thromboxane A_3, a weak platelet aggregator and a weak vasoconstrictor
- an increase in prostacyclin PgI$_3$, leading to an overall total increase in total prostacyclin by increasing PgI$_3$ without a decrease in PgI$_2$ (both PgI$_2$ and PgI$_3$ are active vasodilators and inhibitors of platelet aggregation)
- an increase in leukotriene B_5, a weak inducer of inflammation and a weak chemotactic agent[40,41]

Molecular Aspects and Gene Expression: Beyond the Eicosanoids

The phospholipid class and fatty acid composition and the cholesterol content of biomembranes are critical determinants of physical properties of membranes and have been shown to influence a wide variety of membrane-dependent functions, such as integral enzyme activity, membrane transport and receptor function. The ability to alter membrane lipid composition and function in vivo by diet, even when EFAs are adequately supplied, demonstrates the importance of diet in growth and metabolism.[44]

Complex interactions and displacements of the omega-3 and omega-6 fatty acids take place in plasma and cellular lipids after dietary manipulations. Early steps of cell activation, such as generation of inositol phosphates, are induced by dietary fatty acids.[45] The effects of dietary fatty acids on the inositol phosphate pathway indicate that diet-induced modifications of PUFAs at the cellular level affect the activity of the enzymes responsible for the generation of lipid mediators in addition to the formation of products (eicosanoids) directly derived from their fatty acid precursors. This contributes to the effects of dietary fats on key processes in cell function.

The role of omega-3 and omega-6 fatty acids in the control of gene expression is an area that is expected to expand over the next 5 years as we begin to understand the role of nutrients in gene expression. It is known that nutrients, like hormones, influence and control gene expression and research is now providing more examples.[46] Both omega-3 (EPA and DHA in menhaden oil) and omega-6 fatty acids (AA) inhibit hepatic fatty acid synthase mRNA and thus inhibit lipogenesis.[47] The inhibitory potency of dietary PUFA varies with the degree of unsaturation and chain length.[47]

The greater potency of fish oil is due primarily to its high proportion (greater than 30 percent of 20- and 22-carbon polyenoic fatty acids). Odin and co-workers[48] showed a suppressive effect on hepatic fatty acid synthase and triglyceride synthesis when the membranes of cultured rat hepatocytes were enriched with either AA or EPA.

A sucrose-rich diet stimulates the biosynthesis of very-low-density lipoprotein (VLDL) in rat liver, increases the triglyceride content of hepatic VLDL and changes its apolipoprotein composition. Such a diet has been shown to enhance apolipoprotein E biosynthesis in rat liver in part by stimulating transcription of the apolipoprotein E gene.[49] A high-fat, high-carbohydrate diet that is also high in energy leads to lipogenesis and hyperphagia in animals. Fat deposition, as opposed to fat oxidation, does not have a satiating effect in these animals.[50]

Isomeric Trans Fatty Acids

After World War I, the solvent extraction of oil from seeds came into increased use and the large-scale production of vegetable oils became more efficient and more economic. The hydrogenation process applied to oils in order to solidify them led to the development of margarines. Hydrogenation leads to formation of isomeric fatty acids of both the *cis* and *trans* configuration. Trans fatty acids occur rarely in nature. Although the exact amount of trans fatty acids in the U.S. food supply is not precisely known, it is estimated that they account for about 5 to 7 percent of energy intake in Western countries.[27,28]

Holman and co-workers[51] studied isomeric polyunsaturated fatty acids in liver phospholipids of rats fed hydrogenated oil and concluded:

It is now clear that uncommon isomers of PUFA occur in the lipids of animals fed partially hydrogenated fat and that they inhibit the metabolism of PUFA at many steps in the normal metabolic cascade. It would, therefore, seem wise to avoid foods that contain unusual or unnatural isomeric PUFA or their isomeric monoenoic FA precursors. The latter, both *cis* and *trans* positional isomers of 18:1, occur abundantly in partially hydrogenated vegetable oils now commonly consumed by Western populations. The large-scale hydrogenation of vegetable oils reduces omega-3 and omega-6 EFAs and replaces them by saturated and isomeric 18:1 acids that interfere with the omega-3 and omega-6 metabolism, inducing significant partial deficiencies of EFA. It would seem wise to preserve the essential nutrients and to avoid producing inhibitors of their metabolism by hydrogenation. Evidence is growing for the essentiality of omega-3 PUFA and the occurrence of deficiencies of omega-3 acids in humans under stress conditions. It would, therefore, be wise economy to use oils containing linolenic acid directly as foods and to avoid their hydrogenation.

Trans fatty acids are completely absorbed by the gastrointestinal tract. In rats, the distribution of trans fatty acids in various tissues is influenced by

Table 4. Adverse Effects of Trans Fatty Acids

Increase

       low-density lipoprotein (LDL)

       platelet aggregation

       lipoprotein (α) [Lp(α)]

       body weight

       cholesterol transfer protein (CTP)

       abnormal morphology of sperm (rats)

Decrease or Inhibit

       incorporation of other fatty acids into cell membranes

       high-density lipoprotein (HDL)

       delta-6-desaturase (interfere with elongation and desaturation of essential fatty acids)

       serum testosterone (in male rats)

       cross the placenta and decrease birth weight

the level in the diet and can amount to up to 30 percent of the fatty acid content of phospholipids. Trans fatty acids at about 7 percent of energy intake have a number of adverse effects. They raise LDL cholesterol, triglycerides and lipoprotein a; increase platelet aggregation; and lower HDL[27] (Table 4). Siguel and Lerman[52] determined plasma trans fatty acid levels in patients with angiographically documented coronary artery disease and concluded that dietary trans fatty acids are a cardiovascular disease risk factor.

Koletzko reported an inverse association between trans fatty acid levels in the cord blood and birth weight.[53] Trans fatty acids interfere with elongation and desaturation of essential fatty acids.[54,55] In rat studies, trans fatty acids raise 18:236 while they lower arachidonic acid in tissue phospholipids, indicating an inhibition of delta-6 desaturase.[56] In the same study the fat cell size of rats on diets containing trans fatty acids was significantly larger than that in the control group, despite the fact that the body weights of the animals were the same.[56]

Kuller reported that women who consumed margarine four or more times per week weighed 2.3 kg more, had significantly lower HDL2 and higher total cholesterol and triglycerides than women who consumed margarine less frequently.[57] The difference in weight between the two groups was unexplained since they reported similar energy intake and physical activity. Body weight responds to modest as well as profound alterations in energy intake.[58,59] The rather precise nature of the response suggests that energy intake has a central role in weight homeostasis. Therefore, in Kuller's study the difference in weight is most likely due to the effect of trans fatty acids inhibiting desaturation and elongation of 18:2ω6 and 18:3ω3 (see Figure 4), resulting in lower levels of 20- and 22-carbon PUFAs in cell membranes with subsequent increase in fatty acid synthase, leading to lipogenesis and obesity (Figure 6). In rodents, omega-3 fatty acids are apparently protective against weight gain.[60]

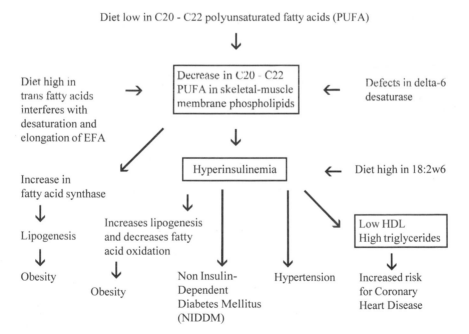

Figure 6. The effects of dietary C20-C22 PUFA on the composition of the C20-C22 PUFA in skeletal-muscle membrane phospholipids and the relation to hyperinsulinemia and chronic diseases (e.g., obesity, NIDDM, hypertension, coronary heart disease).

Fatty Acid Composition of Skeletal Muscle Phospholipids and Their Relationship to Insulin Sensitivity and Obesity

Reduced sensitivity to insulin is the primary metabolic defect from which all other metabolic characteristics associated with obesity follow.[61] It is generally accepted that obesity, particularly truncal obesity, precedes hyperinsulinemia or reduced sensitivity to insulin, but recent studies on insulin sensitivity and body fat distribution in normotensive offspring of hypertensive parents showed that "impairment of insulin sensitivity precedes both the development of overt hypertension and gain or redistribution of body fat."[62] Many studies have shown that hyperinsulinemia and insulin resistance are related to various metabolic disorders such as hypertension, dyslipidemia and non-insulin-dependent diabetes mellitus (NIDDM).[63] These metabolic disorders constitute "syndrome X." In an 8-year follow-up, Haffner and associates showed that high fasting insulin levels or hyperinsulinemia preceded the development of the metabolic abnormalities that constitute "syndrome X." Most importantly, hyperinsulinemia was not related to increased LDL or total cholesterol, but "In multivariate analyses, after adjustment for obesity and body fat distribution, fasting insulin continued to be significantly related to the incidence of decreased high-density lipoprotein cholesterol and increased triglyceride concentrations and to the incidence of non-insulin-dependent diabetes mellitus."[63] This is an important finding because it reinforces the concept that a decrease in insulin sensitivity precedes obesity, including truncal obesity, dyslipidemia and NIDDM. What accounts for this decrease in insulin sensitivity is an area of active investigation because decreased insulin sensitivity, or insulin resistance, is found in patients with NIDDM; is common in patients at increased risk for this type of diabetes; and is found frequently in association with obesity, hypertension, hyperlipidemia and coronary heart disease.

As indicated earlier, the composition of cell membrane fatty acids is determined to a large extent by the dietary fatty acid intake.[9] Increasing the content of PUFA increases membrane fluidity, the number of insulin receptors and the action of insulin,[64-66] whereas saturated fats have the opposite effects.[67] In humans the ratio of omega-6 to saturated fatty acids in serum phospholipids correlates with insulin sensitivity.[68] In rats the insulin resistance resulting from increased saturated fat intake can be prevented by the inclusion of omega-3 PUFA in the diet, particularly DHA.[43]

Modern diets high in saturated fats, in contrast to the diet that man evolved on, and the increase in trans fatty acids with their ability to interfere with elongation and desaturation of essential fatty acids, could account for the decrease in AA serum phospholipids that has been found in some obese individuals and in the genetic Zucker rat.[26,69] In fact, one would favor the hypothesis that current diets, which are low in total 20- and 22-carbon PUFA (cf. Table 3), account for or are the primary factor in the development of impaired insulin sensitivity in those who are genetically predisposed to obesity. The low dietary intake of this total C20-C22 PUFA results in low membrane phospholipids, leading to viscous membranes that interfere with the binding of insulin to its receptors, leading to hyperinsulinemia. Hyperinsulinemia is a compensatory effort to insulin resistance and is considered to be a pathogenetic factor for a number of conditions including obesity.

Variations in the fatty acid composition of skeletal muscle phospholipids have been shown to contribute to variations in insulin sensitivity in humans, "raising the possibility that changes in the fatty acid composition of muscles modulate the action of insulin."[70] In a group of men, mean age 58 ± 8 with coronary heart disease and an average BMI of 26.7 ± 2.4, Borkman and co-workers found that fasting insulin concentration "was negatively correlated with the percentage of individual long-chain PUFA in the phospholipid fraction of the muscle, particularly arachidonic acid; the total percentage of C20-22 PUFAs; the average degree of fatty acid unsaturation; and the ratio of the percentage of C20:4ω6 fatty acids to the percentage of C20:3ω6 fatty acids, an index of fatty acid delta-5 desaturase activity."[70] In the same study, the 18:2ω6 correlated positively with hyperinsulinemia.[70] This is an important finding that the authors did not discuss. It should be pointed out that 18:2ω6 is the most common polyunsaturated fatty acid in the U.S. diet. Therefore, a direct relationship between the level of 18:2ω6 and hyperinsulinemia suggests a role for 18:2ω6 in human obesity (see Figure 6).

In a companion study involving normal men aged 30 ± 11 with a BMI of 23 ± 3 the insulin sensitivity was positively correlated with the percentage of AA in muscle, the total percentage of C20-C22 PUFA, the average degree of fatty acid unsaturation and the ratio of 20:4ω6 to 20:3ω6. The results of this study by the Borkman group are consistent with the studies in isolated cells that have shown direct alterations in the fatty acid composition of the cell membrane to induce changes in insulin responsiveness.[65,67] The remote possibility should also be considered that the changes could be the result of insulin resistance.[71-74] In explaining the mechanisms involved, Borkman hypothesized that the long-chain PUFA could modulate the function of insulin receptors and glucose transporters through effects on the physical properties of the surrounding lipid environment or by acting as precursors for the generation of second messengers such as eicosanoids (cf. Figure 5) or diacylglycerols.[75]

Consequences of Reduced PUFA in Membrane Phospholipids and the Mechanisms Involved

Holman and co-workers[76] reported in their review that nutritional deficiencies of both omega-6 and omega-3 PUFA occur in humans, which lead to abnormalities in the pattern of fatty acids in plasma and tissue phospholipids, including deficiency of essential fatty acids and decreases in membrane fluidity during pregnancy and lactation. Growth, stress, or excessive loss and replacement of tissue all increase PUFA requirements. When EFA deficiency occurs, it is manifested by lower levels of EFA in plasma serum and membrane phospholipids of all cells. All the omega-6 and omega-3 PUFA in membranes are derived from dietary sources. The metabolic conversion by microsomal elongases and desaturases of 18:2ω6 and 18:3ω3 (see Figure 4) controls the relative availability of individual C20-C22 PUFAs for membrane incorporation unless the C20-C22 PUFAs are ingested preformed in the diet. Studies in animals indicate that the fatty acid composition of the diet influences the fatty acid composition of muscles.[43] Measurements of total phospholipids reflect the number of phospholipids in cell membranes. Holman's group also pointed out that significant disturbances in the pattern of PUFAs occur in a number of diseases, including Sjögren-Larsson syndrome, Reye syndrome, alcoholic cirrhosis and multiple sclerosis.[76]

Phinney and associates[26] have reported decreased serum phospholipid AA in obese individuals which rises during very-low-calorie diets, but returns to a low level after weight loss. They have suggested that arachidonic acid plays an important role in the regulation of energy balance by influencing fuel partitioning, that humans vary in their regulation of AA in important tissue pools and that those with reduced membrane AA are predisposed to obesity.[26,69] Phinney favors the hypothesis that the decrease of AA in serum phospholipids is due to increased release of AA from membrane phospholipids as well as its increased catabolism.[77]

Rubin and Laposata have shown that EPA can decrease the catabolism of AA.[78] However, the current intake of EPA in the American diet is only 48 mg/day, much less than that of AA. Therefore, EPA supplementation would be necessary in order to prevent further decrease in AA by inhibiting its catabolism. As indicated earlier, in rats fed high-fat diets, omega-3 fatty acid ingestion prevents insulin resistance.[43] Lower AA in membrane phospholipids could be the result of low dietary intake of AA, which is unlikely in omnivores on Western diets, or a decrease in delta-6 or delta-5 desaturase due to high dietary 18:2ω6 or increase in trans fatty acid intake, a very low EPA,[78] or a genetic defect occurring in one or more steps in AA metabolism (Figure 6).

Any factors that lead to the reduction of delta-5 and delta-6 desaturase activity, whether of genetic or dietary origin, would lead to a reduction of AA and impaired insulin action.[70] In the liver cell, a decrease in AA would not be able to suppress fatty acid synthase, lipogenesis would be enhanced, and the liver would shift carbohydrate calories into the lipid pool at the expense of muscle and liver glycogen (see Figure 6). In such a situation, a high-carbohydrate diet in the presence of low AA would lead to an increase in body weight.

Genetic background largely determines the propensity to become obese, but whether a predisposed person actually becomes obese, and the extent of the obesity depends on the nature of the obesity-promoting factors in the environment and the duration of exposure to those factors.[1-3] Moreover, some genotypes may be much more sensitive than others to the environment. The current food supply provides the perfect environment in which genetically predisposed individuals become obese. As was shown in Table 3, the C20-C22 PUFAs obtained from the diet are very low in comparison to the amounts on which humans evolved. However, omnivores obtain AA from meat, eggs, and milk, whereas the amount of EPA and DHA obtained from fish and poultry is very low in comparison. Trans fatty acids in the form of margarine and shortenings interfere with desaturation and elongation of EFA, which leads to low levels of AA, EPA and DHA in membrane phospholipids, much lower than the amounts present in persons who consume diets consistent with paleolithic nutrition.[10] In addition trans fatty acids are incorporated into cell membrane phospholipids, leading to decreased fluidity of membranes and decrease in the binding of insulin to its receptors, followed by impaired insulin action, insulin resistance and hyperinsulinemia. A low-fat, high-carbohydrate, high-energy diet in this situation will lead to fat deposition from glucose instead of glycogen synthesis and glucose oxidation.[50] In addition the decrease in AA, EPA and DHA of cell phospholipids enhances fatty acid synthase in the liver microsomes, which leads to increased lipogenesis and fat deposition instead of oxidation[47-49] (see Figure 6). The low omega-3 fatty acid intake in the form of EPA cannot come to the rescue of the AA which is catabolized, leading to a further decrease of AA.[78] The general recommendation to eat less fat and more carbohydrates does not help at this point since the carbohydrate is turned into fat in this metabolic labyrinth. Women are particularly susceptible to these metabolic abnormalities since a decreased energy intake is hard to maintain and exercise does not have any effect on the lipogenic enzymes. It follows therefore that dietary changes should include the following:

1. Avoid trans fatty acids (industry should be persuaded to make margarines free of trans fatty acids).
2. Decrease saturated fat intake and replace with monounsaturates.
3. Decrease omega-6 fatty acid intake and increase omega-3 fatty acids in order to maintain a balance of these two families of fatty acids.
4. Decrease carbohydrate intake, particularly high-fructose corn syrup-containing soft drinks and foods.
5. Increase protein intake (see Table 1).

6.   Balance energy intake to energy expenditure by developing lifestyle habits that include 30 min/day of moderate physical activity.
7.   Maintain desirable body weight with a BMI of 20 to 25.

NOTES

1.   Childs B (1988). Genetic variation and nutrition. Am J Clin Nutrition 48:1500-1504.
2.   Simopoulos AP, Childs B, Eds (1990). Genetic variation and nutrition. World Review of Nutrition and Diet, vol 63. Basel: S Karger.
3.   Simopoulos AP, VanItallie TB (1984). Body weight, health and longevity. Ann Intern Med 100:285-294.
4.   Lara-Pantin E (1987). Obesity in developing countries. In E Berry, SH Blondheim, HE Eliahou, et al., Eds, Recent advances in obesity research, vol 5. London: John Libbey.
5.   Chadwick J, Mann WN (1950). Medical works of hippocrates. Oxford: Blackwell.
6.   Eaton SB, Konner M (1985). Paleolithic nutrition: a consideration of its nature and current implications. N Engl J Med 312:283-289.
7.   Simopoulos AP (1992). Dietary risk factors for hypertension. Comp Ther 18(10):26-30.
8.   Leaf A, Weber PC (1987). A new era for science in nutrition. Am J Clin Nutrition 45 (suppl):1048-1053.
9.   Simopoulos AP (1991). Omega-3 fatty acids in health and disease and in growth and development. Am J Clin Nutrition 54:438-463.
10. Sinclair AJ, O'Dea K (1990). Fats in human diets through history: is the Western diet out of step? In JD Wood and AV Fisher, Eds, Reducing fat in meat animals. London: Elsevier.
11. Raper N, Marston R (1988). Content of the U.S. food supply (tables of nutrients and foods). Washington, DC: Human Nutrition Information Service, U.S. Department of Agriculture.
12. Reiser S (1987). Lipogenesis and blood lipids. In S Reiser and J Hallfrisch, Eds, Metabolic effects of dietary fructose. Boca Raton, FL: CRC Press.
13. Hallfrisch J (1990). Metabolic effects of dietary fructose. FASEB J 4:2652-2660.
14. Grundy SM (1986). Comparison of monounsaturated fatty acids and carbohydrates for lowering plasma cholesterol. N Engl J Med 314:745-748.
15. Mensink RP, Katan MB (1987). Effects of monounsaturated fatty acids versus complex carbohydrates on high-density lipoproteins in healthy men and women. Lancet 1:122-125.
16. Garg A, Bonanome A, Grundy SM, Zhang Z-J, Unger RH (1988). Comparison of a high-carbohydrate diet with a high-monounsaturated-fat diet in patients with non-insulin-dependent diabetes mellitus. N Engl J Med 319:829-834.
17. Castelli WP (1986). The triglyceride issue: a view from Framingham. Am Heart J 112:432-437.
18. Simopoulos AP, Norman HA, Gillaspy JE, Duke JA (1992). Common purslane: a source of omega-3 fatty acids and antioxidants. J Am Coll Nutrition 11:374-382.
19. Simopoulos AP (1990). Genetics and nutrition: or what your genes can tell you about nutrition. In AP Simopoulos and B Childs, Eds, Genetic variation and nutrition. World Review of Nutrition and Diet, vol 63. Basel: S Karger.
20. Simopoulos AP (1988). Terrestrial sources of omega-3 fatty acids: purslane. In B Quebedeaux and F Bliss, Eds, Horticulture and human health: contributions of fruits and vegetables. Englewood Cliffs, NJ: Prentice Hall.

21. Simopoulos AP, Salem N (1992). Egg yolk as a source of long-chain polyunsaturated fatty acids in infant feeding. Am J Clin Nutrition 55:411-414.

22. van Vliet T, Katan MB (1990). Lower ratio of n-3 to n-6 fatty acids in cultured than in wild fish. Am J Clin Nutrition 51:1-2.

23. Crawford MA (1968). Fatty acid ratios in free-living and domestic animals. Lancet 1:1239-1333.

24. Hunter JE (1989). Omega-3 fatty acids from vegetable oils. In C Galli and AP Simopoulos, Eds, Dietary ω3 and ω6 fatty acids: biological effects and nutritional essentiality. Series A: Life sciences, vol 171. New York: Plenum.

25. Raper NR, Cronin FJ, Exler J (1992). Omega-3 fatty acid content of the U.S. food supply. J Am College Nutrition 11:304-308.

26. Phinney SD, Davis PG, Johnson SB, Holman RT (1991). Obesity and weight loss after serum polyunsaturated lipids in humans. Am J Clin Nutrition 53:831-838.

27. Nestel P, Noakes M, Belling B, McArther R, Clifton P, Janus E, Abbey M (1992). Plasma lipoprotein lipid and Lpα changes with substitution of elaidic acid for oleic acid in the diet. J Lipid Res 33:1029-1036.

28. Enig MG, Atal S, Keeney M, Sampugna J (1990). Isomeric trans fatty acids in the U.S. diet. J Am Coll Nutrition 9(5):471-486.

29. de Gomez Dumm INT, Brenner RR (1975). Oxidative desaturation of alpha-linolenic, linoleic and stearic acids by human liver microsomes. Lipids 10:315-317.

30. Emken EA, Adlof RO, Rakoff H, et al. (1989). Metabolism of deuterium-labeled linolenic, linoleic, oleic, stearic and palmitic acid in human subjects. In TA Baillie and JR Jones, Eds, Synthesis and applications of isotopically labelled compounds. Amsterdam: Elsevier.

31. Hague TA, Christoffersen BO (1984). Effect of dietary fats on arachidonic acid and eicosapentaenoic acid biosynthesis and conversion to C22 fatty acids in isolated liver cells. Biochim Biophys Acta 796:205-217.

32. Hague TA, Christoffersen BO (1986). Evidence for peroxisomal retroconversion of adrenic acid (22:4n6) and docosahexaenoic acid (22:6n3) in isolated liver cells. Biochim Biophys Acta 875:165-173.

33. Carlson SE, Rhodes PG, Ferguson MG (1986). Docosahexaenoic acid status of preterm infants at birth and following feeding with human milk or formula. Am J Clin Nutrition 44:798-804.

34. Singer P, Jaeger W, Voigt S, et al. (1984). Defective desaturation and elongation of n-6 and n-3 fatty acids in hypertensive patients. Prostag Leukotr Med 15:159-165.

35. Honigmann G, Schimke E, Beitz J, et al. (1982). Influence of a diet rich in linolenic acid on lipids, thrombocyte aggregation and prostaglandins in type I (insulin-dependent) diabetes. Diabetologia 23:175.

36. Simopoulos AP, Kifer RR, Martin RE, Eds (1986). Health effects of polyunsaturated fatty acids in seafoods. Orlando, FL: Academic Press.

37. O'Brien JS, Sampson EL (1965). Fatty acid and aldehyde composition of the major brain lipids in normal gray matter, white matter and myelin. J Lipid Res 6:545-551.

38. Anderson RE (1970). Lipids of ocular tissues. IV. A comparison of the phospholipids from the retina of six mammalian species. Exp Eye Res 10:339.

39. Poulos A, Darin-Bennett A, White IG (1975). The phospholipid-bound fatty acids and aldehydes of mammalian spermatozoa. Comp Biochem Physiol 46B:541.

40. Weber PC, Fischer S, von Schacky C, et al. (1986). Dietary omega-3 polyunsaturated fatty acids and eicosanoid formation in man. In AP Simopoulos, RR Kifer and RE Martin, Eds, Health effects of polyunsaturated fatty acids in seafoods. Orlando, FL: Academic Press.

41. Lewis RA, Lee TH, Austen KF (1986). Effects of omega-3 fatty acids on the generation of products of the 5-lipoxygenase pathway. In AP Simopoulos, RR Kifer and RE Martin, Eds, Health effects of polyunsaturated fatty acids in seafoods. Orlando, FL: Academic Press.

42. Needleman P, Raz A, Minkes MS, et al. (1979). Triene prostaglandins: prostacyclin and thromboxane biosynthesis and unique biological properties. Proc Natl Acad Sci USA 76:944-948.

43. Storlien LH, Jenkins AB, Chisholm DJ, Pascoe WS, Khouri S, Kraegen EW (1991). Influence of dietary fat composition on development of insulin resistance in rats: relationship to muscle triglyceride and 3-3 fatty acids in muscle phospholipid. Diabetes 40:280-289.

44. Galli C, Trzeciak HI, Paoletti R (1971). Effects of dietary fatty acids on the fatty acid composition of brain ethanolamine phosphoglyceride. Reciprocal replacement of n-6 and n-3 polyunsaturated fatty acids. Biochim Biophys Acta 248:449-454.

45. Galli C, Mosconi C, Medini L, et al. (1989). N-6 and n-3 fatty acids in plasma and platelet lipids and generation of inositol phosphates by stimulated platelets after dietary manipulations in the rabbit. In C Galli and AP Simopoulos, Eds, Dietary ω3 and ω6 fatty acids: biological effects and nutritional essentiality. New York: Plenum.

46. Rucker R, Tinker D (1986). The role of nutrition in gene expression: a fertile field for the application of molecular biology. J Nutrition 116:177-189.

47. Clarke SD, Jump DB (1993). Regulation of hepatic gene expression by dietary fats: a unique role for polyunsaturated fatty acids. In CD Berdanier and JL Hargrove, Eds, Nutrition and gene expression. Boca Raton, FL: CRC Press.

48. Odin RS, Finke BA, Blake WL, Phinney SD, Clarke SD (1987). Modification of fatty acid composition of membrane phospholipid in hepatocyte monolayer with n-3, n-6 and n-9 fatty acids and its relationship to triacylglycerol production. Biochim Biophys Acta 921:378-391.

49. Strobl W, Gorder NL, Fienup GA, Lin-Lee YC, et al. (1989). Effect of sucrose diet on apolipoprotein biosynthesis in rat liver. Increase in apolipoprotein E gene transcription. J Biol Chem 264(2):1190-1194.

50. Ramirez I, Friedman MI (1990). Dietary hyperphagia in rats: role of fat, carbohydrate and energy content. Physiol Behav 47:1157-1163.

51. Holman RT, Pusch F, Svingen B, Dutton HJ (1991). Unusual isomeric polyunsaturated fatty acids in liver phospholipids of rats fed hydrogenated oil. Proc Natl Acad Sci USA 88:4830-4834.

52. Siguel EN, Lerman RH (1993). Trans fatty acid patterns in patients with angiographically documented coronary artery disease. Am J Cardiol 71:916-920.

53. Koletzko B, Muller J (1990). Cis- and trans-isomeric fatty acids in plasma lipids of newborn infants and their mothers. Biol Neonate 57:172-178.

54. Siguel EN, Schaefer EJ (1989). Aging and nutritional requirements of essential fatty acids. In J Beare, Ed, Dietary fats. Champaign, IL: American Oil Chemists Society.

55. Siguel EN, Chee KM, Gong J, Schaefer EJ (1987). Criteria for essential fatty acid deficiency in plasma as assessed by capillary column gas-liquid chromatography. Clin Chem 33:1869-1873.

56. Ostlund-Lindqvist A-M, Albanus L, Croon L-B (1985). Effect of dietary trans fatty acids on microsomal enzymes and membranes. Lipids 20:620-624.

57. Kuller LH (1993). Trans fatty acids and dieting. Lancet 341:1093-1094.

58. Garrow JS (1974). Energy balance and obesity in man. New York: American Elsevier.

59. Forbes GB (1984). Energy intake and body weight: a reexamination of two "classic" studies. Am J Clin Nutrition 39:349-350.
60. Pan DA, Storlien LH (1993). Dietary lipid profile is a determinant of tissue phospholipid fatty acid composition and rate of weight gain in rats. J Nutrition 123:512-519.
61. Garrow J (1991). Importance of obesity. Br Med J 303:704-706.
62. Allemann Y, Horber FF, Colombo M, Ferrari P, Shaw S, Jaeger P, Weidmann P (1993). Insulin sensitivity and body fat distribution in normotensive offspring of hypertensive parents. Lancet 341:327-331.
63. Haffner SM, Valdez RA, Hazuda HP, Mitchell BD, Morales PA, Stern MP (1992). Prospective analysis of the insulin-resistance syndrome (syndrome X). Diabetes 41:715-722.
64. Yorek M, Leeney E, Dunlap J, Ginsberg B (1989). Effect of fatty acid composition on insulin and IGF-I binding in retinoblastoma cells. Invest Ophthalmol Vis Sci 30:2087-2092.
65. Ginsberg BH, Chaterjee P, Yorek M (1987). Increased membrane fluidity is associated with greater sensitivity to insulin. Diabetes 36(suppl):51A.
66. Ginsberg BH, Jabour J, Spector AA (1982). Effect of alterations in membrane lipid unsaturation on the properties of the insulin receptor of Ehrlich ascites cells. Biochim Biophys Acta 690:157-164.
67. Grunfeld C, Baird KL, Kahn CR (1981). Maintenance of 3T3-L1 cells in culture media containing saturated fatty acids decreases insulin binding and insulin action. Biochem Biophys Res Commun 103:219-226.
68. Pelikanova T, Kohout M, Valek J, Base J, Kazdova L (1989). Insulin secretion and insulin action related to the serum phospholipid fatty acid pattern in healthy men. Metabolism 38:188-192.
69. Thurmond DC, Tang AB, Nakamura MT, Stern JS, Phinney SD (1993). Time-dependent effects of progressive gamma-linolenate feeding on hyperphagia, weight gain and erythrocyte fatty acid composition during growth of Zucker obese rats. Obesity Res 1:118-125.
70. Borkman M, Storlien LH, Pan DA, Jenkins AB, Chisholm DJ, Campbell LV (1993). The relation between insulin sensitivity and the fatty-acid composition of skeletal-muscle phospholipids. N Engl J Med 328:238-244.
71. Faas FH, Carter WJ (1980). Altered fatty acid desaturation and microsomal fatty acid composition in the streptozotocin diabetic rat. Lipids 15:953-961.
72. El Boustani S, Causse JE, Descomps B, Monnier L, Mendy F, Crastes de Paulet A (1989). Direct in vivo characterization of delta-5-desaturase activity in humans by deuterium labelling: effect of insulin. Metabolism J 38:315-321.
73. Tilvis RS, Miettinen TA (1985). Fatty acid compositions of serum lipids, erythrocytes and platelets in insulin-dependent diabetic women. J Clin Endocrinol Metab 61:741-745.
74. Rizza RA, Mandarino LJ, Genest J, Baker BA, Gerich JE (1985). Production of insulin resistance by hyperinsulinaemia in man. Diabetologia 28:70-75.
75. Stralfors P (1988). Insulin stimulation of glucose uptake can be mediated by diacylglycerol in adipocytes. Nature 335:554-556.
76. Holman RT, Johnson SB, Ogburn PL (1991). Deficiency of essential fatty acids and membrane fluidity during pregnancy and lactation. Proc Natl Acad Sci USA 88:4835-4839.
77. Phinney SD (1993). Paper presented at the National Conference on Obesity and Weight Control. Columbia-Presbyterian Medical Center, New York, April 22-24.
78. Rubin D, Laposata M (1992). Cellular interactions between n-6 and n-3 fatty acids: a mass analysis of fatty acid elongation/desaturation, distribution among complex lipids and conversion to eicosanoids. J Lipid Res 33:1431-1440.

Index

ISBN 0-914783-74-2

54295